SCHEUMANN'S
THE BALANCED BODY

A Guide to the Integrated Deep Tissue Therapy System

FOURTH EDITION

Ruth Werner

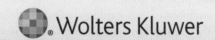
Wolters Kluwer

Philadelphia • Baltimore • New York • London
Buenos Aires • Hong Kong • Sydney • Tokyo

Acquisitions Editor: Jay Campbell
Product Development Editor: Linda G. Francis
Marketing Manager: Leah Thomson
Production Editor: David Saltzberg
Design Coordinator: Stephen Druding
Illustrator: David R. Rini
Prepress Vendor: S4Carlisle Publishing Services

9 8 7 6 5 4 3 2 1

Printed in China

Library of Congress Cataloging-in-Publication Data

Names: Werner, Ruth (Ruth A.), author. | Preceded by (work): Scheumann, Donald W. Balanced body.
Title: Scheumann's the balanced body : a guide to the integrated deep tissue therapy system / Ruth Werner.
Other titles: Balanced body : a guide to the integrated deep tissue therapy system
Description: Fourth edition. | Philadelphia : Wolters Kluwer Heath, [2018] | Preceded by The balanced body : a guide to deep tissue and neuromuscular therapy / Donald W. Scheumann. 3rd ed. 2007. | Includes bibliographical references and index.
Identifiers: LCCN 2016036791 | ISBN 9781496346117
Subjects: | MESH: Massage—methods | Physical Therapy Modalities
Classification: LCC RM721 | NLM WB 537 | DDC 615.8/22—dc23 LC record available at https://lccn.loc.gov/2016036791

RRS1611

This book is dedicated, with gratitude, to Donald Scheumann

About the Author

Don Scheumann began his education in personal growth and transformation as a teenager, when he commenced yoga studies at the Yoga Society of New York. After graduating from SUNY with a BFA in dance, he pursued a career in modern dance in New York City. During this period, he undertook an internship at a major holistic health center, where he studied with many of the premier educators in the human potential movement. This experience led him to move away from the performing arts and devote his career to the exploration of the body as a tool for healing. In 1980, he became a certified yoga instructor, and in 1982 he graduated from massage school. His other certifications in bodywork modalities include polarity, neuromuscular therapy, Reiki, Pfrimmer deep muscle therapy, acupressure, and Zen therapy.

Don was a massage practitioner and instructor for more than 20 years. For much of that time, he taught at the Atlanta School of Massage, where he was a major contributor to curriculum development, creating many of the classes for the Integrated and Deep Tissue Program, as well as classes in the Wellness and Spa Therapies Program.

The *Balanced Body* was first published in 1997, and Don successfully stewarded it through two more editions. In this time, it has become a well-used and much-respected book in the profession. The massage therapy community lost a beloved practitioner and teacher with Don's passing in 2008.

Ruth Werner, BCTMB is a retired massage therapist, and an active writer and educator for massage therapists. Her first book, *A Massage Therapist's Guide to Pathology*, was published in 1998. Now in its 6th edition, it is used all over the world. Ruth is a columnist for *Massage & Bodywork* magazine, and volunteers on several national and international committees for the profession. She was recognized as the Jerome Perlinski Teacher of the Year in 2005—an honor she shares with Don Scheumann, who was recognized in 2001. She served two terms as the president of the Massage Therapy Foundation, and retains a seat on the Board of Trustees. Ruth is fulfilling a lifelong dream of living on the Oregon Coast, where she is daily inspired by her surroundings.

Foreword

By Cindy E. Farrar, LMT, BCTMB

At first glance, you may think *The Balanced Body* is just another deep-tissue-massage text. I am happy to inform you that you would be incorrect and that you are in for a great surprise!

The Balanced Body is a compilation of a lifetime of study, practice, and teaching of deep tissue massage and neuromuscular therapy by Don Scheumann. It is a system of therapeutic massage that takes into consideration the whole client and challenges the massage therapist to bring his or her whole self and focused awareness to each session. It also seeks to expand the self-awareness of the client, leading to the potential for the greatest therapeutic results.

Twenty years ago when I was a massage student, our Deep Tissue Manual was a loose-leaf binder that would serve as the precursor to the initial *Balanced Body* manuscript. Don Scheumann was one of my main instructors. I recall being somewhat in awe as I listened to Don effortlessly relate vast amounts of information across the various curriculum subjects, linking it together as if telling us a story. The only thing that seemed to be more fluid for Don was the manner in which he moved and utilized his body. He was the model of body awareness, alignment, biomechanics, and efficiency. In secret, I called him the "human lava lamp."

Don frequently dropped jewels of wisdom that were especially noteworthy. The extent to which they would play a role in the success and longevity of his many students' practices, we had no way of knowing. Recently, my friend and one of Don's students of 21 years ago, Joan Rau, LMT, shared with me that, to this day, when she is preparing her table and room for her clients she thinks of what Don impressed upon her. "How I presented myself as well as my work space, how I dressed my table was just as important as the work I did with my hands. How will someone feel walking into my space? He was the first to introduce the concept of 'being fully present' with my client during the massage. Being fully present allows me to be open to the conversation between my hands and the tissues underneath them. That concept was a great gift to his students and one I carry with me every time I work on someone."

I would later teach and devise curriculum from the first and second editions of *The Balanced Body*. It was impressive to find that the core of the material remained the same as in the binder manual I learned from 10 years prior. During my time teaching, I would also have the good fortune to be in the classroom alongside Don. While I was in a supervisory position, he remained my teacher. I found not only my teaching skills sharpened, the quality of my massage sessions was also heightened.

Don consistently encouraged his students to see the potential for wellness in our clients. This continues to inform how I interact with my clients today. And that system of Deep Tissue Massage I learned two decades ago (as did scores of others before and after me) has served and continues to serve as the foundation for my massage sessions. In addition, it has assisted countless clients to return to, establish, and maintain a significantly high level of wellness.

It has been a privilege and honor to consult on this revision of *The Balanced Body*. This fourth edition maintains the integrity and enhances the system of Deep Tissue Massage and Neuromuscular Therapy that has stood the test of many decades, therapists, and clients.

Preface

The Balanced Body: A Guide to the Integrated Deep Tissue Therapy System is a comprehensive course in massage from a background of structural integration and neuromuscular therapy. It contains all the elements necessary for a student to become competent in performing this outcome-oriented approach to whole-body function and efficiency.

Many styles of massage have been categorized as "deep tissue" therapy, although the work does not necessarily involve heavy pressure, and it definitely need not be painful. In the context of this text, "deep tissue therapy" refers to a focused approach to accessing structures that are not always on the surface, which allows for the manual alteration of muscular, fascial, and skeletal relationships. This can produce dramatic changes in the efficiency of structural alignment, a reduction of unnecessary muscular tension, and profound changes in a person's physical experience.

The approach presented in this book evolved initially from concepts introduced during Scheumann's training in massage therapy at the Atlanta School of Massage more than 30 years ago. The first edition was written in 1997 as the primary textbook for the deep tissue course taught there. Scheumann continued to develop the book through two more editions before his passing in 2006.

The creation of this fourth edition is undertaken with great respect for the author's original vision and intent, and with enthusiasm for incorporating into his work the advances made in massage therapy from the last decade. It is our hope that new generations of massage therapists may benefit from Scheumann's inspiration, and that his followers and former students and colleagues will find new life in his ideas with this edition.

ORGANIZATION

The book is divided into two parts.
- *Part I:* Chapters 1 to 5 present an overview of integrated deep tissue therapy approach to massage, along with important foundational information for learners. The philosophical underpinnings of integrated deep tissue therapy are found here.
- *Part II:* Chapters 6 to 10 present the technique lessons, each of which is divided into two segments.

- Part I: This section provides essential material about the region of the body being studied, including kinesiology, musculoskeletal anatomy, supplementary exercises, common conditions, and commentary on the holistic integration of this part of the body.
- Part II: The second section is the integrated deep tissue therapy routine for that particular area of the body.

The lessons in Part II are arranged in a recommended order that combines a regional approach to deep tissue therapy with a structural realignment orientation. The progression through the body moves from the central axis to the upper extremity, followed by the lower extremity, the core, and finishes with the neck and head. Finishing this sequence involves many individual sessions that progress through the body.

Scheumann developed this protocol after studying the Rolfing method of fascial manipulation. This approach is designed to reestablish the most efficient and effective relationships between the body and the earth's gravitational forces. When practitioners address body areas in the recommended sequence, they are most likely to succeed in guiding their clients to newfound states of equipoise and freedom of movement.

COMPLEMENTARY MODALITIES

While the primary focus of integrated deep tissue therapy is deep tissue massage, Scheumann found that several complementary therapies helped to enhance the results of his core techniques. This is why the protocol is called *integrated* deep tissue therapy.

The bodywork systems most specifically addressed here include neuromuscular therapy, Swedish massage, connective tissue release, cross-fiber therapy, assisted stretching, and shiatsu. Other techniques may be mentioned, although not specifically expanded upon. These styles are not examined to the same degree as deep tissue therapy, but their use is explained sufficiently to allow students to incorporate them effectively within the context of the integrated deep tissue therapy sessions. Practitioners who adopt this approach to bodywork are extremely well rounded and versatile in their application of massage therapy in general, and deep tissue therapy in particular.

THE ART OF EFFECTIVE TOUCH

This book was designed to help provide a complete educational foundation in the integrated deep tissue therapy system. This foundation includes subtle concepts, including the quality of effective touch: a topic that is neglected in many technique manuals. Part of this skill involves knowing the characteristics of different muscle types, palpation skills, and body mechanics, so these are covered in some detail.

However, the most important discussion of the art of effective touch is found in Chapter 3, in the section titled *Principles of Conscious Bodywork*. Here, readers will find Scheumann's 10 guidelines that succinctly cover the theory and optimal application of all kinds of bodywork, but especially integrated deep tissue therapy. Dedicated study and integration of these concepts will ensure that practitioners have the somatic skills, professionalism, sensitivity, and thoughtfulness to use deep tissue massage effectively.

LESSON STRUCTURE

The chapters in *The Balanced Body* are designed to provide a curriculum for classes in learning this deep tissue therapy technique, and they will be most effective if they are taught in the same order as they are presented in the book. The information covered in the first four chapters may be incorporated into massage theory and history classes. Chapter 5 begins the hands-on training with a discussion of the role of fascia, and it includes a full-body routine of connective tissue techniques. This is the only presentation of a full-body protocol in the text; the rest of the chapters are arranged by body region.

The complete integrated deep tissue therapy protocol is introduced in Chapter 6. Although the body is necessarily divided into segments for learning purposes, the overlying theme expressed throughout the book is that the body is a functional whole. It is important to remember that altering any single part of the body changes relationships throughout the entire structure that may resonate on many levels of a person's experience.

The deep tissue routines are presented in a linear fashion, listing session objectives, muscles to be massaged, strokes to be practiced, and accessory techniques. This orderly method of practice serves more as a learning tool than as a blueprint for actual deep tissue sessions. Although the overall format of each deep tissue routine may be retained as an organizational guide, the expectation is that each therapy session must be customized. Session strategies must be informed by the unique presentation of pain, tension, and limitation in the individual client, and that client's desired goals and outcomes, as discussed before any work begins.

Within the deep tissue routines, deep tissue strokes and neuromuscular therapy techniques are combined. The attachment sites and actions for that muscle are listed first, and then the deep tissue strokes for each muscle are explained. A brief description of the location of common trigger points for that muscle is also included. Being aware of these frequent trigger point sites may assist students in finding and treating these painful areas while applying deep tissue techniques to a muscle.

Special Features, Chapters 6 to 10

Chapters 6 to 10 provide the integrated deep tissue therapy system protocols for each part of the body. Each discussion of body area has these features in addition to the specific routines:

- *General Concepts*—This includes descriptions of the functions of that location, and how it interacts with and affects the body as a whole.
- *Musculoskeletal Anatomy and Function*—This emphasizes the kinesiologic role of the body part through descriptions of the interrelationships of muscles and the bones they move. It is extremely important for massage therapists to have detailed knowledge of the skeleton, including the shapes of the bones and the actions of the joints. Muscles and bones are inextricably related; a concept that often is not adequately emphasized in massage textbooks.
- *Essential Anatomy box*—This provides a list of relevant muscles, bones, and bony landmarks.
- *Endangerment Sites*—This describes the cautions and concerns associated with manipulation of specific body areas.
- *Conditions list*—This offers a brief description of common injuries, diseases, and conditions that are frequently associated with a specific area of the body. These situations are discussed in more detail in Appendix A.
- *Postural Evaluation*—These sections discuss common postural habits that affect various parts of the body. The postural evaluation questions have also been included in the online resources as printable forms for use in the student clinic or session room.
- *Body Reading tables*—These list common postural patterns, and the muscular relationships that may contribute to problems.
- *Exercises and Self-Treatment*—For those whose scope of practice allows it, this section provides the therapist with simple exercises he or she can teach clients to perform at home to reinforce the neuromuscular changes brought about by the deep tissue sessions.
- *Holistic Perspective*—These sidebars introduce students to concepts that are integral to somatic psychology, which examines how beliefs and emotions may contribute to the shapes and tension states of areas of the body.
- *Session Impressions cases*—These descriptions, based on some of Scheumann's actual clients, are examples of how integrated deep tissue therapy protocols may be put to work to help clients achieve their goals.

Online Resources

Students and Instructors may find the following useful resources online at http://thePoint.lww.com/WernerTBB4e:

Student Resources:

- Technique videos featuring the book's original author, Don Scheumann
- Anatomy images from the highly regarded *Acland's Video Atlas of Human Anatomy*
- Image labeling exercises to help reinforce your knowledge of anatomy

Faculty Resources:

- Pre-loaded PowerPoint presentations
- Chapter Objectives tied to the question bank for clear, point-to-point instruction, using the accepted entry-level assessment project (ELAP) standards
- Updated Lesson Plans tied to learning objectives, case studies, and technique videos
- A robust test generator and question bank for building tests and exams quickly and easily
- A complete image bank to support lecture and exam preparation

CONCLUSION

For many years, the massage therapy profession had very few published texts on massage techniques and approaches to bodywork. Now such books are common, but not always usable as stand-alone teaching guides. Texts of this type are no substitute for hands-on training under the supervision of a qualified instructor, and it is the hope of the authors that this book will be used in that way: with the guidance of a teacher who is able to convey in person what the book presents on the page. What makes *The Balanced Body* unique among technique books is its integrated, multidimensional approach to creating the best potential for health and balance through bodywork. Practitioners who use this approach can be sure of bringing their best to the session room, and their clients will be the lucky beneficiaries of their skills.

AUTHORS' NOTES

From Don Scheumann, Original Author

The Balanced Body: a Guide to the Integrated Deep Tissue Therapy System is unique among massage therapy technique books because it provides thorough, up-to-date, fully resourced material on this specialized bodywork approach, and also because it provides both guidance and inspiration to take these bodywork fundamentals and apply them in ways that are customized to meet the needs of each individual client. Every body-area is discussed in the context of a range of bodywork approaches, but the practitioner is encouraged to adapt each session to maximize the effectiveness of the work.

In this age of specialization, many people find benefit in the exploration of approaches to healthcare that view all aspects of a person's being and lifestyle as important health-determining factors. *The Balanced Body* represents my contribution to this holistic perspective within the realm of hands-on bodywork. I hope that the audience this book reaches will find the study of this system of massage as rewarding as I have in the many years I have devoted to practicing and teaching it.

From Ruth Werner, Revision Author

When the publishers at Wolters Kluwer presented me with the idea of updating a beloved technique book with information on pathology and current research, I thought it would be easy. I was wrong. Working on *The Balanced Body* has been one of the most challenging and enriching projects of my career. I have worked hard to keep Don Scheumann's original vision intact, which involved learning and writing about approaches to bodywork that don't resonate with my own point of view. I felt it important to add some explanations and disclaimers about what we currently understand about the phenomenon sometimes called "energy work," but it was imperative to do that without being disrespectful to tradition or to Don Scheumann's vision. I also relished the opportunity to introduce new understandings about fascia and pain science to the discussion, along with updated information about pathologies.

Somehow, largely thanks to the work of my friend and consultant (and Don's student and then colleague) Cindy Farrar, we managed to walk the tightrope and it all got done. We have trimmed away the material that is no longer applicable, and added much that we hope will sustain this text and the practice of integrated deep tissue therapy for generations to come. The result, I hope, is a book that is true to its roots, but is also firmly seated in a modern context. It has been my honor to be a part of it.

User's Guide

Scheumann's The Balanced Body: A Guide to the Integrated Deep Tissue Therapy System provides a complete program for integrated deep tissue therapy, presented in an easy-to-use format. This User's Guide shows you how to put the book's features to work for you.

Part I, Introduction to the Integrated Deep Tissue Therapy System, provides a solid knowledge base and foundation for students to build upon before moving on to the second section. Part II, The Lessons, focuses on hands-on techniques and routines for providing safe and effective deep tissue therapy to massage clients.

You'll find these helpful learning features throughout the text:

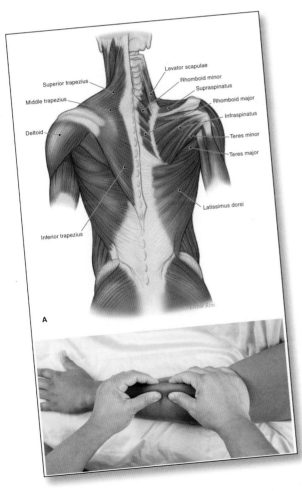

DETAILED ILLUSTRATIONS AND PHOTOGRAPHS (all updated for this edition) bring the techniques to life and clearly demonstrate anatomy and physiology.

HOLISTIC VIEW boxes discuss the relationship between mind and body.

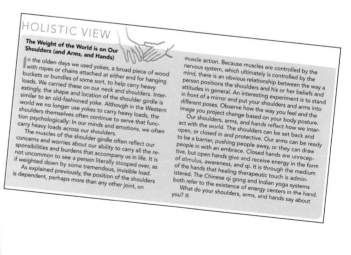

HOLISTIC VIEW

The Weight of the World is on Our Shoulders (and Arms, and Hands)

In the olden days we used yokes, a broad piece of wood with ropes or chains attached at either end for hanging buckets or bundles of some sort, to help carry heavy loads. We carried these on our neck and shoulders. Interestingly, the shape and location of the shoulder girdle is similar to an old-fashioned yoke. Although in the Western world we no longer use yokes to carry heavy loads, the shoulders themselves often continue to serve that function psychologically: In our minds and emotions, we often carry heavy loads across our shoulders.

The muscles of the shoulder girdle often reflect our concerns and worries about our ability to carry all the responsibilities and burdens that accompany us in life. It is not uncommon to see a person literally stooped over, as if weighted down by some tremendous, invisible load.

As explained previously, the position of the shoulders is dependent, perhaps more than any other joint, on muscle action. Because muscles are controlled by the nervous system, which ultimately is controlled by the mind, there is an obvious relationship between the way a person positions the shoulders and his or her beliefs and attitudes in general. An interesting experiment is to stand in front of a mirror and put your shoulders and arms into different poses. Observe how the way you feel and the image you project change based on your body posture.

Our shoulders, arms, and hands reflect how we interact with the world. The shoulders can be set back and open, or closed in and protective. Our arms can be ready to be a barrier, pushing people away, or they can draw people in with an embrace. Closed hands are unreceptive, but open hands give and receive energy in the form of stimulus, awareness, and qi. It is through the medium of the hands that healing therapeutic touch is administered. The Chinese qi gong and Indian yoga systems both refer to the existence of energy centers in the hand. What do your shoulders, arms, and hands say about you? ■

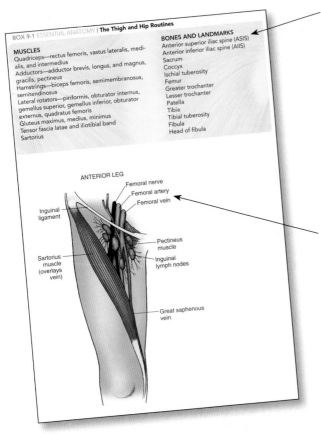

ESSENTIAL ANATOMY BOXES
Boxes list the muscles, bones, and landmarks at the beginning of each section, for easy reference.

ENDANGERMENT SITE figures in all Part II chapters show clearly the areas of caution or contraindication.

ROUTINES for massage practice that focus on the particular body region are outlined in detailed format in each chapter. A variety of techniques are presented. Each routine outlines a sequence, with detailed steps for each muscle set in the sequence. Look for the Trigger Point and Caution icons, shown here, throughout the routines.

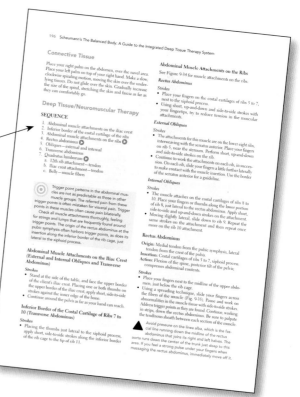

POSTURAL EVALUATION photos and **BODY READING** tables show you how to look, and what to look for, in a client presentation.

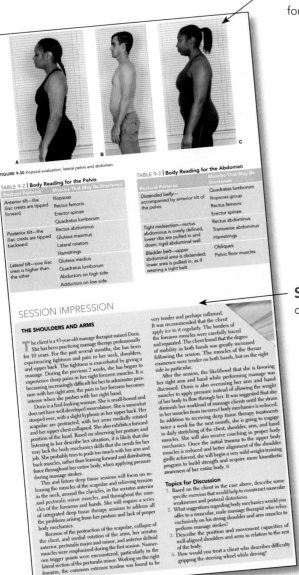

FIGURE 9-30 Postural evaluation: lateral pelvis and abdomen.

TABLE 9-2 | Body Reading for the Pelvis

Postural Patterns	Muscles That May Be Shortened
Anterior tilt—the iliac crests are tipped forward	Iliopsoas
	Rectus femoris
	Erector spinae
	Quadratus lumborum
Posterior tilt—the iliac crests are tipped backward	Rectus abdominus
	Gluteus maximus
	Lateral rotators
	Hamstrings
Lateral tilt—one iliac crest is higher than the other	Gluteus medius
	Quadratus lumborum
	Abductors on high side
	Adductors on low side

TABLE 9-3 | Body Reading for the Abdomen

Postural Patterns	Muscles That May Be Shortened
Distended belly—accompanied by anterior tilt of the pelvis	Quadratus lumborum
	Iliopsoas group
	Rectus femoris
	Erector spinae
Tight midsection—rectus abdominus is overly defined, lower ribs are pulled in and down; rigid abdominal wall	Rectus abdominus
	Transverse abdominus
	Hamstrings
Bladder belt—upper abdominal area is distended; lower area is pulled in, as if wearing a tight belt	Obliques
	Pelvic floor muscles

SESSION IMPRESSION boxes in each chapter provide case studies as well as Topics for Discussion.

SESSION IMPRESSION

THE SHOULDERS AND ARMS

The client is a 43-year-old massage therapist named Doris. She has been practicing massage therapy professionally for 10 years. For the past several months, she has been experiencing tightness and pain in her neck, shoulders, and upper back. The tightness is exacerbated by giving a massage. During the previous 2 weeks, she has begun to experience sharp pains in her right forearm muscles. It is becoming increasingly difficult for her to administer pressure with her right arm; the pain in her forearm becomes intense when she pushes with her right hand.

Doris is a frail-looking woman. She is small-boned and does not have well-developed musculature. She is somewhat stooped over, with a slight kyphosis in her upper back. Her scapulae are protracted, with her arms medially rotated and her upper chest collapsed. She also exhibits a forward position of the head. Based on observing her posture and listening to her describe her situation, it is likely that she may lack the body mechanics skills that she needs for her job. She probably tries to push too much with her arm and back muscles, rather than leaning forward and distributing force throughout her entire body, when applying pressure during massage strokes.

This and future deep tissue sessions will focus on releasing the muscles of the scapulae and relieving tension in the neck, around the clavicles, in the serratus anterior and pectoralis minor muscles, and throughout the muscles of the forearms and hands. She will require a series of integrated deep tissue therapy sessions to address all the problems arising from her posture and lack of proper body mechanics.

Because of the protraction of the scapulae, collapse of the chest, and medial rotation of the arms, her serratus anterior, pectoralis major and minor, and anterior deltoid muscles were emphasized during the first session. Numerous trigger points were encountered, particularly in the lateral section of the pectoralis minor. Working on the right forearm, the common extensor tendon was found to be very tender and perhaps inflamed. It was recommended that the client apply ice to it regularly. The borders of the forearm muscles were carefully traced and separated. The client found that the degree of mobility in both hands was greatly increased following the session. The muscles of the thenar eminence were tender on both hands, but on the right side in particular.

After the session, the likelihood that she is favoring her right arm and hand while performing massage was discussed. Doris is also overusing her arm and hand muscles to apply pressure instead of allowing the weight of her body to flow through her. It was suggested that she diminish her workload of massage clients until the strain in her muscles from incorrect body mechanics is reduced. In addition to receiving deep tissue therapy treatments twice a week for the next month, she is going to engage in daily stretching of the chest, shoulder, arm, and hand muscles. She will also receive coaching in proper body mechanics. Once the initial trauma to the upper body muscles is reduced and better alignment of the shoulder girdle achieved, she will begin a very mild weight-training program to build strength and acquire more kinesthetic awareness of her entire body. ■

Topics for Discussion

1. Based on the client in the case above, describe some specific exercises that would help to counteract muscular weaknesses and postural distortions.
2. What suggestions regarding body mechanics would you offer to a muscular, male massage therapist who relies exclusively on his strong shoulder and arm muscles to perform massage strokes?
3. Describe the position and movement capacities of well-aligned shoulders and arms in relation to the rest of the body.
4. How would you treat a client who describes difficulty gripping the steering wheel while driving?

ICONS in the text refer students to video clips of demonstrations of massage routines ▶ and real-life anatomy footage ▶.

---

thePoint Visit http://thePoint.lww.com/WernerTBB4e and use the scratchoff code on the inside front cover of this book to access the following student resources:

- Technique videos featuring the book's original author, Don Scheumann
- Anatomy images from the highly regarded *Acland's Video Atlas of Human Anatomy*
- Image labeling exercises to help reinforce your knowledge of anatomy

Acknowledgments

When I am asked to sign my books, I usually add this piece of advice to my autograph: *Always be learning.*

This is a guiding commitment in my life, and I am especially grateful when professional opportunities challenge me to live out this principle. Revising Don Scheumann's seminal technique book has been a great example: I have learned so much by becoming immersed in another person's life-work, and I am grateful and humbled by the experience.

I am especially appreciative of the following folks:

- Cindy Farrar, who was a student, and then a colleague of Don Scheumann, who was key to keeping his vision whole and strong. She also provided the beautiful space for our photographs, which provided a lovely return to the Atlanta area and Don's early career as a teacher.
- The models, Bryonna Hall, Chris Lobkowicz, Chris MacHarg, Kenosha Phillips, and Teresa Smith-Hernandez, as well as the other therapists who participated in our photo shoot, and our wonderful photographer, Gene Smith. I am moved by every image. You have enriched every reader with your courage, and your generosity of time and spirit. I know they are as grateful as I am.
- The people at Wolters Kluwer, Jay Campbell, Jonathan Joyce, and Leah Thomson, who thought that my filters of pathology and research might add what was needed to bring this text up to date (I hope I have not disappointed), and Linda Francis, keeper of spreadsheets (that I tend to ignore), unparalleled herder of cats, and poet renowned. I always say "yes" to projects if I get to work with you.

—Ruth Werner

Brief Contents

Expanded Contents

Introduction to the Integrated Deep Tissue Therapy System

Integrated Deep Tissue Therapy System

LEARNING OBJECTIVES

Having completed the reading, classroom instruction, and assigned homework related to Chapter 1 of *The Balanced Body*, the learner is expected to be able to. . .

- Explain the Wellness Model and how it applies to the ways health is described
- Explain the Open System principle and how it applies to the idea of energy and energy-based modalities
- Name some of the pioneers of massage and bodywork who have contributed to the integrated deep tissue therapy system

- Define the term *deep tissue therapy*
- Identify the consequences of muscular imbalance
- List the components of the integrated deep tissue therapy system

The integrated deep tissue therapy system is a specific holistic massage therapy approach to physical well-being that manually accesses both superficial and deep structures. This text is designed for students who have completed an introductory program of basic massage procedures and are ready to expand on what they have learned to incorporate many other ways to address soft tissue dysfunction.

Integrated deep tissue therapy is a method that combines several modalities to address various aspects and qualities of the myofascial system. When combined, these techniques provide a comprehensive protocol for reducing or eliminating many different manifestations of restriction in muscles and fascia. This technique can help to return the body to a healthy, strong, and dynamically resilient condition.

Two premises of understanding human health have heavily influenced the philosophies of the integrated deep tissue therapy system: the Wellness Model and the Open System principle.

The Wellness Model of health was pioneered by Dr. John Travis in the 1970s. Travis and his coauthor, Regina Sara Ryan, viewed wellness as an ongoing, constantly changing process of self-activated participation in a person's health and welfare. According to this perspective, humans are composed of a series of integrated systems that all work synergistically toward optimal health and well-being. This means that our physical, mental, emotional, and spiritual states are vital factors in determining the condition of our bodies, as well as our mental and emotional states. This perspective of mind–body connection and integration has served as starting point for

many complementary healthcare treatment protocols and holistic health centers that have been created since that time.

Dr. Travis' Wellness Model depicts the process of achieving wellness as a journey along a continuum (Fig. 1-1). The midpoint of the scale, labeled neutral, represents an absence of negative signs and symptoms: a condition of moderate well-being in which the individual is capable of functioning in everyday life. For many, this state of health has been accepted as the norm, and maintaining it is considered to be the best-case scenario.

The left side of the scale represents a gradual decline from the neutral state of wellness through a series of signs and symptoms of degenerating health that can eventually lead to disability or even premature death. It is hoped that a person experiencing this slide into dysfunction will seek adequate care and return at least to the neutral point of wellness. The halting of physical and/or psychological breakdown and the rebuilding of health is called the Treatment Model. Most traditionally recognized physical and psychological therapies are based on this goal.

The right side of the scale represents what Travis calls high-level wellness. This half of the continuum describes movement toward expanding states of greater well-being beyond the neutral stage of adequate functioning. These states of more complete fulfillment and happiness are motivated by increased awareness, pursuit of education, and personal growth. Achievement of these states is self-motivated as a person seeks out ways to explore opportunities for expansion of consciousness, creative expression, and productivity.

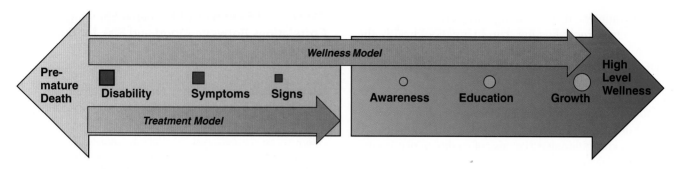

FIGURE 1-1 The Wellness Model. (Reprinted with permission from Travis JW, Ryan RS. *Wellness Workbook*. Berkeley, CA: Ten Speed Press; 1981.)

BOX 1-1 | Wellness: What a Concept!

The concept of wellness as a health-related goal is embedded in the language and provisions of the Affordable Care Act where, for perhaps the first time, incentives for achieving and maintaining health are considered as important as treating illness.[1] Strategies to promote health and well-being are also listed as part of the major goals for the National Center for Complementary and Integrative Health.[2] These government policy statements reflect a major shift in our cultural thinking about what health is and the importance of recognizing and valuing wellness.

[1]Anderko L, Roffenbender JS, Goetzel RZ, et al. Promoting prevention through the Affordable Care Act: workplace wellness. *Prev Chronic Dis.* 2012;9:120092. doi: http://dx.doi.org/10.5888/pcd9.120092.
[2]NCCIH Facts-as-a-Glance and Mission. https://nccih.nih.gov/about/ataglance

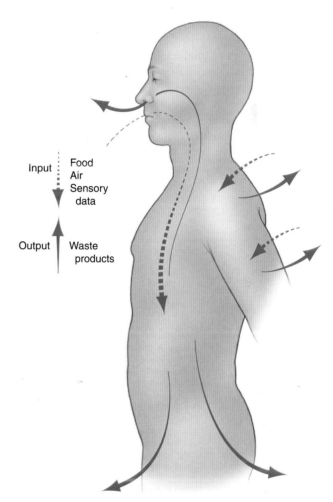

FIGURE 1-2 To maintain a state of health, the body must be able to freely take in and dispel energy.

The Wellness Model describes a potential for personal excellence that we are all capable of achieving. Any method of treatment or intervention that leads a person along the road to health can potentially provide the momentum to motivate that individual to seek the knowledge that will guide him or her to the highest level of wellness that person is capable of manifesting (Box 1-1). The integrated deep tissue therapy system is designed to meet clients in whatever part of the spectrum they inhabit, from fragile to highly functional.

According to Ilya Prigogine's Nobel prize–winning theory of dissipative structures, human beings and all living organisms are examples of an organizing principle known as the open system (Fig. 1-2). An open system operates by taking in energy, metabolizing or converting energy for use, and then releasing or dissipating energy back into the environment. All our vital processes depend on the efficient transformation

of energy for the health and integrity of the human system to remain intact.

The three primary ways that we receive energy are through the air we breathe, the food we eat, and the sensory input we receive through the nervous system and sense organs, including the skin. In a state of health, the physiologic pathways that allow conduction and transformation of energy throughout the body operate effectively and efficiently. When those conduits falter, the stage is set for breakdown and disease.

Research has demonstrated clear correlations between mood disorders (i.e., depression, anxiety) and an increased risk for somatic disorders (i.e., risk of cardiovascular events, pulmonary disease, and others). We also find that focus on resilience promotes both mental and physical health. Put in the context of the Open System principle, it is fair to suggest that as the efficiency of energy conversion (i.e., food, oxygen, and neurologic stimulation) through the body is improved, both psychological and physiologic activities are positively affected. The capacity for adaptation to the environment is stronger, and relationships and mental and emotional outlooks in general are improved when our systems function well. Table 1-1 lists just a couple of examples of research that points in this direction.

Massage therapy provides one option for assistance in the achievement and maintenance of high-level wellness, because it directly or indirectly affects many of the systems that transport

TABLE 1-1 | Examples of Research Showing Correlations Between Mood and Risk for Somatic Disorders

Article Title	Publication
Heart failure and depression	Newhouse A, Jiang W. *Heart Fail Clin.* 2014;2:295–304
Depression is associated with poor prognosis in patients with chronic obstructive pulmonary disease: a systematic review.	Salte K, Titlestad I, Halling A. *Dan Med J.* 2015;62:A5137

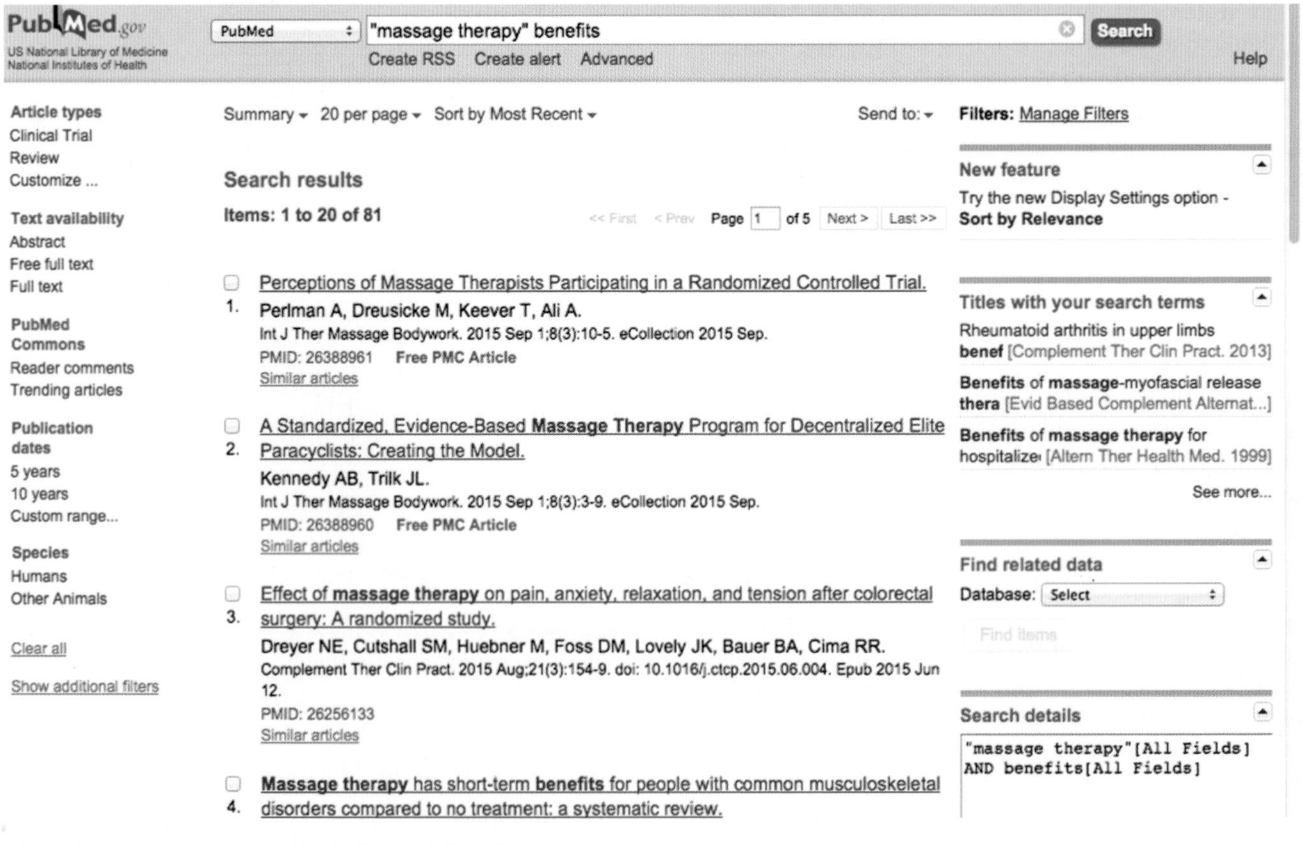

and transform energy within the body. Both clinical experience and formal research suggest that circulatory, respiratory, muscular, endocrine, and nervous system functions can all be supported by massage therapy. This body of knowledge is constantly growing. To see some of the collected evidence, the reader can consult www.pubmed.gov and enter the search terms *massage therapy* and *benefits* (Fig. 1-3).

FIGURE 1-3 Pubmed.gov with search terms *massage therapy* and *benefits*.

The Integrated Deep Tissue Therapy System

The integrated deep tissue therapy system of bodywork encompasses the full spectrum of human experience represented in the Wellness Model, and it works to improve the efficiency of energy conversion as proposed by the Open System principle. This approach to massage therapy does not attempt to replace any form of medical treatment, whether physical or psychological. Massage therapists are not trained to diagnose, treat, or prescribe drugs for any kind of medical condition, nor are they qualified to provide psychological evaluations or counseling. Instead, massage therapists are trained to initiate calming neurologic stimulation of the skin, to work for relaxation and freedom of movement in the myofascial system, and to influence the movement of fluid within the body. To do this well, massage therapists, especially those who practice integrated deep tissue therapy, need to be familiar with the factors that lead to soft tissue dysfunction, including postural abnormalities and movement habits that can result in misuse, abuse, and injury to the body. They must also understand the role of the mind and emotions in creating heightened activity of the sympathetic nervous system that can lead to muscular tension and increased sensitivity to pain.

A person who practices integrated deep tissue therapy may be viewed primarily as an educator. Through manipulation and realignment of the body's soft tissues, the therapist teaches the client to experience the benefits of becoming more relaxed, balanced, and pain free. The client may then feel motivated to pursue the lifestyle changes that will assist him or her in sustaining this higher state of well-being. These adjustments may include receiving regular massage therapy, instituting a fitness program, improving nutrition, and learning meditation or other forms of stress reduction.

Integrated deep tissue therapy incorporates viewpoints and methodologies from both Western and Eastern approaches to health. Many of the soft tissue techniques used here were developed within the context of the Western rehabilitative therapy model. A primary goal of these techniques is to improve overall function through:

- Enhancement of oxygen and nutrition levels within tissue cells
- Reduction of the effects of scar tissue and other adhering factors in the myofascia
- Decreasing pain sensations by minimizing irritation to nerve endings

The perspective on health provided by the Wellness Model and advocated by the integrated deep tissue therapy system is decidedly holistic. The holistic perspective views all aspects of a person—including the body, mind, spirituality, and relationships—as important factors contributing to the overall state of health. For this reason, the integrated deep tissue therapy system incorporates some Eastern perspectives on health, some of which are more capable of a holistic approach to wellness than the conventional Western rehabilitative system.

ORIGINS OF THE INTEGRATED DEEP TISSUE THERAPY SYSTEM

In embracing both the rehabilitative and holistic perspectives in healthcare, the integrated deep tissue therapy system follows in the tradition of many bodywork approaches that have been developed or promoted since the 1960s. A variety of sources have contributed to weave the tapestry that makes up this comprehensive style of body therapy.

The overriding goal of integrated deep tissue therapy is to establish an environment in which energy (food, oxygen, neurologic stimulation) may be taken into the body, utilized, and dispersed back into the environment in a fluid, efficient manner. It approaches this goal through identifying and minimizing restrictions in the myofascial system, which manifest as shortened or adhered areas within the muscles and fascia and result in limited range of motion, reduced function, and pain. As the physical body is restored to a condition of optimal function, many signs and symptoms of breakdown may resolve: Breathing becomes easier, movement is freer, and the mind may be clearer. An improved sense of self-efficacy and a more positive outlook toward life in general often accompany this improvement in physical well-being.

One of the first people to develop a method of bodywork based on this concept of comprehensive, overall body assessment and realignment was Dr. Ida Rolf (Fig. 1-4). Her style of therapy is commonly known as Rolfing. Dr. Rolf was a biochemist who began to formulate some principles and techniques of bodywork during the 1940s. She developed a 10-session series in which the fascial network is manipulated to realign the vertical axis of the body to the earth's gravitational field. Many styles of specific massage therapy and myofascial work, including structural integration, are at least partially derived from Dr. Rolf's pioneering concepts.

Neuromuscular therapy, or trigger point release work, rests on a foundation laid by Dr. Janet Travell (Fig. 1-5). Dr. Travell was a cardiologist who served two presidents as the White House physician. She did much research in the area of muscular involvement in pain causation and relief. Her two-volume work, *Myofascial Pain and Dysfunction: The Trigger Point Manual*, coauthored with David Simons, MD, serves as the seminal guide in this field.

Polarity therapy is a comprehensive, holistic bodywork concept that includes physical manipulations performed

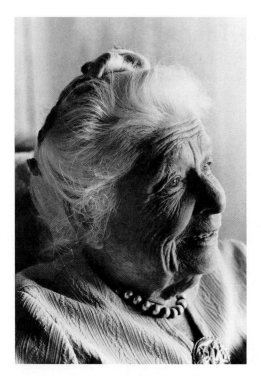

FIGURE 1-4 Ida Rolf, PhD. (Reprinted with permission from the Rolf Institute.)

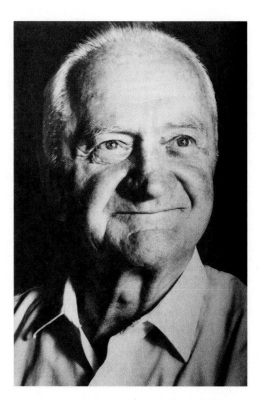

FIGURE 1-6 Dr. Randolph Stone. (Reprinted with permission from the American Polarity Therapy Association.)

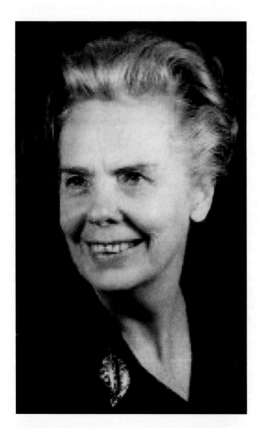

FIGURE 1-5 Janet Travell, MD. (Reprinted with permission from Virginia P. Street.)

while the patient is on a massage table. It was developed by Dr. Randolph Stone (Fig. 1-6) and was based on his years of studying traditional healing systems worldwide. The basic premise of polarity therapy is that health is built on freeing blockages in the underlying energetic pathways (see Box 1-2) that provide organizational templates for the physical and psychological structures. Dr. Stone's writings and work have a broad interface with many styles of bodywork, including structural integration, acupressure, craniosacral therapy, myofascial release, and therapeutic touch.

This list of pioneers whose works have informed the integrated deep tissue therapy system is only a partial one. Many other talented individuals have also participated in the design and refinement of techniques in this fluidly adaptable synthesis of massage modalities. Their contributions are acknowledged and much appreciated.

▶ COMPONENTS OF THE INTEGRATED DEEP TISSUE THERAPY SYSTEM

The techniques included in the integrated deep tissue method are depicted on a wheel (Fig. 1-7) rather than in a list. This is done to illustrate that they need not always be applied in a predetermined sequence; instead, they can be blended and mixed as required by the specific situation.

BOX 1-2 | What Does "Energy" Mean?

The term *energy* is introduced in this chapter in the context of the Open System principle, where it refers to the chemical and electrical reactions that are exchanged and dispelled when we breathe, eat, think, metabolize, and otherwise interact with our environment. Energy in this context is consistent with what we understand about the physical universe. It is observable and predictable.

The term *energy* in the context of "energetic forms of healing" refers to something that is neither objectively observable nor predictable. As we use it here, the word "energy" is a metaphor for an as yet not agreed-upon phenomenon that can occur with or without the component of touch. At this time, research suggests that what we see in this setting may be some combination of the results of positive expectations from both client and practitioner, the power of ritual in a person's experience of being cared for, and other factors not yet identified. This phenomenon can be a powerfully positive part of the massage therapy interchange, regardless of the style of bodywork that is employed.

This book incorporates some types of "energy work," including polarity, shiatsu, and reflexology. These techniques are woven into the integrated deep tissue therapy system in a way that may maximize their positive effects. This is a reflection of the author's many years of experience, rather than because a strong evidence base supports these techniques.

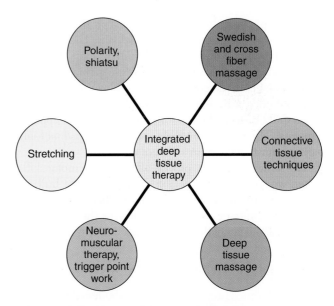

FIGURE 1-7 The integrated massage wheel.

In each lesson of this text, the techniques are described in a prescribed order that is suggested as a general protocol for approaching the body. This sequence opens the body progressively, beginning with preparatory contact between the therapist and client, warm-up of the tissues, and then work on the deeper layers. This basic structure allows much room for adaptability by moving through the techniques on the wheel according to the unique needs of the individual.

Deep Tissue Therapy

The muscles with the most influence on posture are those closest to our core: the deep muscles. The center of the integrated deep tissue therapy system is, naturally, massage to those deep and important soft tissue structures. Specifically, this means addressing superficial muscles first and then accessing tight muscles through the softened superficial tissues. The primary goal of this focused, precise type of massage is to reduce the level of pain and inefficient movement that occurs when muscles and fascia are overly tight, or overly stretched. This is done through the application of slow, compressive, and lengthening procedures to the involved muscles and fascia. Note that "deep tissue therapy" does not always mean deep pressure, nor must it be painful to receive.

Deep tissue therapy is designed to return the body to a state of ease and balance by eliminating the uneven pulls on the skeleton caused by contracted muscles and constricted fascia, and restoring functional relationships to counterbalanced forces. These areas of imbalance and restriction may be observed by watching how a person stands and moves. Manual testing of the degree of movement available at the joints also helps to determine which muscles are shortened or contracted and which are lengthened and weakened. After recognizing the patterns of distortion, the therapist then systematically addresses the shortened muscles to allow them to relax and return to a neutral length and works to loosen the constricted fascia to re-establish freedom of movement.

MUSCLES: COUNTERBALANCING FORCES

A primary function of muscles is to provide movement for the body. This happens when a motor impulse from the central nervous system signals a muscle to contract by pulling on its attachments.

Each muscle has synergists (partners that help in a particular movement) and antagonists (muscles that do the opposite movement). For any given action, the prime mover—the main muscle enlisted to move a part of the body—and its synergists interact. For instance, when we bend our elbow to take a sip of tea, the prime mover is typically the biceps brachii and a major synergist is the brachialis: These partners contract by pulling their bony attachments closer together. For this to happen, the antagonist—the triceps brachii—must perform an eccentric contraction that allows it to lengthen in a controlled way, and all of this must happen smoothly, or we spill our tea. Then to lower the teacup, the opposite happens: The triceps contracts, and the biceps/brachialis partners must lengthen in a controlled way.

The same interactions provide all of our fine motor skills. When we write, chop vegetables, change a light bulb, or do massage, the intrinsic muscles in our hands and fingers alternately contract and relax to allow us the freedom of movement and strength we need to accomplish these tasks.

EFFECTS OF MUSCLE IMBALANCE

Muscles become chronically tense and shortened for a lot of different reasons, but the end result is usually a dysfunctional relationship between a prime mover and its antagonists. The consequences of living with unnecessarily tense muscles are many:

- Inhibition of fluid movement. Circulation of blood and lymph is inhibited both locally at the cellular level and at a larger level that can inhibit flow through major vessels. In an open system, energy exchange must be efficient for the body to function well, and chronic muscle tension can interfere with this.
- Nutrient/waste turnover is impaired. Muscles rely on a steady intake of oxygen and nutrients to provide the fuel necessary for muscular contraction and relaxation to occur. They also rely on the efficient removal of the by-products of work: carbon dioxide and other wastes. These are released into the lymph and venous blood supply to be processed for removal from the body. If this cycle is disrupted, the muscles can no longer perform their job effectively.
- Local neuron irritation. Wastes within and around muscle cells can irritate nerve endings, resulting in pain. Poor circulatory turnover can interfere with the function of motor neurons and the neuromuscular junction, resulting in weakness. Tight muscles may also put mechanical stress on nerves. Altogether, the interruption of energy exchange at the muscle cell level creates a scenario for pain, inefficient function, unnecessary work, and a risk of injury.
- Asymmetry and imbalance. Muscles that are chronically contracted disrupt the symmetry of balanced forces acting on the skeleton (Fig. 1-8). They hold bones out of their best position, causing postural distortions that result in structural and functional inefficiencies. Tissue integrity is compromised when the body is not in balance in relation to gravity: Muscles tighten, fascial sheaths may thicken, and cartilage, tendons, and ligaments bear shearing stress for which they are not designed. Ultimately, even the bones may change shape to adapt to long-term changes in weight-bearing load.

- Increased risk for injury. When one group of muscles is chronically tight and shortened, it is likely that their antagonists are also tight, but lengthened and weak. Lengthened muscles have poor weight-bearing capacity, and any sudden demand for rapid, forceful movement may cause them to tear. These muscle strains happen most frequently at the tenoperiosteal junction, or at the musculotendinous junction. Then the body compensates further for these injuries, leading to states of greater dysfunction and pain.

APPLICATION OF DEEP TISSUE THERAPY

Muscle spindles and Golgi tendon organs (GTOs) are special sensory neurons called proprioceptors that are found in muscles, tendons, and joints (Fig. 1-9). Muscle spindles wrap in a spiral around individual muscle fibers and convey messages to the central nervous system about how long or short those fibers are, as well as how quickly they change shape. GTOs are located mostly in tendons, and they are stimulated by the mechanical distortion that happens when a tendon bears weight. They convey messages to the central nervous system about how hard a muscle-tendon unit is working. Together these proprioceptors allow us to sense muscle tension, movement, and resistance. They create a highly complex feedback loop with motor neurons that respond to their messages with just the right amount of **motor unit** recruitment to do the desired task. In short, proprioceptors help to determine muscle tone (see Box 1-3).

Unfortunately, our proprioceptors are adaptable to our movement and postural habits. With enough long-term stimulus, they come to accept inefficient tightness or length as normal, even if it is not optimal. This is how people can come to develop a forward-head posture, or a tendency to raise their shoulders without knowing it. Consciously overriding the proprioceptors to correct these habits feels difficult and clumsy at first, but the proprioceptors can be "retrained" into accepting more efficient levels of muscle tension as normal.

If a muscle is stretched very far and very quickly, the muscle spindles lengthen rapidly and the motor response is to contract. This mechanism is known as the **stretch reflex.** This protective device prevents muscles and tendons from being torn by sudden overstretching. If, however, a muscle is stretched slowly, so the muscle spindles also lengthen slowly, the stretch reflex is not elicited. In this case, the motor response from the central nervous system allows the muscle to relax and lengthen further.

The goal of the slow, compressive strokes applied along the length of a muscle is to help recalibrate the muscle spindles so that they allow a chronically contracted muscle to relax. Slow stretching of the muscle after the deep tissue strokes are applied is intended to activate the GTOs, with the intention that they will help to reset the muscle's resting tone at a more efficient, relaxed level.

Long, specific strokes are also performed along the borders of adjacent muscles to address fascial adhering and any

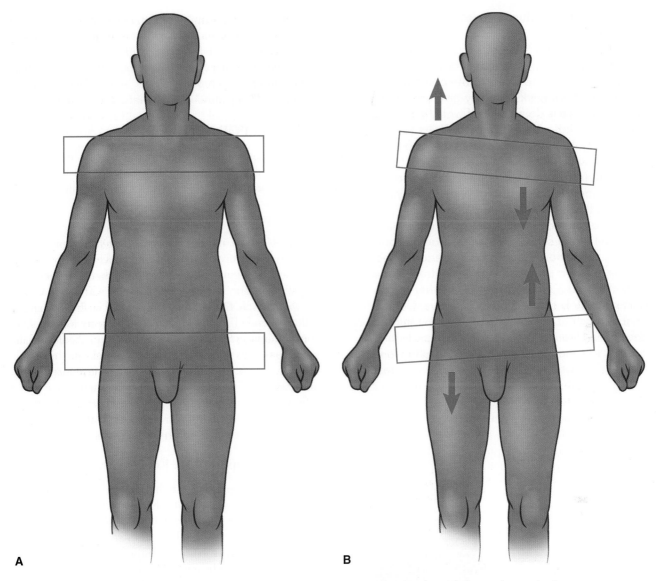

A   B

FIGURE 1-8 A. Normal muscle balance resulting in body symmetry. **B.** Uneven muscle relationships contribute to body assymetry.

accumulation of scar tissue that may prevent the targeted muscles from moving independently of each other. In some cases, it may be possible to loosen or undo adhesions; in others, the best goal may be to simply soften the fascia with the heat and improved local nutrition and hydration that massage supplies. In deep tissue therapy, muscle groups are freed in layers, from superficial to deep, to allow each individual muscle to perform its actions without restriction. Reducing or removing these glitches from the musculature can help to restore full movement capacity.

BENEFITS OF DEEP TISSUE THERAPY

As the soft tissues of the body are realigned and muscular balance is restored, the entire organism can function more efficiently. With better posture and freer movement, the risk of injury is decreased. Coordination between synergists and antagonists is also improved, so less effort is needed to accomplish simple tasks. Minimizing tension around joints reduces the risk of joint irritation, osteoarthritis, and ligament tears as well. Improving tone in the muscles of respiration means that breathing can become more effortless. The overall level of vitality and oxygen/carbon dioxide turnover promotes clearer thinking. All the body's systems benefit from having more metabolic energy available to fuel them.

Neuromuscular Therapy

Neuromuscular therapy is a specialized form of work that addresses a specific manifestation of muscular dysfunction known as **trigger points**. Trigger points are tiny areas of irritation

BOX 1-3 | **What Is Muscle Tone?**

Many bodywork professionals have their own way of describing muscle tone. For our purposes, the term muscle tone refers to the percentage of fibers that are working at any given moment. When a muscle is doing a lot of work, it is appropriate for a high percentage of its fibers to be contracting. But when it is at rest, it is appropriate for a much lower percentage of fibers to be activated. (A *fully* relaxed muscle with *no* contracting fibers is a sign of central nervous system damage; this is called flaccid paralysis.)

Muscle tone for work or for rest is determined with the help of sensory messages from proprioceptors about how much force is needed in the moment. This is processed in the central nervous system, and the motor response is either to contract or to stop contracting muscle fibers. The goal of much of the deep tissue therapy that is described here is to encourage those proprioceptors to send messages that will result in lower muscle tone when the targeted muscle is at rest.

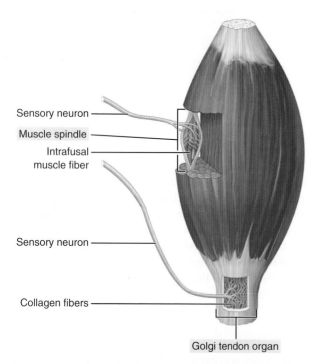

Sensory neuron ———

Muscle spindle ———

Intrafusal muscle fiber ———

Sensory neuron ———

Collagen fibers ———

Golgi tendon organ

FIGURE 1-9 Proprioceptors: muscle spindles and Golgi tendon organs. (From McConnell TH, Hull KL. *Human Form, Human Function.* Philadelphia, PA: Wolters Kluwer; 2010.)

that form within strained bands of muscle tissue. They refer sensations of pain, weakness, or numbness to surrounding or distant areas of the body. Trigger points are common factors in chronic muscular pain. They appear to develop in areas where muscles are chronically tight, and chronic tightness is often a result of painful trigger points: a vicious circle.

TRIGGER POINT THEORIES

Although these common phenomena have been documented for several decades, the precise mechanism of how trigger points come about is still an issue of some debate.

Waste Products and Nerve Irritation

Dr. Janet Travell and her associate Dr. David Simons were pioneers in identifying, mapping, and treating trigger points. Dr. Travell's original theory is that these points formed when the constant presence of waste products within a damaged group of muscle **fibrils,** apparently produced by unrelenting cellular metabolism in that section of the muscle, stimulates nerve endings in the area to send amplified input into the spinal cord. This stimulus is then thrown back into the peripheral nervous system through weakened or **facilitated nerve pathways**. The impulses traveling along these nerve routes activate pain sensations in a specific portion of the muscles stimulated by those particular nerves. The areas affected by trigger points are called **referred pain zones.**

Adenosine Triphosphate Energy Crisis

A more recent theory suggests that damage occurs at the neuromotor junction where **acetylcholine** is released, setting up a chain reaction that results in calcium flowing constantly within portions of muscle cells. This causes continual contraction of sets of **sarcomeres** so that adenosine triphosphate (**ATP**) is used up and cannot be renewed. This situation is sometimes called an ATP energy crisis. The presence of ATP is necessary to provide energy for all the cell's activities, including the return of calcium to its storage compartment, the sarcoplasmic reticulum, thus allowing the sarcomeres to resume a resting state. Without access to ATP, the affected fibers cannot relax.

This theory suggests that manual pressure on the trigger point provides the stimulus to pump ATP into the damaged cells and deactivate the positive feedback loop between the acetylcholine and calcium. The flow of nerve impulses to the trigger point's referred pain zone thus ceases. Pressure on the trigger point may also instigate the release of **endorphins** and **enkephalin,** two of the body's natural pain fighters.

Current Pain Science

The most recent research on trigger points challenges both of the previous theories. Some scientists who specialize in pain doubt the mechanisms that have been so far proposed. The reasons for this are beyond the scope of this discussion,

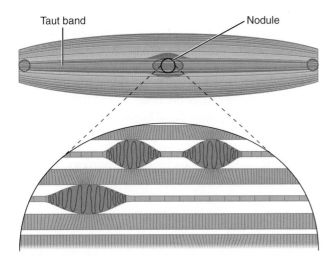

Taut band — Nodule

FIGURE 1-10 A trigger point is embedded within a taut band of muscle fibers. The contraction knots within the trigger point represent portions of a muscle fiber where the sarcomeres are fully contracted. (Reprinted with permission from Simons D, Travell J, Simons S. *Myofascial Pain and Dysfunction: the Trigger Point Manual.* Philadelphia, PA: Lippincott Williams & Wilkins, 1999:70. *Upper Half of Body*; vol 1.)

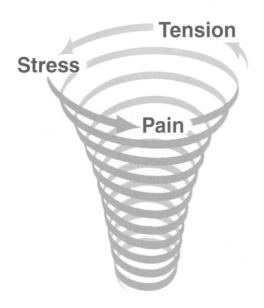

Tension

Stress

Pain

FIGURE 1-11 The stress-tension-pain cycle generates a self-perpetuating, downward spiral of dysfunction that often requires therapeutic intervention to be halted.

but the controversy calls into question the best treatment options for clients who are affected by trigger points. Although the traditional approach to trigger points is static manual pressure for 8 to 12 seconds, this appears to be less effective than gentler manipulation that does not cause the client to withdraw, tighten muscles elsewhere, or change breathing patterns to tolerate. Interestingly, the original Travell recommendations appear to follow this guideline; it is only through generations of interpretation that the deep painful pressure approach to trigger point treatment has become the standard approach.

TRIGGER POINT SYMPTOMS

Regardless of their cause, trigger points have some predictable palpatory patterns: They are hard, hypertonic "knots" or "taut bands," always in muscle tissue, and they often cause a short involuntary contraction or fasciculation when they are palpated (Fig. 1-10). A small amount of pressure on an active trigger point can cause pain that is far beyond what would be expected, and that pain may radiate to distant areas in the body. For some patients, their primary symptom is this referred pain from a trigger point: a headache stemming from a trigger point in the neck, for instance.

Trigger points can be self-perpetuating. They accompany a phenomenon called the **stress-tension-pain cycle** (Fig. 1-11). Stress can be generated by a number of factors, including physical pain, emotional turmoil, trauma, or other issues. The result is areas that feel sore or weak.

The body attempts to isolate areas of weakness through **muscle splinting.** This protective mechanism causes muscles

around the injured area to contract to isolate the weakness and prevent movement that could lead to further damage. Fascia may thicken in this area, and taut, unyielding muscle cells may train the proprioceptors into maintaining this high level of tone. The lack of local circulation, along with the cellular damage that results from trauma, maintains the tension-pain cycle.

Active trigger points are painful. Living with pain invariably raises a person's general perception of stress and interferes with several important functions, including the ability to get good-quality sleep. This leads to more tension and increased pain sensitivity, which foster the conditions that increase pain, and thus the cycle is perpetuated.

TREATMENT OF TRIGGER POINTS

Neuromuscular therapy attempts to interrupt the stress-tension-pain cycle by locating trigger points and altering the signals that maintain them. Manual pressure at the trigger point, often with a pumping action, is intended to change the flow of nerve impulses that provide the sensation of referred pain. Done in such a way that does not cause more pain for the client, this therapy can help trigger points to resolve and stop causing pain altogether.

To reduce the possibility that a trigger point may reactivate, the muscle fibers in the area need to be as relaxed as possible. It is important to stretch the affected muscle after treating it and instruct the client to continue to stretch that area on a regular basis.

Neuromuscular therapy works best when it is accompanied by other modalities that help the muscles to lengthen and relax, thus reducing the likelihood of future trigger point formation and activation.

SWEDISH MASSAGE

Swedish massage is classified as a circulatory style of massage. Its broad, sweeping strokes promote increased blood flow through muscle tissue, which facilitates metabolic efficiency. The Swedish style may also induce relaxation in the body by enhancing parasympathetic nervous system activity. It is often performed as a full-body massage, which helps to bring a sense of wholeness, continuity, and integration to the recipient.

Within the integrated deep tissue therapy system, Swedish techniques are used to warm up the tissues in preparation for more specific work. Swedish strokes may also suggest the proper directions for the myofascial tissues to follow to eliminate stress-producing misalignment. The massage therapist can utilize these strokes almost like a sculptor, shaping and remolding the body into a better-organized configuration of muscle and bone.

Integrated deep tissue therapy is primarily a nonverbal form of communication with the body's nervous system and soft tissue components. It is designed to reeducate proprioceptive **reflex arcs** to produce more effective movement patterns. The relaxing, pleasurable, lengthening sensations generated by Swedish massage strokes are the perfect vehicle for introducing sensations of ease and comfort.

CROSS FIBER MASSAGE

Cross fiber massage techniques are incorporated along with Swedish strokes to further relax the muscle groups and assist in the elimination of myofascial restrictions. The application of strokes perpendicular, rather than parallel, to the direction of muscle fibers is the distinguishing characteristic of all styles of cross fiber manipulation.

The cross fiber massage used in the integrated deep tissue system is performed symmetrically and bilaterally. This means that strokes are applied across the muscle fibers in both directions, forward and backward, rather than in one direction only. The procedure consists of rolling bundles of muscle fibers over each other using either the fingers or the broad side of the thumb. The intention of cross fiber massage is to reduce or eliminate the effects of adhered myofascia that may interfere in optimal efficiency of movement.

CONNECTIVE TISSUE TECHNIQUES

Connective tissue techniques are designed to address the fascial membranes that surround and permeate the musculature. The fascial component of muscles is both strong and flexible and is responsible for providing support to all the body's structures.

The degree of fascial mobility is an important factor in determining a person's physical health and resilience. Fascial restrictions may be minimized through slow stretching and low-force compressive movements, and a renewed sense of expansiveness and freedom can be reintroduced to the body.

Many varieties of connective tissue work have been developed. The specific strokes offered here have been chosen for their focus on spreading fascial membranes in conjunction with deep structure massage. Improving the quality of myofascia around constricted muscles allows deep tissue massage to be more effective.

STRETCHING

Lengthening the soft tissues through stretching movements serves several important functions. The therapist stretches the recipient's muscles during a massage treatment for those muscles to better assimilate the neuromuscular changes that have occurred during the session, and the client stretching on his or her own after receiving an integrated deep tissue therapy session is highly encouraged. Maintaining muscle length through stretching reduces the overall level of stress in the body and helps to minimize many of the muscular imbalances that can result in pain and injury.

Receiving massage is mostly a passive activity. During the session, the client's body is manipulated and moved, primarily by the therapist. But for the changes brought about by this kind of bodywork to last, the client must repeatedly use the recalibrated proprioceptive reflex arcs achieved in the session. The client can do this through voluntary movement based on the body's new alignment. Otherwise, the previous, dysfunctional muscle patterns may soon return, and progress toward greater body function will be slowed or interrupted.

ENERGY WORK

Techniques of energy balancing are based on the premise that the body is formed and nourished by currents that determine the state of health and vitality of the individual. When these pathways flow freely, all the body's systems are fortified and continued growth and development are assured. Weakening or blockage of the currents eventually leads to dysfunction. A reminder: the term *energy* in this context refers to the positive responses that can occur when one person receives the caring attention of another, with or without the component of touch.

The two methods of energy balancing that are included in integrated deep tissue therapy are polarity and shiatsu, and reflexology is frequently called for in the sections on accessory work. These are systems of bodywork and healthcare that require extensive specialized training to learn in their entirety. Practitioners of this integrated style of deep tissue therapy cannot be considered to be experts in any of these modalities unless they have acquired the education to meet the necessary requirements. The techniques from these systems are included here because they enhance the effects of the whole integrated deep tissue therapy system.

Polarity

The theory behind polarity therapy likens the body's energy currents to the flow of magnetic forces, with positive and negative poles (Fig. 1-12). Balance between these two poles is mediated by a third, or neutral, pole. Blockage through any

of these three poles weakens the natural flow of energy. This inhibition of energy flow may manifest physically as myofascial restriction. Most of the polarity procedures described in these lessons consist of contacts wherein the therapist places his or her two hands on the client's body at locations corresponding to this flow of energy, with the intention of enhancing the body's natural healing abilities.

In this text, we include polarity therapy as a respected historical reference. It is an approach to educated touch that has low risk for adverse events and a potential benefit as introductory touch at the beginning of a session. Although scientific evidence does not support the proffered mechanisms of polarity, the technique can be a valuable part of integrated deep tissue therapy. It can provide a pause: a gentle transitioning touch that provides time to help the therapist to focus on his or her intention, to help the client tune in to what he or she is experiencing, and to make the techniques that follow more welcomed, and therefore more beneficial.

Polarity procedures are usually applied at the beginning of the session to help induce relaxation and a state of readiness on the part of the client. The simple polarity holds described here are intended to induce a parasympathetic state, allowing the client's body to assimilate the effects of the massage treatment more effectively. Sustained, quiet contact to open a session, along with the innately nurturing quality of this kind of work, helps to build a bond of confidence and trust between the therapist and client: This is the foundation for the therapeutic relationship.

Shiatsu

Shiatsu is a Japanese style of bodywork that intends to encourage the flow of the life energy, or **qi**, through a series of energy channels known as **meridians** (Fig. 1-13). It is administered through a combination of compressive strokes and stretching of the body along these pathways. The shiatsu procedures described in this course were chosen because the author's experience supports their inclusion to achieve the best benefits of integrated deep tissue therapy.

Reflexology

Many of the massage routines in Chapters 6 to 10 end with a brief reflexology component meant to enhance work to a particular part of the body. The reflexology protocols offered here are derived from the work of Eunice Ingham who, during her career as a physiotherapist, observed and documented that pressure to specific areas of the foot seemed to lead to improvements in physical function. More on Ingham's work can be found in her books, *Stories the Feet Can Tell* and *Stories the Feet Have Told (Ingham Publishing, St. Petersburg, FL).*

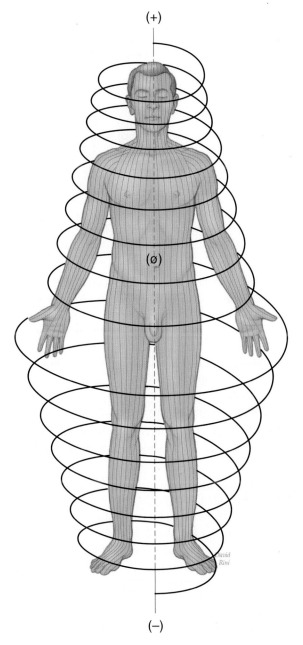

FIGURE 1-12 Polarity energy currents.

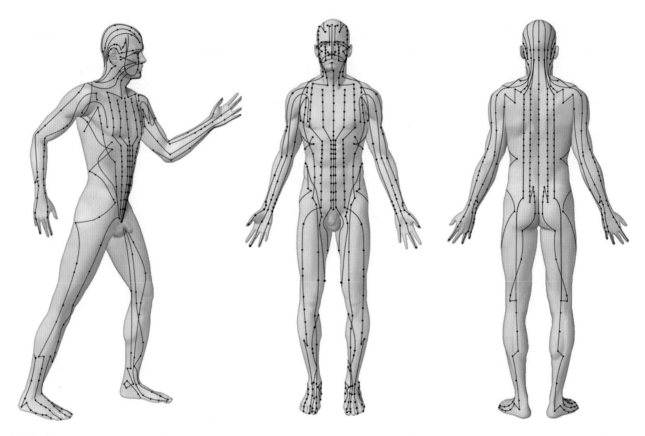

FIGURE 1-13 Direction of meridian flow. (From: Williams A. *Massage Mastery*. Philadelphia, PA: Wolters Kluwer; 2013.)

REVIEW QUESTIONS

Level 1

Receive and Respond

1. In the integrated deep tissue therapy paradigm, an ongoing dynamic participation in a person's health is described as...
   a. the Wellness Model.
   b. the Open System principle.
   c. the mind–body continuum.
   d. holistic perspective.

2. An organism takes in energy in the forms of fuel and stimuli and disperses it in the forms of work or intellectual activity. This is a description of...
   a. holistic perspective.
   b. the Open System principle.
   c. the mind–body continuum.
   d. the Wellness Model.

3. Which is the list of contributors to the origins of integrated deep tissue therapy?
   a. Farrar, Rolf, Travell
   b. Hanna, Upledger, Stone
   c. Travell, Lowe, Quintner
   d. Rolf, Stone, Travell

4. What is the best description of "deep tissue therapy?"
   a. Massage or bodywork applied in a way that redistributes stress or weight-bearing force through the core
   b. Massage or bodywork applied to target muscles that support the core
   c. Massage or bodywork applied to any muscle below the most superficial layer
   d. Massage or bodywork applied in the context of the integrated deep tissue therapy system

Level 2

Apply Concepts

1. Inhibition of local fluid movement is a consequence of muscular imbalance because...
   a. fascial restrictions inhibit the dilation and constriction of the major lymphatic vessels.
   b. chronic muscle tension interferes with lymphatic or circulatory turnover.
   c. tight muscles exert external pressure on major blood vessels, driving up blood pressure and interfering with oxygen delivery systems.
   d. irritated nerve endings cause lymphatic and circulatory capillaries to dilate.

2. Nutrient/waste exchange is impaired at a cellular level when. . .
   a. irritated nerve endings cause the local circulatory and lymphatic capillaries to constrict.
   b. the pumping action of muscle contraction and relaxation is interrupted because of chronic muscle tightness.
   c. pro-inflammatory chemicals flood the tissues at areas of chronic muscle tightness.
   d. major blood and lymphatic vessels are restricted by excessive connective tissue resistance.

3. Chronic muscle imbalance can contribute to a risk for injury because. . .
   a. when muscles are chronically tight, then nearby ligaments degenerate, raising the risk of sprains.
   b. chronically tight muscles ultimately degenerate and are replaced with connective tissue that has less weight-bearing capacity.
   c. lengthened and weakened muscles have reduced weight-bearing capacity and are vulnerable to damage with sudden demands for work.
   d. the bony attachments of chronically tight muscles are likely to develop avulsion fractures.

4. Local neuron irritation becomes a problem when. . .
   a. irritated nerve endings cause lymphatic and circulatory capillaries to dilate.
   b. pain leads to inefficient muscle function and an increased risk for injury.
   c. irritated nerve endings cause the local circulatory and lymphatic capillaries to constrict.
   d. neurons become exhausted and signals fail to travel appropriately to the central nervous system.

Level 3

Problem Solving: Discussion Points

1. The components of the integrated deep tissue therapy system include neuromuscular therapy and the treatment of myofascial trigger points. Discuss the current understanding of myofascial trigger points and how new understanding has changed the traditional approach to their treatment.

2. The integrated deep tissue therapy system includes some elements of "energy work," specifically in the forms of polarity and shiatsu. Using the Open System principle, discuss how the term *energy* might be applied in the context of bodywork.

Learning the Work

The latter portion of this book consists of the integrated deep tissue therapy lessons. Each lesson contains information essential for learning and understanding this system of deep tissue therapy. While learning the work, the lessons should be read and practiced in the same order as they are presented in the book. The lessons have been organized to teach the student a logical, sequential approach to mastering the concepts of integrated deep tissue therapy. This book is not to be considered a self-teaching guide. It is best used as a supplement to teaching with an experienced instructor who has extensive experience in the system, and who can give the student important guidance and feedback.

The routines given in the lessons do not represent exact reproductions of specific bodywork sessions that would actually be performed with a client. Rather, they outline a general sequence of possible choices for a given session.

Each routine describes techniques for addressing most of the muscles associated with that particular part of the body. Although an integrated deep tissue therapist needs to know all these techniques, he or she would probably not use every procedure described here on any single client.

The student will practice all the techniques in each lesson with a partner in class, and then exchange roles; this is done so that both students can learn the material effectively and experientially. Having students change partners for each lesson is optimal, so they can work with as many different bodies as possible. It is not possible to determine which techniques would be most beneficial for any individual without assessing that person for his or her particular needs, but the more people students work with while under supervision, the better preparation they will have as they take these techniques into their professional lives.

Format of the Lessons

Each lesson is divided into two parts. The first portion presents information and assessment tools that provide the foundation for acquiring the skills of an integrated deep tissue therapist. The second portion describes the techniques that are used in the integrated deep tissue system based on its six components.

The first part of each lesson is divided into the following sections:

▶ GENERAL CONCEPTS

This section presents foundational information pertaining to the area of the body under discussion. It acquaints the

student with the overall design of this segment, and it introduces the anatomical relationships students will find in this part of the body.

▶ MUSCULOSKELETAL ANATOMY AND FUNCTION

This portion of the lesson expands on the information mentioned in the General Concepts section. The material discussed here focuses on the anatomy and movement capabilities of the targeted muscles as they pertain to integrated deep tissue therapy.

▶ ENDANGERMENT SITES

Areas that require special caution or concern with bodywork are described and illustrated.

▶ CONDITIONS

These are problems, diseases, and cautions for bodywork that the therapist may encounter. It is not a comprehensive list; it is designed to point out common situations that prompt clients to seek massage, most of which primarily affect the musculoskeletal systems. The learner is encouraged to pursue further information in this area as needed.

▶ HOLISTIC VIEW

The whole-person scope of the work is discussed in this section. Students are introduced to concepts involving the relationship between thoughts, beliefs, and emotions, as well as cultural associations connected to various parts of the body as they influence the physical state of the client.

▶ POSTURAL EVALUATION

An outline for a full analysis of the body segments being studied is included in this section. Postural evaluation is one of the major assessment tools of the integrated deep tissue therapist. It provides much of the necessary information to outline a plan of bodywork for an individual client. It also serves as a baseline assessment, to track changes in the client's body resulting from the application of integrated deep tissue therapy.

▶ EXERCISES AND SELF-TREATMENT

This section focuses on exercises the client can do on his or her own that will stretch and strengthen the muscles that have been treated in the sessions. These exercises can be taught to clients so that they can be performed between massage sessions and will enhance and prolong the results of the deep tissue therapy. Be aware that teaching exercises to clients is not within the scope of practice for all massage therapists, so this section may not apply to all readers.

▶ QUICK REFERENCE BOXES/TABLES

1. *Essential Anatomy.* This box lists the muscles, bones, and bony landmarks that will be referred to and/or addressed during the lesson.
2. *Body Reading for the Area.* This chart outlines the most common muscles involved in certain postural deviations.
3. *Range of Motion.* Most of the possible movements for each major joint are listed, along with the muscles that perform those actions. Examining range of motion lets the therapist know if the client has soft tissue restrictions, and requires additional work on the muscles and fascia involved.

▶ SESSION IMPRESSIONS

These are descriptions of real-life interactions with clients that demonstrate how the principles of integrated deep tissue therapy may be put to work. These cases are followed by a series of discussion questions that allow learners to explore the recommended strategies.

Lesson Sequence

The order of presentation for the integrated deep tissue lessons has been planned to give the learner a clear understanding about the organization of the body according to structure and function. The author is indebted to the pioneering work of Dr. Ida Rolf, who conceived a unique vision of the body's design and created a logical, effective plan to realign the soft tissues in reference to the field of gravity in which we live.

The integrated deep tissue therapy system is not considered to be a form of structural integration in the Rolfing tradition, and it does not follow the progressive, 10-session series plan that is characteristic of that style of bodywork. The overall layout of the lesson plans in this book does follow, in a very general way, the sequence of treatment that Dr. Rolf advocated, because this is an effective order in which to perform

a series of deep tissue therapy sessions with a client over a period of time. The sequence exemplifies the eighth guideline in *Principles of Conscious Bodywork*, "seek to re-establish balance" (see Chapter 3).

The order of the lessons is as follows:

▶ THE TRUNK

- *Chest.* The chest houses our breathing mechanism, and one of the first manifestations of anxious feelings is restricted respiration. Intense feelings and patterns of emotional holding often reflect in shallow or rapid breathing. Reducing tension in the muscles of the chest helps to ease the flow of air in and out of the body. Improving efficiency of the breathing mechanism is crucial for the rest of the deep tissue work to be fully effective. The increased oxygen intake acquired by full, deep breathing is necessary to support the metabolic changes that are brought about by this therapy.

- *Spine and Back Muscles.* The spine supports the weight segments of the upper half of the body, and it must be aligned properly to perform this function properly. When the vertebrae are in best relationship, the nerves passing through the spinal column are unimpeded. Lengthening soft tissues around the spine also helps to support and balance the chest area in the anterior side of the trunk.

▶ THE UPPER EXTREMITY

Treatment moves from the proximal portion of the arm to the distal portion.

- *Scapula.* This is the root of the upper extremity. Many of the muscles that attach the arm to the body are anchored on the scapula. Improving the freedom of movement of the scapula allows more complete function of both the upper arm and the rib cage.
- *Shoulder and Upper Arm.* Reducing unnecessary tone in the rotator cuff muscles and other shoulder muscles helps to reposition the arm and improve alignment of the upper body.
- *Forearm and Hand.* The muscles that control the hand are the smallest of the upper extremity. Re-establishing efficient refined movement of the hand helps to strengthen its connection to the brain, and contributes to the reduction of tension throughout the body.

▶ THE LOWER EXTREMITY

The progression of the sequence on the lower extremity is from distal to proximal, from the foot to the pelvis.

- *Foot, Leg, and Knee.* The foot forms the foundation for vertical support of the entire body; it is our primary interface with the force of gravity. The knee has to transfer multidirectional forces of rotation and lateral pressure into a narrow range of motion of mostly flexion and extension. These complex joints and muscles need to function optimally to stay injury-free, and to accommodate and support the shifts that occur when the upper body has already been treated.

▶ THE THIGH, HIP, ABDOMEN, AND PELVIS

Work on the thigh muscles helps to support changes in tone of the core muscles of the trunk and elsewhere. Several of

the thigh muscles attach on the pelvis, and they greatly affect pelvic positioning and overall body alignment.

- *Posterior Thigh and Hip.* The posterior thigh muscles draw the base of the pelvis downward and flex the knees. They counterbalance the actions of the quadriceps muscles on the anterior thigh. The hip muscles control the outward rotational movements of the femur, which aligns the rest of the leg. Hip rotators are often very tight, which can resonate in the knee and foot.

   The pelvis forms the body's center of gravity. Muscles that attach to the pelvis tie the upper and lower portions of the body together. Integrated deep tissue therapy can help to increase sensory awareness in the pelvic region, which facilitates well-coordinated, full-body movement.

- *Abdomen and Intestines.* The muscles of the abdominal wall provide support for the lower spine, and assist in holding the viscera in place. The body's ability to reach its full potential for health and vitality is greatly enhanced when this area moves freely.

   The abdominal wall muscles connect the chest to the pelvis, and control the motions of the trunk and pelvis. The rectus abdominus muscle assists the hamstrings of the posterior thigh in pulling the base of the pelvis anteriorly. The quadratus lumborum, which is the deepest abdominal muscle, forms the posterior wall of the abdominal cavity. It counterbalances the rectus abdominus by elevating the iliac crests and moving the pelvis posteriorly.

   When a person has poor digestive motility, energy in the form of fuel and potential work is not readily available to them. Wastes in the colon may accumulate, and the effect on the whole organism is a sense of sluggishness. But when the intestines function well, the body is more highly functional and more able to adapt to changes that integrated deep tissue therapy brings about.

- *Lateral Thigh and Medial Thigh.* Balancing the lateral and medial thigh muscles helps to reduce lateral shifting of the pelvis and supports the healthy function of the knee joint.
- *Anterior Thigh and Iliopsoas.* The abdominal muscles and thigh muscles should be addressed before work on the iliopsoas complex is attempted. Both the rectus femoris and psoas muscles tilt the pelvis anteriorly, in opposition to the hamstrings and rectus abdominus, which tilt the pelvis posteriorly. The psoas is the deepest core muscle, and arguably a keystone in upper and lower body integration. It has superior extensions that interdigitate with the diaphragm, so it is involved in breathing as well as in pelvic tilt and thigh flexion. Improving iliopsoas function can have profound effects on the entire body.

▶ THE UPPER POLE—HEAD AND NECK

The head and pelvis are the two weighted segments that are positioned on either end of the spine, and they serve to counterbalance each other. The head and pelvis have a direct biomechanical relationship to each other. Work on the upper pole is most effective after balance of the pelvis has been achieved. That said, it is often a good idea to invest a few moments into relaxing the neck area at the beginning of each massage session to set the stage for more effective work with the rest of the body.

- *Neck and Head Extensors.* These muscles prevent the head from tipping forward. They are called into use often, and they tend to accumulate inefficient levels of tension. It is difficult to restore healthy muscle tone in the rest of the body until the neck has been addressed.
- *Neck and Head Flexors.* The anterior portion of the neck is seldom addressed in standard massage sessions, but it is extremely important that it receive the same attention as the rest of the body. These muscles counterbalance the often-overused extensor muscles at the back of the neck, and they are subject to damage and chronic pain from neck-related injuries.
- *Head, Face, and Jaw.* Massage to the cranial, facial, and particularly, jaw muscles completes the balance of the upper pole, and helps to integrate the head to the neck. Relaxation of this area promotes parasympathetic activity, reducing mental agitation, and diminishing perceived stress. Treating the neck and head completes the process of total body re-education, allowing the client the opportunity to fully embrace the changes produced by the experience of integrated deep tissue bodywork.

Designing a Session

The lesson plans outline the full scope of the integrated deep tissue system, but they do not provide the step-by-step details of actual massage sessions. The therapist must construct the plan for each bodywork session, with input from the client.

Four parts comprise an integrated deep tissue therapy session:

- The presession interview
- Client assessment
- The session
- The postsession interview: homework, recommendations, and follow-up

▶ THE INTERVIEW

1. *Talk to the Client.* A massage therapist and client need to get to know each other a bit before their work together is likely to be productive. Find out why this person has come to receive bodywork. What are his or her expectations? Take a brief history of the client's previous experience with massage. Emphasize that the client is in charge of the session, and has the right to stop the session at any time.
2. *Ask Questions.* Elicit as much information as possible from your client about his or her state of health, and any factors that might affect receiving massage. Use a good intake form to gather information about previous injuries, surgeries, medical conditions, current medications, and so forth. This form will also serve as a guide to asking questions that will fill in the details of the client's health. Don't expect the client to know what the most important factors are; that's your job.
3. *Talk About How the Client Is Feeling.* Within appropriate boundaries, gather information about the client's emotional state. Is she stressed about work? Is he worried about whether his knee will heal? What factors are affecting their emotional state? Remember that people are not bringing just their bodies to the massage table — they are bringing their whole selves. Factors affecting a client's general well-being are important for the massage therapist to know.

Feelings are a major component of how we experience ourselves through our bodies. The client's emotional state will play a part in the design of the sessions, and it may color the therapist's approach. For instance, if a person expresses sadness, then a nurturing style of touch might be more appropriate and beneficial than a more forceful, fast-moving approach.

4. *Establish Goals with the Client.* It is vital the therapist discuss with the client what their mutual goals are for the session. What are the client's expectations and desired outcome from the session(s)? What does the therapist propose to accomplish during the session? And what session design supports both of their goals? This makes the client an active participant in the process: he or she can align with the goals, modify them, or add to them.

▶ CLIENT ASSESSMENT

1. *Observe the Client.* The most important assessment tool the integrated deep tissue therapist uses is postural and movement analysis. A client's posture and movement can reveal what the body's major tension patterns are. Then the therapist can guide the client to more effective use of the body, reducing the likelihood of future problems and discomfort.

Postural evaluation is also used to monitor changes occurring throughout a sequence of sessions. Take time to observe the client before, during, and after the session to assess the effects of the work. The body may respond differently than anticipated, and some modifications may need to be made.

2. *Use the Charts.* The range of motion and condition charts provided in the lessons can help to determine which muscles are contracted, based on the information gathered from the body reading. For example, if the client rolls his or her left shoulder forward, the therapist would check the range of motion chart for the shoulder joint and find which muscles medially rotate the shoulder. The client could also perform the same movements with his left and right arms to check for restriction in range of motion of both shoulder joints.

3. *Assess Other Factors.* Facial expressions, vocal tone, and gestures can all be indicators of a person's general state of being and can help in assessing the person's reaction to the bodywork, both while receiving it and afterward.

▶ THE SESSION

There are two levels of organization within the integrated deep tissue therapy method presented in the lessons: a sequence for each individual session, and a sequence of sessions to address the whole body.

The first level deals with the order of application for the six components of the integrated system within a single massage session.

To work effectively, a suggested sequence of treatment is to do the following:

1. *Open* the session with still, quiet touch and focus on breathing. This helps to relax the body and create a level of trust and good will that will make the rest of the session more effective. The two techniques used to accomplish this are polarity and shiatsu.

2. *Warm up* the muscles and fascia and enhance metabolic functioning by increasing local fluid flow. Swedish and cross-fiber techniques serve this purpose.

3. *Reduce* restrictions within and between fascial components of the soft tissues so that the muscles can lengthen more freely and work more efficiently. The connective tissue techniques are designed for this purpose.

4. *Decrease* tension held in chronically shortened muscles. Deep muscle strokes work toward this result.

5. *Interrupt* cycles of pain generated by trigger point formation in the muscles. Neuromuscular therapy targets this phenomenon.

6. *Teach* the muscles and the nervous system to incorporate (see Box 2-1) the newfound freedom that is created by the application of all these techniques. Stretching serves this purpose.

This is a highly effective sequence that can yield excellent results. After the initial sequence has been applied to an area, the techniques may be interwoven into the rest of the massage as dictated by the client's response. This intermingling of the massage components gives a rich dynamic to the sessions, and it allows the therapist to tailor the approach to be maximally effective.

BOX 2-1 | Incorporation: More than a Business Idea

The word "incorporate" has many meanings, but in the context of massage and bodywork it is an especially rich term.

In the business world, "incorporation" means to legally declare a corporate entity as separate from its owners—it is meant to protect the owners' assets from the company's liabilities. It denotes separation between ownership and operations.

By contrast, the massage context of "incorporation" means to weave together: to magnify and amplify the interconnectedness of every aspect of being alive, from muscles and fascia to heart rate and emotional state. When we work with the muscles and nervous system, it is important to incorporate—to merge into our *corpus*, or body—the changes that massage therapy brings about.

The second level of organization of the integrated deep tissue therapy method deals with the order in which the areas of the body are addressed over a series of sessions. The recommended protocol is to progress in the following sequence:

1. The trunk—chest and back
2. The upper extremity—shoulder, arm, and hand
3. The lower limb—foot, leg, and thigh
4. The core—abdomen and pelvis
5. The upper pole—neck and head

This list refers to the order in which each body segment is emphasized over a series of bodywork sessions. Following this sequence uses the counterbalancing relationships of the segments to help create the best results. The number of sessions required to bring satisfactory full-body integration varies. The therapist may choose to focus on any one segment for several sessions in a row, and may return to that area again in future sessions.

We have deliberately omitted a detailed, recipe-like treatment plan, because the inherently organic nature of this style of bodywork requires practitioners to be flexible and responsive. The therapist is encouraged to monitor the client's progress and adapt the session to match his or her individual pattern of unfolding.

In the integrated deep tissue therapy system, a single session emphasizes one specific body segment, but other areas of the body are also addressed. The principle of working with counterbalancing relationships applies not only over a series of bodywork sessions, but also within each individual session. This means that a degree of whole-body symmetry and integration is sought with each treatment.

Some suggestions for creating a whole-body experience of integrated deep tissue therapy include:

- Follow the suggestions listed in the lessons under the category Accessory Work. They present useful ideas for creating complete bodywork sessions.
- Include some work on the head, neck, and the feet in each session.
- The suggested order in which to process the body over a series of treatments can also be applied within an individual session. In other words, in a 60- or 90-minute time span, the therapist may progress through the five segments of the body, selecting the appropriate type of work and amount of time to spend on each.

▶ HOMEWORK AND FOLLOW-UP

After the massage session, the therapist may choose to show the client some exercises and self-care treatments he or she can do to further facilitate the changes that took place in the session, as long as such recommendations are within the therapist's scope of practice. The activities described in the lessons were chosen specifically for this purpose. It is helpful to demonstrate the activity for clients first, and then watch them perform it, offering guidance on proper form and execution. This can also be done in subsequent sessions, to make sure the stretches and exercises are being done accurately.

Integrative deep tissue therapy sessions can affect more than muscles and fascia. Encourage clients to take the time to relax and reflect on their feelings and sensations after receiving bodywork. Some clients may use a personal journal to record their experience. This can also enhance the effects of the massage by providing a means for the client to acknowledge consciously any internal differences that he or she notices during the process of receiving this work.

It is important for clients to know that they can reach out with questions or concerns that may arise in the days following their sessions. The therapist may also want to check in, but it is important to ask permission before assuming that the client will welcome this contact. Follow-through on the part of the therapist will affect the communication and trust-building that will help future sessions to be more effective.

▬▬▬▬ REVIEW QUESTIONS ▬▬▬▬

Level 1

Receive and Respond

1. What feature of the text can best help with the client assessment portion of the session?
   a. Holistic View discussions
   b. Postural evaluation charts
   c. Essential anatomy boxes
   d. Endangerment site illustrations

2. The sequence of sessions recommended in the integrated deep tissue therapy system is based on the work of. . .
   a. Ida Rolf.
   b. John Barnes.
   c. Thomas Hanna.
   d. Randolph Stone.

3. The integrated deep tissue therapy sequence recommends which order of treatment?
   a. Lower extremity; trunk; head and neck; thigh, hip, and pelvis; upper extremity
   b. Trunk; upper extremity; lower extremity; thigh, hip, and pelvis; head and neck
   c. Thigh, hip, and pelvis; trunk; upper extremity; lower extremity; head and neck
   d. Head and neck; upper extremity; trunk; thigh, hip, and pelvis; lower extremity

4. A typical integrated deep tissue session includes what components?
   a. Presession interview; client stretches; treatment; postsession assessment
   b. Client stretches and exercises; assessment; treatment; postsession stretches
   c. Client assessment; treatment; postsession interview; exercises and stretches
   d. Presession interview; client assessment; treatment; postsession interview

Level 2

Apply Concepts

1. Why is it important to open an integrated deep tissue therapy session with a still, quiet touch?
   a. This helps prime the nervous system for the challenging work that is to follow.
   b. This helps preserve the therapist's energy so he or she can have better stamina.
   c. This helps to create a space for the client to relax and build trust.
   d. This helps the therapist become more centered.

2. In integrated deep tissue therapy, it is important to. . .
   a. be flexible and willing to customize each session to the client's needs.
   b. adhere to the established protocol for best results.
   c. observe the client doing the recommended exercises to be sure they are done correctly.
   d. assess the client immediately before and after each session.

3. How many integrated deep tissue therapy sessions are needed to create balance and restore function?
   a. Ten to begin, followed by at least five follow-up sessions
   b. It varies from one client to another
   c. Twelve sessions provide a whole-body sequence, but it is recommended to follow up as needed
   d. Twenty sessions are needed to address the body completely

4. The postsession interview in integrated deep tissue therapy is likely to include what topics?
   a. Recommendations for stretches, exercises, and self-care
   b. Options for payment and scheduling a follow-up appointment
   c. Emotional processing of feelings brought up during the session
   d. Dietary recommendations so that the client may have a holistic approach to treatment

Level 3

Problem Solving: Discussion Points

1. The scope of practice for massage therapy varies from one area to another. What are the rules in your area about massage therapists recommending stretches and exercises? What guidelines must you follow in order to practice within your scope, but also to give your clients the best possible care?

2. Read Box 2-1, "Incorporation—More than a Business Idea." Discuss what problems might occur if a therapist neglects this important aspect of bodywork?

3. Part of the presession interview is establishing or reviewing the client's goals. Can you imagine a situation where a therapist's goals might differ from a client's goals? What does that look like? How might it be resolved?

Guidelines for the Integrated Deep Tissue Therapist

LEARNING OBJECTIVES

Having completed the reading, classroom instruction, and assigned homework related to Chapter 3 of *The Balanced Body*, the learner is expected to be able to. . .

- Identify the main components of massage therapy ethics, including professionalism, integrity, boundaries, communication, and education
- Recognize the signs of emotional release, and describe the appropriate role of a massage therapist in that setting
- Describe and explain each of the 10 principles of conscious bodywork

Ethics

Massage therapy is increasingly recognized by the medical community and by the population at large as a viable and popular adjunct to conventional stress reduction and rehabilitative healthcare. The intimate nature of touch therapies demands that massage therapists be very clear about what services they provide to assure protection and clear boundaries for both the clinician and the client. Therefore, it is important to maintain a strict code of ethics. Ethics are rules of behavior that define the parameters of effective interactions between people. Adherence to accepted rules of conduct and protocol will help to assure that massage therapists are afforded the respect this profession deserves.

The American Massage Therapy Association, Associated Bodywork and Movement Professionals, and the National Certification Board for Therapeutic Massage and Bodywork have all published a set of ethical guidelines that members agree to abide by (Table 3-1). Many states also have ethical expectations built into their licensing laws or rules. A few topics from these codes are of special importance, however, and are discussed below.

▶ PROFESSIONALISM

One way to think about professionalism is that with each interaction you are representing the whole massage therapy field, including your colleagues. Your clients, their primary care providers, all of your business-related contacts, and the public at large will judge the rest of the massage therapy field by what they see in you.

A consummate professional projects an image of impeccable, healthy appearance and demeanor. Massage therapists should wear clothing that is neat, clean, does not drape onto their clients, and is appropriate to their activities and setting. As healthcare role models, they should "walk the talk," of good self-care, especially in public settings.

Timeliness is a vital aspect of professionalism. The therapist must be fully prepared for each client before the scheduled appointment time. The session room should be clean, quiet, and have an appropriate temperature; the massage table should be dressed with clean sheets and set at an appropriate height; and any notes pertaining to the client should be reviewed ahead of time and readily available.

It is important that scheduled appointments begin and end on time. It is unprofessional to give some clients extra time at the risk of short-changing others. If it becomes clear that a client needs a longer session, this needs to be discussed in the moment—including any conversation about extra fees. Alternatively, the session can be concluded on schedule, but the prospect of longer future sessions can be brought up during the closing interview.

Fees for all services should be clearly stated and strictly followed. While it is certainly the option of each therapist to make individual payment arrangements in special situations, maintaining consistent pricing for all clients helps to minimize the risk of disagreements, misunderstandings, and boundary violations.

TABLE 3-1 | Massage Therapy Codes of Ethics

Organization	Web Address
American Massage Therapy Association (AMTA)	https://www.amtamassage .org/About-AMTA /Core-Documents/Code-of-Ethics.html
Associated Bodywork & Massage Professionals (ABMP)	https://www.abmp.com /abmp-code-ethics
National Certification Board for Therapeutic Massage & Bodywork (NCBTMB)	http://www.ncbtmb.org /code-ethics

▶ INTEGRITY

If professionalism is how we represent our field to others, integrity is how we represent ourselves. A person with high integrity is trustworthy and dependable. Her or his choices are made based on internal values, not on whether someone is watching. This applies to how he or she handles finances, business relationships, and messaging on social media.

A massage therapist must be reliable and accountable. Treating every client with the same focus and consideration—the last of the day as well as the first—is imperative to maintaining a respected practice.

A massage therapist must operate from a position of personal and professional integrity. This creates an environment of safety and trust that allows clients to be fully receptive to the benefits of massage therapy.

▶ BOUNDARIES

Establishing clear personal boundaries strengthens the therapeutic relationship, and protects both client and therapist from inappropriate interactions. Adherence to the following guidelines will help therapists to maintain appropriate boundaries in their practice:

- Always provide adequate draping for the client. Let the client choose the level of undressing he or she prefers, and be aware that this level of comfort may vary from one appointment to the next.
- Invite feedback, and always respect a client's request to change the manner in which a technique is being applied, or to stop work all together if the client so desires.
- Maintain a strictly professional relationship with clients. Do not date or socialize with clients. Many state laws legislate this issue and mandate a minimum amount of time between ending a client–therapist relationship before starting a personal one.
- Do not discuss a client's sessions or private information with other people, including those close to the client.

For instance, do not discuss a husband's session with his wife, even if she is the one paying for it. The exception to this rule is when your client signs a waiver allowing you to share information with his or her medical team or other people.

The topic of boundaries in massage therapy goes far beyond these few points, but for the context of integrated deep tissue therapy, these are the most essential. This topic is rich and complex, however, and many good resources are available for further exploration.

▶ COMMUNICATION

Ethical relationships rely on honest interactions. Two areas of interactions with clients are especially important for building trust: communication about the understood benefits and mechanisms of massage therapy, and communication about scope of practice, and referring out to other professionals.

Benefits and Mechanisms

We have seen, and research confirms, that massage therapy can be beneficial for many situations, including pain, stress, mood disorders, and many types of injury rehabilitation. But massage therapy is not a cure-all, and it is not appropriate in every situation.

It is vital for both personal integrity and professional representation that massage therapists are realistic and truthful about predicted outcomes of therapy, and the anticipated amount of time that might be required to achieve those goals. To make unsupportable claims, or to overstate the value of massage therapy, only weakens our reputation.

Further, it is important for massage therapists to be forthright in sharing what we know and what we are still learning about how massage therapy works. Some clients are curious and eager to learn what is happening when we stretch a muscle, or access a deep layer of fascia. They may want to know more about trigger points, or about why gentle touch seems to help them feel more peaceful. While it is appropriate to share answers to some of these questions about massage mechanisms with statements that begin, "the traditional understanding is. . ." or, "I was taught. . .," it is also important to acknowledge the fact that much of what we know about how massage therapy acts on health and function is new, and we are adding to our understanding every day. Therefore, what we learned in school or in a continuing education class that was acceptable at that time, may no longer be considered accurate now. And when we repeat what our teachers taught us as fact, without being sure that those mechanisms are supported by science, we risk for perpetuating myths that ultimately weaken our entire field.

Scope of Practice, Referring Out

Massage therapists must be diligent about staying within the scope of their legal status, education, and abilities when working with clients. When it becomes apparent that a client requires treatment that the therapist is not qualified to offer, we are obligated to recommend other sources for that treatment. It is a good idea to build a network of qualified healthcare providers that specialize in the kinds of conditions that you see frequently with your clients. Clients generally have much more respect for and loyalty to therapists who are honest about the limits of their skill, and they appreciate referrals to other healthcare providers that come with a personal recommendation.

▶ EDUCATION

Massage therapy is a field that affords the opportunity for lifelong learning and expansion. One could dedicate an entire career to exploring massage, and still not exhaust all the possibilities. Massage therapists who invest in their own growth as practitioners through continuing education are more likely to find new sources of inspiration and excitement that keep them engaged in this career, while those who do not expand their skills and interests are less likely to flourish.

We have an obligation to stay informed of new developments in our field. This is an evolving challenge, as information about health, wellness, and high-quality massage therapy research is being generated at an unprecedented rate. Nonetheless, baseline skills, even for entry-level massage therapists, now include being able to find, read, evaluate, and apply research in their practice. Without this, we cannot promise to create the pathways for our clients to achieve the best possible outcomes.

BOX 3-1 | **Staying Up-to-Date**

Trade journals for massage therapists are often associated with a professional organization or malpractice insurance provider. They are also often available online and subscription free. At this time, this list includes *Massage Therapy Journal*, *Massage and Bodywork*, *Massage Today*, and *Massage Magazine*. Each of them carries articles on techniques, and a regularly appearing research column, in which a research finding is interpreted for broad application.

To access the original research, it is necessary to go to an academic journal. As of this writing, two scholarly journals are published quarterly with peer-reviewed research articles about massage therapy. The *International Journal of Therapeutic Massage and Bodywork* is open sourced and subscription free, and the *Journal of Therapeutic Massage and Bodywork* charges a subscription fee, but it is also possible to access and pay for individual articles. Articles about massage therapy frequently appear in a wide range of other scholarly journals as well, according to the nature of the research. The best way to find these is through the search function at www.pubmed.gov.

Staying up to date on massage therapy research and innovations can be accomplished by reading good-quality periodicals (see Box 3-1), participating in continuing education classes, and pursuing your own points of interest through searches in PubMed and other health science databases.

Incorporating the Holistic Aspect of Integrated Deep Tissue Therapy

▶ THE NATURE OF TENSION

One of the primary values of massage therapy is its effectiveness for relieving tension in the body. Tension manifests physically as chronically contracted muscles, and it contributes to many problems, including pain, irritability, and diminished function. The manifestations of tension are often what prompt a person to seek massage therapy.

The mechanical techniques of massage therapy address tension directly, through lengthening and relaxing contracted muscle fibers with a combination of pressure and movement.

These results can be short lived, however, because when the client is again confronted with stress-producing experiences, the tension and its ensuing problems often return. For longer lasting results, it may be necessary for clients to explore the nature and sources of tension more fully, so that they are capable of neutralizing its effects on mood and physical function.

Tension is a form of resistance. It is the body's attempt to defend itself against a perceived threat. Mild short-term tension, which accompanies low-level stress reactions, can be a useful response. The increased muscular tone and heightened activity of the sympathetic nervous system that accompany mild stress can improve a person's ability to respond to a threatening situation. For example, the tension we feel when driving in traffic, although not necessarily making us feel very good, does improve our reflexes and mobilize our senses, letting us react to potentially dangerous events quickly and effectively. Stress becomes a problem when it is overbearing and unyielding, or when we cannot move back into a state of equilibrium. Long-term experiences of stress produce chronic muscle tension and a host of other physical challenges.

▶ EMOTIONS AND TENSION

Psychological and emotional sources of stress can be as devastating as physical ones. Very often, people are unaware that the condition of their mind has a direct impact on their body, and vice versa. When worry, fear, anger, and other highly charged emotional states are unrelenting, they can impact foundational health. As long as these emotional prompts are present, the body cannot maintain an environment that promotes good health and equilibrium.

To complicate matters, patterns of chronic muscle tension may have been initiated by emotional stimuli that occurred years before. If a perceived threat is strong enough, or has a sustained duration, or both, it can create an area of muscular tension that becomes ingrained by the proprioceptors that determine our muscle tension. That level of tightness becomes the norm, and to break that pattern can feel disorienting, unsteadying, and even unsafe.

This type of unrelenting muscular tension was labeled "armoring" (Fig. 3-1) by psychologist Wilhelm Reich, who suggested that these patterns work as a protective device against an unwanted or unacceptable feeling. There are many sources for these blocks, but the result is always the same—an area of pain or even numbness, caused by muscular restriction that may be linked to an emotional trigger.

In this view of human function, armoring may develop in childhood, before a person has acquired the resources that allows him or her to deal effectively with intense emotional experiences. This paradigm suggests that an invisible matrix of memories and emotions that are reflected in muscle tension patterns is simply part of the human condition. This is common and usually not pathologic. But in some cases, these patterns may become problematic because they interfere with optimal function, and raise the risk of injury. Integrated deep tissue therapy can reveal places where tension has become habitual, and work to relieve unnecessary and inefficient levels of muscle tone, fascial thickening, and movement inhibition.

As muscles and fascia soften during integrated deep tissue therapy sessions, some therapists and clients find that the underlying feelings that initiated a pattern may resurface. In some instances, the client may choose to explore these feelings. If this is the case, the therapist must recommend that the client talk to a qualified psychological counselor;

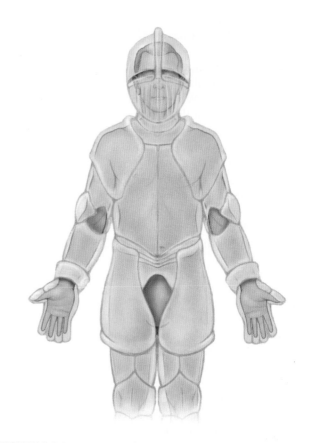

FIGURE 3-1 Armoring: muscle tension begins as a protective adaptation, but ultimately it inhibits our ability to function. (From Greene E, Goodrich-Dunn B: *The Psychology of the Body.* 2nd ed. Philadelphia, PA: Wolters Kluwer; 2013.)

the massage session room is not the place to process these intense emotional experiences. But sometimes these episodes occur so quickly that they must be addressed in the moment.

▶ WHAT IS AN EMOTIONAL RELEASE?

Muscles that are chronically tense often generate pain signals. The contracted cells prevent fresh blood, which is loaded with oxygen and nutrients, from reaching them. Chemicals that irritate nerve endings may accumulate, and local sensory neurons may be trapped and compressed. All in all, the exchange of energy in the form of nutrition and stimulation is blocked.

Over time, people with this pattern may feel lethargic, or trapped in unproductive patterns of behavior, but it all accrues so slowly and quietly that they may not notice or realize how far from true vitality they have come. The physical and emotional pain that generated these patterns has not gone away; it is still reflected in these unproductive muscular and fascial patterns, which can influence posture, movement, and even mood at an unconscious level.

As bodywork frees tissues from their constant gripping, some clients may experience a sudden loosening of blocked emotions along with the muscular change. Depending on the source of the original inhibition, an emotional outpouring can manifest in a number of ways, including crying, laughing, a feeling of great relief, or a flash of insight regarding the nature of the physical–emotional pattern. Massage-induced muscular relaxation and emotional release are similar in many ways. Both signify a new consciousness of our physical state and how it influences our emotional state; both represent the potential to let go of restrictive patterns that may involve the nervous system, the emotional mind, and the musculature.

Signs of Emotional Release

The signs of an emotional response to bodywork are many and varied. Therapists need to be aware of them so that they will know how to respond appropriately should this happen during a session.

- A change in breathing pattern: He or she may begin to hold the breath, or he or she may take deeper or more rapid breaths.
- Skin changes: The client may flush, or the skin may become paler.
- Temperature changes: The therapist may feel a change in the temperature level on the surface of the client's body.
- Muscle tension: Tightness, particularly in the jaw, chest, and abdomen, may suddenly increase.
- Behavior changes: The client may begin to fidget or become unusually subdued.
- Rapid eye movement: If the client's eyes are closed, the therapist may notice rapid movement under the eyelids.
- Staring: The client may suddenly open his or her eyes and begin to look around or stare off into space.
- Communication: A person who has been talkative and becomes uncharacteristically quiet, or one who was quiet and unexpectedly begins to converse, may be experiencing the surfacing of feelings.

Many other signals may suggest a possible emotional outpouring, or he or she may seem to "check out" and become removed or detached, because an experience is too intense. Therapists must be attentive and note any changes in a client's demeanor that might indicate strong feelings are rising.

How to Manage an Emotional Release

What is the best course of action if a client should experience an emotional release? First, the therapist needs to check with the client to make sure his or her needs are being met. Every massage session room should be equipped with tissues, extra blankets, and water in case the client requires them. Beyond making sure that the client feels safe and comfortable, the therapist does not need to do anything except to be present and nonjudgmental.

Therapists should not push the client to express his or her feelings, nor should the therapist discourage an honest outpouring of emotion if it should spontaneously occur. It is important that the therapist stay calm and centered while the client is experiencing an emotional release. Any attempt to actively suppress or encourage emotional expression by the client can heighten the feelings of shame and embarrassment that many people experience when revealing suppressed feelings.

Integrated deep tissue therapists deal with emotional release in very much the same manner as we deal with a tight muscle that relaxes. We acknowledge the opening, give the client space to fully experience and absorb it, and offer any neutral assistance or support that may be required. Most of the time, providing a compassionate and nurturing presence is all that the client requires from the therapist to process these feelings.

Another form of emotional processing that may happen during a massage therapy session occurs when a client becomes detached from the moment and the location. This is seen most frequently with people who have been through some kind of psychological or physical trauma. In this situation, a client consciously or subconsciously experiences a trigger that causes him or her to emotionally withdraw, because the feelings that are being evoked are simply too intense. In other words, the client's consciousness attempts to separate from his or her body. If this happens, it is important that the massage therapist interrupts the session to gently re-establish verbal contact, and help the client re-orient to the setting. This helps to reset the sense of safety and presence that is vital for every bodywork session.

Many people—therapists and clients alike—are fearful of emotional reactions in the session room. Feelings may be suppressed because a person is anxious about expressing them. That fear may resurface as the client becomes conscious of his or her restricted emotions, and how they are connected to muscular holding patterns. Many clients feel a great relief when suppressed feelings are expressed, as if a huge burden has been lifted, and this may also be reflected in reduced muscle tension and a sense of renewed energy. It is important to remember, however, that it is not the massage therapist's job, nor is it within our scope of practice, to guide clients through emotional processing.

When a client has a complicated emotional situation, especially when a history of trauma may be a factor, it is important to refer out to a skilled professional counselor or psychologist. To do this, it is necessary to find out if the client has a support system in place. If not, it is a good idea for a massage therapist to develop a network of physicians and other healthcare providers to whom they can refer. In any case, the client must grant written permission for communication between their massage therapist and their doctor or counselor to occur.

Principles of Conscious Bodywork

The following principles provide guidelines that yield the best results of integrated deep tissue therapy. They encapsulate many of the concepts discussed in this book, and they serve as important checkpoints for maintaining the highest standards of ethics and excellence when performing integrated deep tissue therapy. Therapists would do well to commit these principles to memory, and strive to embody them in all of their massage therapy interactions.

1. *Respect the Client.* When a client chooses to receive bodywork, that person is entrusting his or her body to us, with all the vulnerability that implies. Our responsibility is to honor and care for that person to the best of our ability. Every opportunity to work with someone in this manner is a privilege. Let us honor our clients for their desire to grow, and for allowing us to grow with them. Each individual is unique and precious. The gift that conscious bodywork offers is the reminder that we are all unfolding into our own perfection.

2. *Be Attentive.* For us to be sensitive to the process of opening that occurs within each session, we must be present and focused. Clients are also more open to change if he or she feels that the therapist is attentive and responsive. Communication takes place continually between the therapist and client; it is critical that we are sensitive to the messages being conveyed through touch, breath, observation, and words. These messages must be interpreted correctly for us to make appropriate choices and responses with our touch.

3. *Move Slowly.* A single integrated deep tissue massage may use many variations of pressure, speed, and flow within a single session. When the goal is to change the condition of myofascial structures, the pace must be slow to be effective. Connective tissue massage, deep tissue massage, neuromuscular therapy, and stretching techniques are all performed at a slow rate. Patience is required for the tissues to respond to the stimulus being applied; if we rush, the body responds through protective and tightening reflexes, and this is how injuries occur and clients can feel overwhelmed. When we move slowly, however, we can reduce this risk. A slow pace is also more conducive to the process of self-awareness that fosters transformational growth for the client.

During a massage, the client can become especially sensitive to what the therapist conveys. The therapist's quality of breathing, pace, and state of mind are reflected in the quality of each touch. A slow, fluid quality transfers a deeper feeling of integration and deep relaxation to the recipient. This helps to create the space for growth and healing that people seek from deep tissue massage.

4. *Never Force the Tissues.* There is an old saying that a blossom will open on only when it is ready, and any attempt to pry the flower open early only ruins the flower. The same is true with the body. An effective massage therapist learns how to listen and interact with the soft tissues in such a way that they are encouraged to relinquish their holding patterns willingly. When the body opens freely, the therapist experiences a melting sensation under the fingers as they sink into the tissues, and an invitation to move along the tissues, as if the hands were a boat being carried by moving waters.

When we encounter resistance, the best tactic is to wait patiently for resolution before moving further. Resistance is a natural defense against invasion. It is the body's way of protecting itself against what it perceives as an intrusion, whether physical or emotional. Pushing against resistant tissues sets up a tug-of-war situation between the therapist and recipient. We might plow through the blockage with assertive force, and we may even succeed in creating an opening, but all the effort and pain produced during the attempt neutralizes the benefit, and may cause increased resistance and pain as the body further protects itself. Matching force with force is never fruitful if the goal is to bring someone around to your point of view, and the same is true with muscles. Kindness, patience, and understanding are much more effective means to melt resistance.

5. *Look for "The Edge."* This guideline is closely related to the previous one. This describes an approach to soft tissue manipulation that creates the most productive environment for change to occur. Working on the edge means that the therapist has found the pace, pressure, and rhythm that provide the ideal stimulus for the client's tissues to release tension patterns and move into dynamic equilibrium. In other words, transformation happens here.

When the qualities of pace, pressure, and rhythm are not in cadence with the client's tissues, the massage is likely to be less productive. Using pressure as an example, the client will not feel the muscles and fascia lengthening if the depth of the stroke is too light and, consequently, will not feel tension melting in the tissues. But if the pressure is too deep, pain signals may block any other stimulus to the nervous system and a local pain and inflammatory response may build, inhibiting the positive benefits of the work. When the pressure is just right, the client's experience is that the body becomes freer, and he or she has the experience of profound wholeness and the restoration of a sense health and vitality.

6. *Always Move Toward Greater Ease.* During any body-work session, the therapist must be sensitive to the state of tension in the client's muscles and then, through the manipulation and positioning of the body, create the greatest degree of comfort. The client can then experience easy, pleasurable movement, giving him or her the opportunity to embrace and consciously incorporate it.

   Often, changing the position or angle of a body part on the table will relax the muscles around it and increase the effectiveness of any techniques applied to those muscles. Pads and bolsters can be used to change the alignment of the body on the table for more effective muscle relaxation. Good positioning creates efficient pathways of movement for the muscles and fascia to follow as they move toward their optimal relationships.

7. *Elongate Shortened Muscles, and Strengthen Stretched Muscles.* Most deep tissue massage techniques are designed to bring balance to the body by lengthening shortened muscle fibers and the fascial sheaths that surround them. Muscles act in pairs. When a muscle contracts, its opposing partner is stretched. If the muscle stays contracted, the antagonistic muscle remains in a lengthened position, which may weaken it. Therefore, once the shortened muscles have reduced tone, the stretched muscles need to be strengthened with specifically targeted exercises.

   Muscles must be free to contract and lengthen without resistance so the body can respond and adapt to stimulus. To bring harmony and coordination to muscular relationships, the massage therapist evaluates where tissues are shortened through observation and palpation, and then elongates them through a combination of compression and stretching techniques. When the shortened muscles regain their ideal length, the pull on the opposing muscles is reduced, and these muscles also return to a resting state. This allows the reflex arcs that establish muscle tone to function more efficiently, and the body's full capacity for adjustment returns.

8. *Seek to Establish and Re-establish Balance.* As stated above, muscles operate in counterbalancing relationships. The body as a whole operates in the same way: when part of the body shifts in one direction, the rest of the body compensates to maintain some sort of functional integrity. Anyone who has tried to balance a stack of blocks knows that when one block is moved out of position, the whole stack has to be readjusted to prevent the blocks from falling into a pile. Practitioners must be conscious of the body's counterbalancing nature and work accordingly. This means that massage sessions take into account the body's oppositional relationships. In practical terms, this means that when we focus on the top of the body, we must also do some work to align the bottom half of the body with it. Juxtapose work on the back of the body with work on the front. Integrate the right side of the body with the left side. Balance the deep, inner muscles with the more superficial muscles, and so forth. Approaching the body in this manner within each session provides longer lasting and much more profound results.

9. *Pursue Ease of Flow.* A healthy body is analogous to a flowing river. The water in a river is constantly moving, finding its way along the path of the riverbed. The surface of the water may at times appear to be still, yet underneath, deep currents are always moving. The river exhibits a quality of fluidity and ever-changing dynamics amidst a backdrop of constancy. When the body is unified in harmonious balance, it exhibits the same ease of flow and adaptability as a rushing river. An ease of movement appears to be almost liquid in nature. The tissues seem to ripple with a sense of aliveness.

   When the body is viewed with this image in mind, blocks to the ease of flow become readily apparent. The breath may appear uneven or shallow, and muscles seem knotted in stiffness and immobility. Structural misalignment radiates obvious tension and inefficient effort. The role of the massage therapist is to observe these areas of blockage, and to remove or minimize them, in much the same way one would remove a log that is damming the flow of water in a stream.

10. *Keep a Perspective of Wholeness.* The words *heal* and *whole* are derived from the same linguistic root. Therefore, *to heal* means *to make whole*. The ultimate goal of integrated deep tissue therapy is to help guide a person to a state of completeness, or wholeness. The body is the vehicle used for this healing to take place.

    In the process of learning various massage techniques, we discuss the body as parts to be labeled and analyzed. The student learns how atoms make up molecules, which combine to create cells, which build all the physiologic systems. Muscles are delineated in the same manner. Bundles of muscle tissues are given special names and are described as performing specific actions. When massaging the body, the therapist may also compartmentalize his or her work by addressing individual systems with techniques designed to facilitate their specific functioning. However, a person is not just the sum of all these systems. We do not experience ourselves internally as a collection of distinct parts. A human being is a locus of consciousness that transcends all individual facets: the whole is very much greater than the sum of its parts. It is this expansive quality that allows us to go beyond our limitations and expand our abilities. Conscious bodywork offers the potential to tap into this experience of finding and expressing our unique qualities and individual natures.

SESSION IMPRESSION

CONSCIOUS BODYWORK

The subject is a 28-year-old man named Brian who works as a medical technician. He received a series of massage sessions several years ago and enjoyed them. He now wants to experience massage therapy again, because he is feeling out of touch with his body and thinks that receiving bodywork will help to bring him more physical awareness. Another reason he would like to achieve greater physical presence is that Brian has been experiencing problems with low self-esteem. He contends that a lack of assertiveness is causing problems at work and with his relationships. As a result, he feels weak and ineffective. As well as beginning massage therapy sessions, Brian has bought a health club membership and started a weight-training program to build himself up as part of his program to increase self-confidence.

Physically, there is a lack of symmetry between Brian's upper and lower body. His torso is well developed, with good muscular definition in the chest and arms. The abdominal region appears to be overly contracted. The lower ribs are drawn inward toward the midline, creating compression in the solar plexus region. This restriction is partially the result of tightness in the rectus abdominus.

Viewing Brian from the side, his back appears to be overly straight. Shortness in the abdominal wall has caused the pelvis to be drawn into a posterior tilt, causing a reduction in the lordotic curve. His midsection seems restricted and tense. The cervical curve is also reduced, and Brian's jaw is slightly retracted. The sternocleidomastoid muscles are clearly visible, with both tendons being prominent at the base of the anterior neck. His lower body lacks the definition of his upper body. His hips are broad, and the quadriceps muscles lack tone. His ankles are thick, and both feet are turned out. The piriformis and hamstring muscles appear to be contracted.

One of the initial goals in working with this client is to help him feel more supported by his legs and feet. He seems to control his body from the waist up, creating areas of tension in the torso and neck. When he walks, he throws each leg forward rather than swinging the thigh freely from the hip. Each step lands flat, on the entire plantar surface of the foot, rather than rolling smoothly from heel to toe to cushion the impact. In addition to receiving deep tissue therapy, Brian is encouraged to perform exercise activities in which he must use his legs and feet actively and with awareness. Tai chi classes and walking daily are recommended.

The plan for the first session was to begin the process of balancing the musculature of the legs. The initial contact was a polarity head hold followed by Swedish massage on the neck, with deep tissue strokes along the lamina groove in the cervical region. Next, the feet were addressed. Some time will be spent on the feet in each session to increase their mobility so that they become more active during walking actions. Freeing restrictions in the feet will also enhance Brian's feeling of being grounded and help build awareness through the lower body.

After the work on the feet was completed, focus was shifted to the right tibialis anterior and peroneal muscles. These muscles were quite tense, contributing to a lack of fluidity throughout the feet. Next, the quadriceps muscles were massaged. This sequence was then repeated on the left leg.

As the quadriceps were reached on the left side, the client began to complain of an uneasy feeling in his abdomen, almost a feeling of light spasm. With Brian's permission, the therapist moved to the abdominal area to explore the feelings being generated there. The therapist lightly placed his right hand on Brian's abdomen while his left hand cradled the back of Brian's head. Brian was encouraged to breathe deeply into his abdomen, trying to push up the therapist's hand by expanding his abdomen as he inhaled and allowing the therapist's hand to sink toward his spine as he exhaled.

After a few rounds of deep breathing, Brian's breathing rhythm became choppy, especially on exhalation. He began to complain of tightness rising into his upper chest. The therapist asked him if he wished to continue. Brian responded that he would, so the therapist removed his left hand from behind Brian's head and placed it on the upper chest, just below the clavicles. Brian took a few breaths and began to clench his jaw. His neck and face were becoming flushed. The therapist asked if Brian was aware that he had begun to grit his teeth. Brian said no, he had not realized it and was only aware that it was a little difficult to take a deep breath, but he wanted to continue. The therapist asked him to open his mouth slightly and allow his lower jaw to drop. Brian did so, and at that point, he began to cry. The therapist removed his hand from Brian's chest, reached for a tissue, and put the tissue in Brian's hand. Brian said he was not sure what was happening but felt comfortable staying with the work. He closed his eyes and continued to breathe slowly and deeply. The therapist's right hand remained on his abdomen while the left hand lightly touched his shoulder in a reassuring manner. Soon, his body started shaking as waves of movement began to ripple through his trunk and legs. The crying became deeper.

After several minutes, the movement in his body calmed, and the crying subsided. Brian lay there for a while continuing to breathe rhythmically but more slowly. The therapist gradually removed his hands from Brian's abdomen and shoulder and asked him how he felt. Brian began to smile and said he could sense a buzzing, tingling sensation across his forehead and in his hands. He then related that his breathing felt much easier and that the tension in his abdomen was totally gone. He was very aware of the sensations in his body as he lay on the table. He said it felt as if a tight, heavy belt had been removed from around his waist, allowing him to sense his legs and feet much more fully. The therapist asked Brian if he would like to try to sit up on the table, and Brian answered that he would. The therapist helped lift him to a sitting position, with his legs hanging off the side of the table, and then brought him a glass of water, which Brian slowly sipped. When the therapist was sure that Brian was all right, he left the room to allow Brian to get dressed.

Upon entering the room again, the therapist encouraged Brian to walk around a little and describe how he felt. Brian said his legs felt much freer and easy to move, and he could sense himself land lightly on each foot as he took a step. When he walked, he was also more aware of the movement of his arms coordinated with the swinging of his legs. He said he felt as if a huge amount of bottled-up tension had been released during this session. Brian is now looking forward to continuing to become better acquainted with his body through deep tissue therapy. ■

Topics for Discussion

1. How would you describe to a client the possibility that emotional release can occur as part of a deep tissue therapy session?
2. Explain appropriate actions you should—and should not—take with a client who is experiencing emotional release.
3. Describe some potential situations in which it might be necessary to refer a client to a psychological counselor.
4. What would you say in a follow-up conversation or phone call to a client who has experienced an emotional release?

REVIEW QUESTIONS

Level 1
Receive and Respond

1. Which is the best description of the concept of tension?
   a. The body's attempt to defend itself against a perceived threat
   b. The absence of equipoise
   c. The result of a lifetime of toxic exposures and unresolved emotional pain
   d. The body's response to mental challenge

2. "Walking the talk" of self-care, timeliness, and being open and transparent about fees are all part of what quality?
   a. Honesty
   b. Integrity
   c. Professionalism
   d. Communication skills

3. Unrelenting muscular tension that dates back to an early history of trauma is sometimes referred to as. . .
   a. posturing.
   b. defending.
   c. protecting.
   d. armoring.

Level 2
Apply Concepts

1. It is important to work on both sides of the body: anterior and posterior; left and right; medial and lateral. What principle of conscious bodywork does this address?
   a. "Be attentive"
   b. "Seek to establish and re-establish balance"
   c. "Never force the tissues"
   d. "Move slowly"

2. When an integrated deep tissue therapist encounters resistance in the tissues, this is a sign that. . .
   a. the client is holding onto an emotional response; the tissues would not relax until that is released.
   b. it is time to back off and address another area of the body while that one recovers.
   c. it is necessary to meet force with force so that the tissues can finally relax.
   d. it is necessary to slow down and allow the tissue to incorporate the changes being brought about.

3. Why is it important to stay informed about massage therapy research?
   a. So we can work in clinical settings, which pay better than recreational settings
   b. So we can represent what is understood about the science of massage therapy accurately
   c. So we can speak with authority to our clients
   d. So we can defend our profession when other people are disrespectful

Level 3

Problem Solving: Discussion Points

1. While you were working on his thigh, your client unexpectedly burst into tears on your table. It soon subsided, and he asked you to continue as usual. After his session, he seemed embarrassed. He did not make eye contact or schedule another appointment, and he left as quickly as possible. Discuss with a classmate how you might initiate a conversation with this client to help him feel more comfortable.

2. Your client is a middle-aged woman who feels she is very overweight. She asks you for advice on weight loss supplements; her friend's massage therapist actively markets products specifically for this purpose. What is your most appropriate response?

Integrated Deep Tissue Therapy System Techniques

LEARNING OBJECTIVES

Having completed the reading, classroom instruction, and assigned homework related to Chapter 4 of *The Balanced Body*, the learner is expected to be able to. . .

- List the three major steps of an integrated deep tissue therapy session in correct order
- Explain the concepts of tonic and phasic muscle relationships
- Demonstrate familiarity with the modalities discussed in integrated deep tissue therapy, specifically: polarity, shiatsu,

Swedish massage, cross-fiber massage, connective tissue therapy, deep tissue therapy, and neuromuscular therapy
- Apply the five-question body mechanics checklist to his or her own practice
- Describe strategies for therapist self-care

The integrated deep tissue therapy system, while incorporating many facets of stress-reducing relaxation styles of massage, embraces a broader vision of high-level wellness. It provides a precise method for normalizing the muscular system, thereby reducing unbalanced pulls on the skeleton that lead to the loss of structural integrity and, eventually, to physical breakdown. This system supports healthy muscular relationships, efficient movement, and the potential for improved metabolic functioning. This can happen on a microscopic level with the well-organized turnover of chemicals in the cells, and in larger ways with the interventions of stretching, exercise, and soft tissue manipulation.

The integrated deep tissue therapy system is designed to reduce pain and promote well-being on a physical level and

beyond. An important consequence of a relaxed, stress-free, pain-free body is a calm and powerful mind. Excessive firing of nerves brought about by the effort of holding muscles in distorted positions disturbs both physical and mental equilibrium, and stimulates random mental chatter in the brain. As the body is brought into a state of dynamic equilibrium and poise through the integrated deep tissue therapy techniques, the nervous system is able to return to its optimal, efficient state of function. The subconscious mental static that accompanies chronic low-grade pain and postural inefficiencies subsides, and we can enter into an improved state of mental processing and mindfulness.

The Integrated Deep Tissue Therapy System: a Three-Step Approach

Openness, presence, patience, and lack of agenda are qualities that distinguish integrated deep tissue therapy. The skilled therapist creates pathways for improvement, and then allows the client to explore those pathways in whatever ways he or she can assimilate. This can be done with consistency when we use a three-step process of observation, planning, and implementation. Applying these procedures with each client provides both a working strategy, and an ongoing means of evaluating progress. It is important to emphasize that the assessment of progress never stops; this is part of every decision

in every session. This allows modification of the plan to be made at any time in response to the client's ability to derive benefit from the session.

▶ STEP ONE: OBSERVE PATTERNS OF MYOFASCIAL COMPENSATION

The first step that the integrated deep tissue therapist must master is the ability to observe and recognize the unique patterns of muscular compensation brought about by distortions in the myofascial system of each client. The characteristics of an individual's posture and movement are largely determined by the limitations imposed by restricted soft tissues. After the therapist has evaluated these patterns, he or she must determine which ones are most detrimental (i.e., causing pain, producing wear and tear on joints, creating imbalances in posture or muscle tone, straining ligaments and muscle tissue, or leading to fascial build-up and bracing).

Integrated deep tissue therapy sessions are built around minimizing dysfunctional patterns of distortion in posture and movement. Because every person's muscular relationships are unique and ever changing, no two deep tissue therapy sessions are exactly the same. Each treatment is designed to address the counterproductive soft tissue patterns that are generating problems, as observed on that particular day.

Observations can occur through the visual assessment of posture and movement, and also by way of palpation.

Palpation

Palpation is the art of sensing the status of the tissues, and changes that occur as we work. It is a critical part of the observations that inform a plan of action.

Conscious palpation must happen alongside the massage strokes to generate an instantaneous feedback loop. In other words, to gauge the effectiveness of a technique, a massage therapist must be sensitive to the reaction of the client's tissues in that moment. Good palpation awareness informs us of how the client is receiving the massage: whether it is welcomed or threatening. If necessary, the therapist can make adjustments to the stroke in terms of pace, pressure, or intention to yield the desired outcomes: a decrease of pain and tension, with increased freedom of movement.

Our hands are extremely sensitive instruments for performing massage—particularly the fingertips, because they contain a high number of sensory receptors. Fingers are capable of perceiving temperature differences, textural qualities and variations, degrees of hardness or softness, moisture, degrees of depth, and minute movements. The ability to register all this information allows us to tune into the client's tissues at a very subtle level.

Skill in palpation develops through practice. With experience, the brain develops the capacity to become aware of more and more input from the nerve receptors, increasing the ability of the practitioner to distinguish and analyze all the signals coming through sensory neurons. This happens most easily with the richly innervated fingers and palms. But palpatory proficiency with knuckles, forearms, and elbows can also be developed through regular, concentrated practice. Developing these skills can add to the longevity of a career in massage therapy, but it is important, as the practitioner develops this sensitivity, to remember that the skin on the

knuckles, forearms, and elbows is always less perceptive than that of the palms and fingertips, so attention must be paid to much subtler sensory signals.

Accurate palpatory assessment requires that we clearly visualize the soft tissues that we work with. Therefore, a thorough knowledge of anatomy is necessary to train the hands to move through the layers of the body both accurately and safely. The therapist must be able to palpate and interpret the condition of the skin and the underlying layers of adipose and fascia—and then the layers of muscles beneath. Being aware of the qualities of the skin can yield useful information about the underlying tissues. An unusually warm area on the skin may indicate inflammation in the soft tissues beneath it, and skin that feels tight and cannot slide easily over the underlying tissues may indicate binding in the superficial fascial layers.

Fascial structures have different palpatory qualities, depending on where they are found. Healthy superficial fascia is usually elastic, with some stretchiness and quick rebound. Deeper or thicker layers of fascia, like that found in the lumbodorsal area, is more likely to be dense, with less yield, and more resistance to pressure. Fascia can convey a thick, dense feel, or a dried out, crunchy texture.

To palpate the muscles accurately, the therapist needs to be familiar with their shape, the directions of their fibers, and their points of attachment on the bones (Fig. 4-1). The therapist must also be able to distinguish the differences between normal and abnormal muscle tissue. A normal muscle that is free of tension and restrictions has a springy, resilient quality. It yields to pressure, and it maintains even tone. Healthy muscles do not resist palpation. Deeper tissues can be felt through them. Touch does not elicit pain in a healthy muscle, even when deep pressure is applied.

Abnormal muscle tissues embody the effects of strain and imbalance. They can be weak and flaccid, or they can be dense and tough. Their fibers are often more pronounced than those of healthy muscles. They may feel stringy or ropy, and they may have a crunchy texture when rolled across. Highly contracted muscles feel thick and hard. They are not elastic when pressed; rather, they are resistive. Muscles that are unnecessarily tight, or that are weak and lengthened, can feel like taut cable wires. Touch may elicit a pain response, but the area may also feel numb or deadened, particularly if the abnormal condition is long-standing. With experience, the various states of muscle health can be palpated accurately, and appropriate techniques can be applied to counteract the effects of strain and improper usage.

Knowledge of the shape and function of the skeleton is equally as important as the ability to visualize muscles when palpating the body. Most muscles initiate movement by pulling their bony attachments closer together. Much of the damage done to muscles through trauma and stress occurs at their attachments to the bones. Tracing the contours of the bones is an extremely important aspect of deep tissue therapy. Addressing damage at the tenoperiosteal junction may help

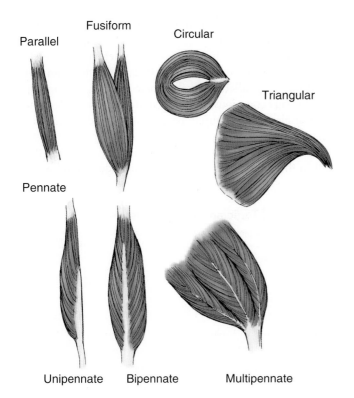

Parallel

Fusiform

Circular

Triangular

Pennate

Unipennate   Bipennate   Multipennate

FIGURE 4-1 Examples of common shapes and patterns of skeletal muscles.

to reduce much of the pain that people experience as a result of injured muscles.

▶ STEP TWO: CREATE A PLAN OF ACTION

The second step in the integrated deep tissue therapy system involves the ability to envision the client's progression to a balanced state by organizing a logical, effective plan of treatment. It takes time and patience to undo the effects of years of trauma and dysfunctional postural and movement habits. The therapist's job is to guide the client to the capability of pain free, unrestricted movement through a combination of progressive integrated deep tissue therapy treatments and supplemental stretching and strengthening recommendations.

In Chapter 2, we introduced an effective sequence of sessions. To review, the trunk and upper extremity are attended first, followed by the lower extremity. Lower extremity sessions begin with the feet, because they form the structural foundation of the vertical body. The sessions then progress upward to the body's core, which consists of the abdominal cavity and pelvis: the lower pole of the spine. After the function of the core architecture is addressed, work concludes at the upper pole of the spine: the neck and head region.

Part of mastering integrative deep tissue therapy is acquiring the ability to recognize myofascial aberrations, and choosing which techniques might work best to address them. Just as a mechanic uses an assortment of specialized tools to perform specific tasks, massage therapists may use a variety of techniques to address a full range of muscular qualities and conditions.

The relative tone of prime movers and their antagonists may be easier to identify when the client is on the table and as relaxed as possible. This is also true when we compare the tone of superficial and deeper muscles. When we have a full picture of the client's holding patterns during movement and rest, then we have the information we need to design a treatment strategy that will help restore ease and efficiency throughout the myofascial system.

The plan of action for an integrated deep tissue therapy session or series of sessions must be built on the goal of establishing equilibrium between counterbalancing forces in the body. Examples of these dynamic relationships include the equilibrium of the pelvis and the head: two poles of the spine; the tension between prime movers and their antagonists; relationships between superficial and deep layers of tissue; and between slow-moving postural muscles and their associated fast-moving phasic partners. Working toward functional, healthy relationships between these opposing forces is the heart of integrated deep tissue therapy. The sequences provided in the following chapters give readers practical knowledge of how the naturally counterbalancing relationships in the body may manifest.

▶ STEP THREE: IMPLEMENT THE PLAN

The third step in the integrated deep tissue therapy system involves using the results of observation and planning to begin the work of re-establishing balance between opposing myofascial forces.

Slow compressive strokes are applied along the length of contracted muscles, from attachment to attachment, covering the tendons and muscle bellies. Shorter, focused strokes are then used to treat smaller sections of the muscle that may need attention. These strokes may be applied parallel to or across the muscle fibers, depending on the nature of the restriction. They are also used on the tendinous attachments to the bones to aid in minimizing scar tissue formation and to stimulate the Golgi tendon organs to send messages through the nervous system to direct the muscle to soften and relax.

Remember that the primary goal of integrated deep tissue therapy is to re-establish the most functional, efficient relationships between muscular and fascial forces around the skeleton. This is accomplished by lengthening chronically contracted muscles, loosening constricted fascia, helping the client to strengthen weakened muscles, reducing irritation to nearby sensory receptors, and addressing other restrictive conditions, like scar tissue and trigger points, that inhibit full and pain-free movement.

Superficial and Deep Muscles

Integrated deep tissue therapy addresses the muscular system in layers, from superficial to deep. The therapist must have a thorough knowledge of muscle anatomy to distinguish the layers of muscles that are being accessed. None of the layers should be neglected in an integrated deep tissue session. Each has unique characteristics, and tends to react to tension differently.

The superficial layer of muscle is the level that is most affected by the external environment. It, along with the skin and adipose tissue, forms a barrier between the external world and the internal body. The superficial layer of fascia and muscle are most vulnerable to invasions from the environment, such as exposure to extreme temperatures, or trauma resulting from accidents or falls. Tension patterns sometimes appear to migrate from the surface of the body to the deeper levels. Sometimes it is tempting to skip or short change the superficial layers of muscles to get to what seems like more exciting work. But if the deep layers of muscle are overemphasized while the superficial layers are neglected, the origin of many tension patterns that originate at the surface may be easily overlooked. In other words, "deep tissue therapy" is not exclusive to the deep muscles: superficial muscles are equally important.

The deeper layers of muscle, which are often called on for maintaining postural positions, tend to adopt inefficient tension patterns from trauma, faulty habits of movement, and psychological conditioning. The ropy, knotted fibers that are characteristic of tense muscles, along with trigger points, often manifest at this level. Relieving these patterns while addressing the superficial layer of muscle brings longer lasting results than addressing superficial tissues alone. Imbalances between superficial and deep layers of soft tissue distort the body, and the compensations they demand create tension and inefficient movement and breathing. When the soft tissue layers of muscles and fascia move freely and in balance with each other, the body can become more functionally integrated throughout.

Postural (Tonic) and Movement (Phasic) Muscles

Understanding the characteristics of skeletal muscles helps the therapist to anticipate the types of problems that are likely to be encountered in specific muscles. Skeletal muscle serves two important functions: support and movement. Skeletal muscles support the position of the bones in relation to each other against the force of gravity to maintain postural integrity. The skeletal muscles also move the human structure through space. They exhibit an extraordinary dynamic range, capable of producing large bursts of motion that propel the body against the force of gravity, or controlling tiny, subtle movements that allow the fingertips to trace the contours of a single strand of hair.

To carry out these functions, two distinct types of skeletal muscle have evolved. The muscles that are mostly responsible for support are called postural or **tonic** muscles. The muscles that provide conscious, voluntary movement are called **phasic** muscles. These muscle types have some distinguishing characteristics that may influence strategies for the integrated deep tissue therapist. A list of major muscles and where they fall in the tonic/phasic categories is provided in Table 4-1,

TABLE 4-1 | Tonic and Phasic Muscles

Postural (Tonic) Muscles	Phasic Muscles
Face and neck muscles	
Masseter	Deep cervical flexors
Temporalis	
Scalenes (these have characteristics of tonic and phasic muscles)	
Shoulder girdle and upper extremity	
Pectoralis major (sternal fibers)	Trapezius (middle)
Levator scapulae	Trapezius (lower)
Trapezius (upper)	Rhomboids
Biceps brachii	Serratus anterior
Subscapularis	Triceps brachii
Suboccipitals	Supraspinatus
Wrist and finger flexors	Infraspinatus
	Deltoid
	Wrist and finger extensors
Trunk	
Lumbar erector spinae	Thoracic erector spinae
Cervical erector spinae	Rectus abdominus
Quadratus lumborum	Internal and external obliques
	Transversus abdominis
Pelvis and thigh	
Hamstrings	Vastus lateralis
Iliopsoas	Vastus medialis
Rectus femoris	Gluteal muscles
Short (crossing one joint) hip adductors	
Piriformis	
Tensor fasciae latae	
Leg and foot	
Gastrocnemius	Tibialis anterior
Soleus	Fibularis muscles
	Toe extensors

but be aware that this is not a comprehensive list, not every expert agrees on every item, and some muscles engage in both tonic and phasic activity.[1,2]

CHARACTERISTICS OF TONIC MUSCLES

- Postural, or tonic, muscles support the body against the force of gravity. They are referred to as the workhorse or antigravity muscles, because they have to be able to perform for long periods, sustaining a semicontracted state to support the skeleton.
- These muscles have a high percentage of slow-twitch red fibers, which have a plentiful blood supply, so they can do a lot of work over a long period of time.
- These muscles maintain a high level of stamina, because their fibers do not contract in unison but, rather, in turns. The motor units in the fibers work by taking turns, like blinking holiday lights. As group of muscle units contract, others relax and re-fuel. Because the fibers contract in relay fashion, these muscles do not tire quickly and, therefore, can offer long-term support to the body.
- Tonic muscles are slow to respond to a reflex stimulus. They cannot contract and relax as quickly as phasic muscles can.
- These muscles tend to cramp easily if called on to move quickly or exhibit great strength.
- When a person's posture is distorted, the postural muscles have to brace misaligned joints, and they tend to become hypertonic: a higher percentage of fibers are working than is necessary or efficient.
- This permanent, highly contracted state of muscles is associated with the formation of trigger points.
- The body also produces additional connective tissue in these muscles, possibly to bolster their bracing capability. The overabundance of connective tissue confines the muscle in its shortened state, preventing it from being able to lengthen fully. Thus, the body becomes locked into a distorted shape. The built-up connective tissue is dense and unyielding, so the person cannot easily or consciously move the body into optimal alignment. Slow, focused stretching exercises that are practiced over time may help to improve range of motion in these constricted muscle and fascial tissues. In addition, connective tissue therapy may help return the body to its natural, relaxed, and lengthened state.

CHARACTERISTICS OF PHASIC MUSCLES

- The phasic muscles are responsible for moving the body through space.
- These muscles are made up predominantly of fast-twitch red fibers, which contract and relax rapidly in response to stimulus. They can move the body quickly to adapt to unanticipated events, like stepping off an unseen curb, or withdrawing from a dangerous stimulus.
- The fast-twitch fibers of phasic muscles fatigue quickly. Although the phasic muscles have more short-term strength than the postural muscles, they tire much faster and need more recovery time than do tonic muscles.
- Because the phasic muscles often have to make quick adjustments, their fibers are prone to microtearing. This tearing often occurs at the musculotendinous junction. The constant pull of the muscles against the attached bones can lead to damage at the tendon; this is tendinitis when it is acute, and tendinosis when it is a long-term problem.
- Phasic muscles can also become hypertonic. Repetitive use of certain muscle groups for a specific activity, such as hammering nails, can lead to chronic contraction of those muscles. The quick changes in length that are sometimes required of movement muscles to stabilize the body's equilibrium can lead to spasms and permanently contracted states.

Tonic muscles, the postural muscles that keep us upright, often become hypertonic and shortened. The counterbalancing phasic muscles then have a tendency to become stretched and weak. A good example of this is the relationship between the scalenes and pectoralis minor, and the rhomboids: the tonic anterior muscles contract and are often abnormally shortened, and the phasic rhomboids get stretched and weakened. Alternatively, a person with hypertonic erector spinae muscles in the low back is likely also to have weakened abdominal muscles on the anterior side. Because the deep tissue compressive manipulations are designed to lengthen contracted muscles, the postural muscles are often the focus of integrated deep tissue sessions. As postural muscles are addressed, the musculoskeletal relationships become more integrated, and the phasic muscles naturally become normalized. If particular tonic muscles remain weak even after treatment, additional strengthening exercises may be recommended to improve their function.

Using the Lesson Material

When a therapist uses the three steps of observation, planning, and implementation, he or she can perceive the continuum of myofascial influences that act on the client's body. The information presented in the following lessons and the deep tissue routines provides the necessary foundation to use these steps to be an effective integrated deep tissue therapist. Then the practitioner's job is to adapt each routine to fit the specific requirements of the client based on the three steps of treatment design.

For step one, observing the client's patterns of muscular tension and compensation, the therapist uses the postural evaluation outline, along with the charts for range of motion and conditions.

Step two, planning a strategy, relies on the sequence of the routines presented in this book. Part of planning a strategy involves engaging the client in the process. This is to confirm that the client's goals and the therapist's goals are in alignment, that their expectations are realistic and achievable, and also to be sure that whatever the therapist plans is acceptable to the client. This conversation needs to begin before bodywork starts, and it may need to be revisited periodically throughout the session. A special "permission" icon ⚠ appears in the lessons where massage that may require special sensitivity is described, but it must be understood that the client can stop or change the session at any time.

Step three, implementing the plan, involves the hands-on work. It is a good idea to discuss with the client the number of sessions you think might be needed to bring his or her body to a state of better functioning, so that a level of commitment to your work together is agreed on from the start. Most people experience some improvement in their state of health and well-being within three to five sessions, and substantial improvement beyond that point. If they do not, it may be that the therapist is on the wrong track and needs to re-evaluate his or her strategy.

An integrated deep tissue therapy session is generally scheduled in a 60- or 90-minute format, depending on the preference of the therapist and the needs of the client. Each session is structured as follows:

- Presession interview: postural assessment and discussion of session strategies
- Opening: polarity and shiatsu
- Warm-up: Swedish and cross-fiber techniques
- Connective tissue therapy
- Deep tissue and neuromuscular therapy
- Stretching
- Accessory work
- Closing: reflexology or polarity
- Postsession interview: client feedback is received; stretches, self-care tips, or other recommendations may be suggested if this is within the therapist's scope of practice; and plans for the next session may be made

Table 4-2 provides an approximation of the amount of time spent on each section. Remember, this is applied to a specific area of the body, not to the whole body.

This timeline is very flexible. It is only meant as a general guideline to help structure the session time efficiently. The large

TABLE 4–2 | Timing an Integrated Deep Tissue Therapy Session

Sequence	60-Minute Format	90-Minute Format
Opening	3 min	3 min
Warm-up	5 min	7 min
Connective tissue therapy	5 min	5 min
Deep tissue and neuromuscular therapy	38 min	65 min
Stretching	2 min	2 min
Accessory work	5 min	6 min
Closing	2 min	2 min

block of time given to deep tissue and neuromuscular therapy allows the therapist to intersperse techniques from the other sections as needed. In addition to the time given to work on the massage table, the therapist must factor in the time spent with the client both before and after the session, which could add up to an additional 30 minutes to the appointment time.

Each routine contains instructions for deep tissue massage of all the muscles in that particular body region. It is not necessary to address all the muscles listed in a routine within a single session. Contracted muscles are chosen for focus based on the therapist's observation of the client's unique patterns of distortion. The therapist must also take into account the client's history of traumas and reported areas of pain when he or she decides which muscles to target for deep tissue massage and neuromuscular therapy treatment.

The illustrations that accompany the descriptions of the strokes demonstrate the full technique performed with a willing recipient. In this way, the student can see the completed application.

It is always important to take into account the client's level of comfort in receiving massage, both for depth of pressure and for draping. Some clients may need adjustments so that less of the body is exposed, or some strokes may need to be stopped before the therapist reaches the muscle attachment, particularly in the pelvic region. Alternatively, some strokes may be done through the drape or clothing, which may help some clients to be more comfortable and receptive. This conversation should happen before the session begins, as described above, so that the client can be confident that his or her boundaries are respected.

Guidelines for Performing the Modalities

▶ ENERGY WORK

The goal of these styles of bodywork is to allow a more effective flow of energy. Whether one thinks of "energy" as an immeasurable subjective experience of life force, or as a way of describing the body's internal activities as described in Chapter 1, opening each session with some time spent in conscious, nonmoving touch is a powerful way to create a space for positive changes to happen and to prepare for the work that is to follow. This practice establishes an important bond between the therapist and client, and enhances the level of receptivity in both parties.

Sample holds or maneuvers from polarity and shiatsu are recommended for the beginning of each deep tissue therapy session. These help to prepare the client for the massage work that is to follow. The initial contact between client and therapist defines the quality of their interaction. It allows the client time to relax, to become accustomed to the therapist's touch, and to begin to tune in to his or her body. The therapist can use this time to establish rapport and to build an environment of trust and safety.

Polarity

The polarity protocol described here is derived from the work of Dr. Randolph Stone, who used principles of magnetism, that is, positive and negative poles, to describe the direction of the flow of energy through the body. In this context, polarity serves as an introduction to each integrated deep tissue therapy session, because it creates a separation of space and time from normal routine. Polarity techniques are described at the beginning of each routine for the part of the body being emphasized in that lesson.

Touch in a polarity treatment is very soft and is usually administered with full, open hands. The therapist places the hands on the client's body slowly and lightly. The therapist's palms and fingers touch the surface of the body with just enough pressure to make contact with the client's skin. A useful image is to imagine placing your hand on a leaf floating on the surface of a pond. Use only enough pressure to feel the leaf against your palm without submerging it in the water. Directions for appropriate placement of the therapist's hands are given in the description of each polarity position in the lessons.

After the therapist establishes contact with the client's body, the polarity position is generally held for 1 to 2 minutes. During this time, the therapist sits or stands upright in a relaxed, receptive stance, and his or her pattern of breathing should be even and calm. This allows the client to take the cue for calm, tension-free breathing as well. The therapist is fully sensitive to the sensations in his or her hands. Feelings of warmth or mild vibration in the therapist's palms and fingers while contacting the client's body are common sensations, as is heightened attunement to the client's various rhythms. The therapist may also become aware of subtle shifts and movements in the client's body. This may feel like softening, or giving way. Clients often report becoming deeply relaxed and more in tune with the sensations in their body as a result of the focused contact. This opportunity to be aware of inner sensations—promoting **interoception**—is an important component of integrated deep tissue therapy.

No conscious analysis is necessary for this part of the treatment to be effective. The therapist's focus is on being receptive to, and in tune with, the client.

To release the polarity hold, the therapist very slowly removes his or her hands from the client's body while maintaining focus on the client's comfort and welfare. It is helpful to time the release of the hands to the client's inhalation, as if the client is gently pushing the therapist's hands off the surface of the body as it expands to take in a breath.

Shiatsu

The shiatsu techniques are performed after the polarity hold is released. A few easy-to-perform options have been chosen from the vast repertoire of shiatsu procedures. These suggestions come from the traditional practice of shiatsu, but have been chosen specifically to augment the effectiveness of the integrated deep tissue therapy as a whole.

As explained in Chapter 1, the premise of shiatsu is that it enhances the flow of qi, or life force, through a complex series of channels, or meridians, that run through the body. Tradition suggests that this is accomplished by applying a series of compressive moves that trace the course of the channels. Whereas traditional shiatsu techniques move very specifically along the path of a meridian, often with the client on the floor, the techniques suggested for integrated deep tissue therapy are more general, administered on a massage table, and usually covering several channels at a time.

The shiatsu techniques incorporated in the lessons involve compression moves done with the hands along the length of a limb, moving proximal to distal. To begin the sequence, the therapist faces the client's body and holds the limb with both hands. The thumbs are placed on the lateral side of the limb, the palms cover the center of the limb, and the fingers wrap around the medial side. A combination of compression, squeezing, and slight medial rolling of the limb is used in coordination with both therapist and client exhalations. The stroke begins by pressing the thumbs into the lateral side of the limb. The stroke is continued by pressing down on the top of the limb with the palms. As the thumbs maintain contact, the therapist adds a squeezing action with the fingers to embrace the limb fully with the hands. The stroke is completed by rolling the limb slightly medial while maintaining the pressure on it with the hands.

Unlike the polarity segment, this application of shiatsu incorporates the therapist's whole body, not just the hands. The weight and motion of the body into the stroke, not the strength of arm or hand muscles, supply the necessary compressive force. The correct body motion for the move described above begins with the stance (Fig. 4-2). The therapist's feet are placed a little wider than hip-distance apart and separated from each other lengthwise by the distance of a comfortable walking stride. Both knees are slightly flexed, with awareness

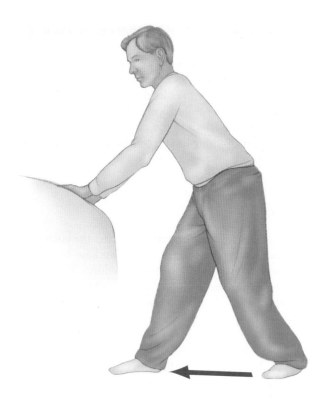

FIGURE 4-2 Proper body position for the application of shiatsu strokes.

focused on the pelvis as the initiator of movement. At the beginning of the stroke, about 70% of the body's weight is on the back foot. As the stroke continues, the weight is shifted forward, timed with the pace of the stroke and with exhalation. At the completion of the stroke, about 70% of the therapist's weight is on the front foot. The spine stays long, and the shoulders, arms, and hands remain relaxed throughout the entire stroke. The therapist slides the hands a little further down the limb, shifts his or her weight back to the back foot, and begins the compression sequence again. The therapist continues in this manner to the wrist or ankle. When this technique is well executed, it feels complete and satisfying to receive, and practically effortless to deliver.

▶ SWEDISH MASSAGE

The Swedish strokes are introduced after the polarity and shiatsu techniques. Swedish massage offers excellent transition and smoothing strokes that may be woven throughout the session at the therapist's discretion. The goal is to induce a sense of fluidity and continuity to promote a quality of integration throughout the soft tissues. More than any other technique, Swedish massage generates a sense of unity or "incorporation" in the body, and it enhances the benefits of every other modality.

Swedish massage contains a huge repertoire of strokes. The three basic Swedish techniques—effleurage, petrissage, and

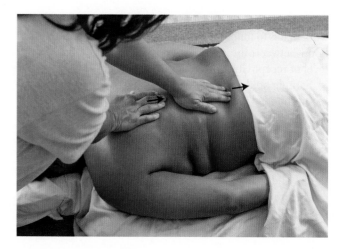

FIGURE 4-3 Shingles stroke.

friction—are utilized in the integrated deep tissue therapy system to warm up the tissues, enhance local circulatory turnover, and create a unifying bridge between the other modalities.

Effleurage

Effleurage strokes are smooth, gliding strokes that are executed over the surface of the skin. One or both hands may be used, depending on the particular pattern of the stroke. Effleurage is used to warm up the tissues, soothe the nervous system, and relax tense muscles. Various degrees of pressure may be applied depending on the purpose of the stroke and the preference of the client. Lubricant is used to ease movement over the skin. Although the palmar surfaces of the hands are the most commonly employed tools, other parts of the hand or arm may be used as well, including the knuckles, thumbs, and forearms.

Basic effleurage patterns should cover the entire length of the muscles. Effleurage strokes are used to delineate muscular arrangements to the client's nervous system, promoting relaxation-inducing sensations of length. An effleurage stroke that is stopped before it reaches a muscle's bony attachment tends to create a sense of shortness and tightness that is counterproductive to the goal of massage.

The following are descriptions of effleurage-style strokes used in this course that may not be familiar to all readers:

- *Shingles* is an effleurage variation in which one hand replaces the other by gliding under it every 2 or 3 inches throughout the length of the stroke (Fig. 4-3). It creates a pattern reminiscent of overlapping roof shingles.
- *Swimming* is a forearm variation of effleurage that is commonly performed on the back or thighs. The therapist places both forearms parallel to each other on the midback or midthigh (Fig. 4-4). The therapist simultaneously shifts

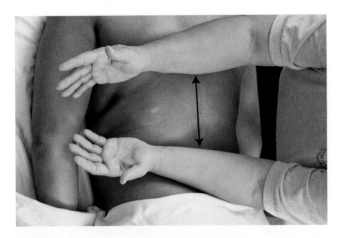

FIGURE 4-4 Swimming stroke.

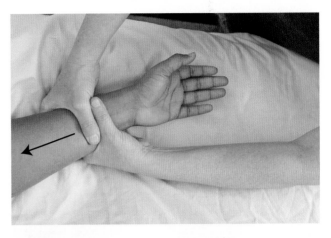

FIGURE 4-6 Draining stroke (shown on the forearm).

his or her weight forward and slides and rolls the forearms apart, allowing them to glide over the skin until they are shoulder-width apart. At that point, the therapist draws the arms back together, without losing contact with the skin, to begin the stroke again. The motion is somewhat similar to the arm movement used by swimmers in the breaststroke.

- *Thumb gliding* is an effleurage stroke incorporating the full lengths of the thumbs. The thumbs alternately glide over the skin in an overlapping pattern similar to the path of windshield wipers (Fig. 4-5). This stroke is commonly used on smaller body parts, such as the palm of the hand, the plantar surface of the foot, and around the knee.

- *Draining* is a two-handed effleurage stroke that is performed on either the arm or the leg, moving from the distal to the proximal end. Both hands are wrapped around the extremity at either the ankle or the wrist, with the fingers embracing the sides of the extremity while the thumbs cross each other over the midsection (Fig. 4-6). The webbing between the thumb and index fingers of both hands makes full contact with the central, rounded contour of

the limb. Light pressure is maintained as the hands glide up the limb toward the proximal end. Upon reaching the proximal end, the hands separate and slide down the medial and lateral sides of the limb to begin the stroke again. Contact with the skin is never broken.

Petrissage

Swedish petrissage strokes are used to further relax muscles and improve local blood and lymph circulation with grasping, lifting, squeezing motions of the hands. One- or two-handed variations are commonly employed (Fig. 4-7A and B). Knuckle kneading is a form of petrissage that uses the knuckle side of an extended-finger fist position. The knuckles are rolled back and forth over a small section of the body at a comfortable pace and pressure (Fig. 4-8).

Friction

Friction strokes are used to relax contracted muscle fibers and address adhesions and scar tissue. The therapist presses into the client's tissues, pinning the skin directly under the fingers or palm to the underlying muscle and fascia. When friction is used to address deeper tissues, the skin and muscle may be moved as one unit. The pressure is firm so that the therapist's hand does not glide over the skin, as this can cause irritation. Friction strokes are performed in circular motions, in line with muscle fibers, or in back-and-forth, cross-fiber patterns (Fig. 4-9).

▶ CROSS-FIBER THERAPY

Cross-fiber therapy techniques form a bridge between traditional relaxation styles of massage therapy and deep tissue therapy. They are meant to address and loosen adhesions in

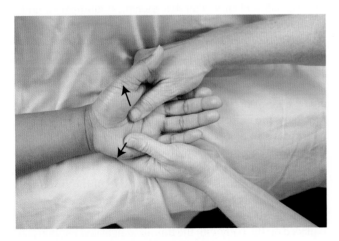

FIGURE 4-5 Thumb gliding stroke.

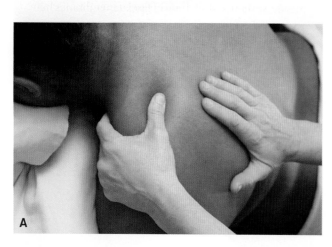

FIGURE 4-7 Classic petrissage.

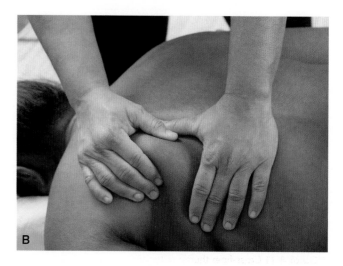

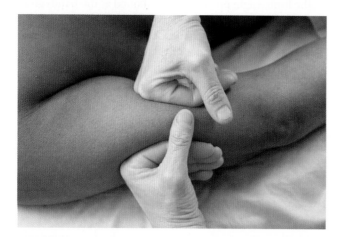

FIGURE 4-8 Knuckle kneading.

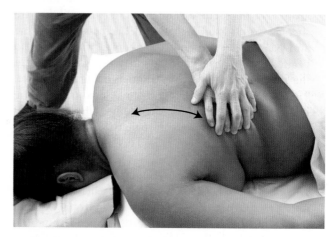

FIGURE 4-10 Cross-fiber fingertip raking stroke.

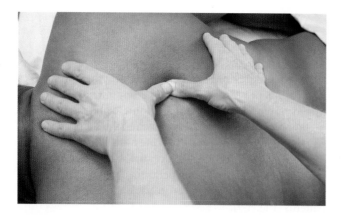

FIGURE 4-9 Cross-fiber friction, supported thumb.

bundles of muscle fibers. Adhesions can interfere with healthy function. They may obstruct local fluid flow, restrict range of motion, and bind up local sensory neurons, which may elicit pain and impair proprioception. The goal of cross-fiber therapy is to minimize these problems.

The two cross-fiber strokes incorporated in the integrated deep tissue therapy system are fingertip raking and a rolling technique using the full length of the thumb. These techniques are based on the work of Therese Pfrimmer, one of the originators of cross-fiber style therapy. Both strokes require enough lubricant to provide a smooth, back-and-forth, gliding motion across the muscle fibers, but not so much that access to the inter-fiber adhesions is missed.

Fingertip raking is executed with a hand position formed from a cupped palm and curved fingers that are spread slightly apart. One or both hands may be used. The fingertip pads roll across the muscle at a 90° angle to the direction the fibers are running in a continuous, back-and-forward motion that progresses along the full length of the muscle between its two attachments (Fig. 4-10).

The rolling stroke uses the broad side of the thumb all the way from its tip to the thenar eminence on the palm. To execute the stroke, the entire palmar surface of the hand is placed on the body with the thumb straight and comfortably extended from the hand in its natural position, an approximately

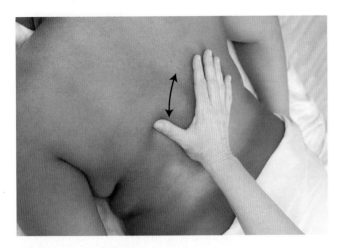

FIGURE 4-11 Cross-fiber thumb rolling stroke.

60° angle (Fig. 4-11). The length of the thumb lies parallel to the direction the muscle fibers are running. As the hand glides back and forth across the muscle, the thumb rolls over the muscle fibers. This causes the bundles of fibers to slide against each other, spreading them and loosening fascial restrictions that may be keeping them bunched together. A helpful image in performing the stroke properly is a rolling pin being rolled back and forth across a ball of dough, flattening it out.

Both cross-fiber strokes are performed at a moderate pace. The therapist should be able to cover the entire length of an average-sized muscle in five or six back-and-forth strokes. Because they roll across muscle fibers, cross-fiber strokes allow the therapist to feel the condition of the fibers more effectively than strokes that run parallel to the fibers. Stringy or ropy fibers are signs of tightness, and may need more attention than their softer neighbors.

Cross-fiber strokes should not be performed over the same section of muscle for more than five or six passes in a row, or they can be irritating to the skin. If the underlying tissues still feel dry and stringy after several passes, the therapist should move on, perhaps returning to that section of fibers later to recheck it.

▶ CONNECTIVE TISSUE THERAPY

The goal of working with the body's fascia is threefold: to change local fluid dynamics and make the ground substance more fluid, at least temporarily; to loosen the collagen bonds that cause muscle sheaths to adhere to each other or to other structures; and to improve the function of the many sensory neurons located in fascia that provide us with our sense of movement and position in space. The techniques that are used to spread and separate fascial membranes often incorporate slow stretching and pulling actions.

Steady, sustained stretching of fascial membranes helps to free restricting links that form within the collagen mesh. The key to successful fascial loosening is the ability to sense the limit of the tissue's ability to stretch, and then hold the stretch until a yielding or lengthening sensation is felt. The tissues are never forced with more pressure or stretch than they can comfortably accommodate—to do so is perceived as threatening at a subconscious level, and may result in involuntary guarding from nearby muscles, along with possible injury.

Application of Connective Tissue Strokes

1. *Fascial Lift and Roll Technique.* This is a skin and muscle rolling technique designed to loosen adhered areas in the superficial fascia. Both hands are used. The thumbs are placed end to end on one side of the tissue to be rolled, and the fingers are positioned on the other side. The tissues are lifted and pressed toward the fingers with the thumbs. They are then rolled between the fingers and thumbs (Fig. 4-12). If the skin can be lifted easily off the underlying tissues, it may be rolled independently. Otherwise, the skin, adipose, superficial fascia, and muscle tissue may all be lifted and rolled. Always move slowly and deliberately. Adhered areas may be tender. Begin the rolling action on a section of tissue that is relatively easy to lift, and gradually move toward the more resistive areas. Never force the tissues, and be aware that it may take more than one session to achieve the best results.

2. *Myofascial Spreading.* This stroke may be executed using fingers, knuckles, or the base of the palms. A very small amount of lubricant may be used. The therapist's hands should be able to stretch the client's skin without slipping over it. Press into the midline of the section of tissue to be softened until slight resistance is felt. Allow

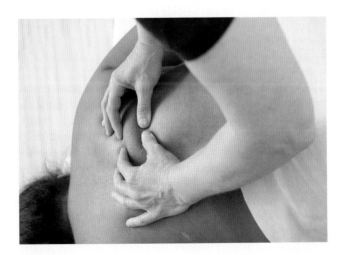

FIGURE 4-12 Fascial lift and roll technique.

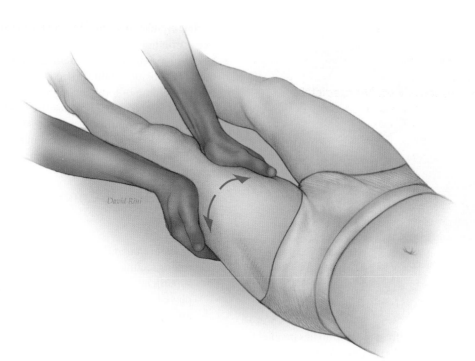

FIGURE 4-13 Myofascial spreading.

the hands to draw apart evenly until the client's tissue will not stretch any further. Hold at that point until the resistance yields and your hands can slide further apart (Fig. 4-13). This stroke is designed to reduce binding in the fascial membranes.

3. *Myofascial Mobilization.* The fingers, knuckles, palm, or forearm may be used for this stroke. The myofascial tissues are rolled against the underlying muscles and bones with a back and forth or a circular movement (Fig. 4-14). This technique is used to improve movement in myofascial tissue that is adhering to itself. The goal is to re-establish the ability of tissues to slide freely over each other.

▶ DEEP TISSUE THERAPY

The term *deep tissue therapy* has many connotations. It may be interpreted as the application of deep pressure to muscles, or as therapy to the deeper lying muscle groups in the body. For our purposes, the most accurate description of deep tissue therapy is that *it is therapy that has a deep impact for the client*. At its core, deep tissue therapy is transformative in nature. It can transform the dysfunctional characteristics of the body's soft tissues to minimize pain and stress. In doing so, deep tissue therapy can enhance function on many levels. To accomplish these goals, firm pressure on the tissues may be required at times. However, the pressure of strokes should never feel painful or intrusive to the client (see Box 4-1).

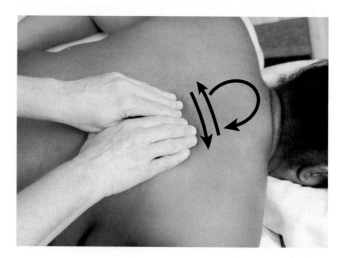

FIGURE 4-14 Myofascial mobilization.

Application of Deep Tissue Therapy Strokes

After the warm-up phase of the session is completed, the client is ready for deep tissue therapy. The lessons provide descriptions of the application of the strokes to specific muscles. They do not give details about the pace, depth, or number of repetitions of each stroke, because those factors are variable, depending on the needs of the client. Palpatory

BOX 4-1 | "Deep Tissue" Massage and the Nature of Pain

All pain is subjective, and pain related to touch and pressure is especially so. No predictable, measurable amount of pressure causes the same response in every person, or even in the same person on different days.

Pain is usually experienced as coming from somewhere in the body, but the actual interpretation of a nerve signal into the phenomenon that we understand as "pain" happens in the brain. Our connective tissue and muscles are well supplied with sensory neuron extensions that convey messages about pressure, position, and potential damage. Massage stimulates these neurons, and the signals they send to the brain are then construed as welcome (pleasure) or threatening (pain). If pain is the interpretation, this is followed by the secretion of local pain-promoting chemicals from the irritated nerve endings. These local chemicals exacerbate the threatening stimulus, and essentially eradicate any possible benefit from further pressure-based massage therapy.

What determines whether a person will experience touch—deep or superficial— as painful or pleasurable? This depends on many factors, including the degree of tension in the tissues, the status of local injuries, the person's attitudes and expectations about massage, and the person's interpretation of the quality and intent of the touch. To be able to relax and painlessly welcome deeper gradations of pressure, the client must feel sure that the therapist is completely present, compassionate, sensitive, confident, and knowledgeable. The therapist must be capable of making the necessary adjustments to prevent his or her touch from becoming harmful, or intrusive—in short, from causing pain. The consequence of a mistake here is that pain is unnecessarily increased, and the client guards against the therapy instead of benefiting from it.

The dynamic nature of the interaction between the therapist and client during a deep tissue session requires constant vigilance and sensitivity for the therapy to be productive.

The overall goal of the deep tissue strokes is to help contracted muscles to relax. This is accomplished by the application of slow, compressive force into the muscles, accompanied by gradual movement of the stroke along the length of the muscle. This compressive force slowly lengthens the fibers in the muscle belly and in surrounding fascial sheaths, similar to sustained stretching of a muscle. This pressure with torsion or shearing (i.e., stretch) is especially good to access the proprioceptors that communicate with the central nervous system (CNS) to lower muscle tone.

Deep tissue strokes that are designed to lengthen shortened muscles are performed parallel to the muscle fibers. In this book, they are referred to as elongation strokes. They must be performed very slowly; otherwise, the stroke will activate the stretch reflex, causing the muscle to contract even more, and defeating the purpose of the deep tissue therapy.

When an elongation stroke is performed at the appropriate pace, the tissues feel as if they are yielding, or melting, under the therapist's touch. If resistance is encountered while stroking along the muscle, the therapist must stop at that point and hold the stroke steady until the resistance melts. The therapist may need to lessen the pressure being used to achieve the requisite softening of the muscle tissue before continuing the stroke.

Muscle Layers

Muscles are addressed in progression from the surface to the deeper layers. The therapist must be thoroughly familiar with the musculature and able to picture the muscles' shapes and positions in relation to each other so that he or she knows when a particular muscle is being reached. Deeper muscles cannot be palpated directly. Their fibers are felt *through* the layers of muscle superficial to them. If the surface muscles are contracted and tense, their fibers are not pliable enough for the therapist to feel through them to the deeper layers. Therefore, the surface layers must be softened before the deeper layers are accessible.

As the therapist applies pressure, he or she sinks into the tissues only to the level of mild to moderate resistance. The feeling of resistance is a result of the muscle's contracting to defend itself against potentially harmful pressure. Deep tissue strokes may be applied with more pressure than other strokes, but never to the point at which the client tightens the muscles against the pressure. As soon as the soft tissues contract to defend themselves, tension is reintroduced into the body, and deep tissue therapy is counterproductive.

▶ DEEP TISSUE STROKES

On Muscle Bellies

assessment and ongoing verbal communication with the client are necessary to offer the best application of the deep tissue techniques. The approach to deep tissue therapy will be different with every individual, and even the same client will require varying degrees of pressure on different muscle groups, or even on different days.

1. *Elongating/Lengthening.* This stroke is a slow, gliding, compressive movement that is performed parallel to the muscle fibers, from origin to insertion (Fig. 4-15). The

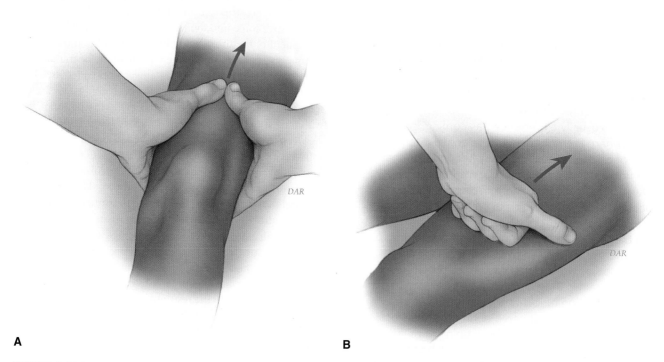

A   **B**

FIGURE 4-15 A. Deep tissue elongation stroke using both thumb pads. **B.** Deep tissue elongation stroke using knuckles.

fingers, knuckles, base of the palm, thumbs, elbow, or forearm may be used. It is the primary technique used to return a contracted muscle to its resting length.

2. *Spreading.* These techniques are used to palpate aberrations in small sections of muscle fibers. They are incorporated within taut bands of fibers to locate trigger points precisely (Fig. 4-16).

The fingers, thumbs, knuckles, or elbow may be used. Although the thumb pads are the most sensitive part of the body used for delivering deep tissue strokes, it is best to perfect the use of these other body parts to save wear and tear on the thumbs.

- *Up-and-Down.* Move parallel to the muscle fibers, covering 1-inch sections at a time.
- *Side-to-Side.* Move perpendicular to the muscle fibers using back-and-forth motions in 1-inch segments.
- *Combination.* Perform up-and-down and side-to-side strokes on the same section of muscle, creating a 1-inch square.
- *Fanning.* The hands spread apart from each other in an arc pattern 3 to 4 inches wide (Fig. 4-17). This stroke stretches fascial membranes.

3. *Static Compression.* Lean directly into the muscle tissue at a 90° angle to the surface of the body (Fig. 4-18). Thumbs, fingers, knuckles, or elbows may be used. This stroke is used on extremely contracted sections of muscle fibers. It is also used to treat trigger points and acupressure points.

4. *Sifting.* This is a cross-fiber style stroke. Grasp a section of muscle tissue between your fingers and thumb, and then roll the fibers to loosen adhering factors and locate trigger points within taut bands of tissue (Fig. 4-19).

On Tendons

The following deep tissue procedures are used to treat tendons:
1. Stroke on the tendon toward the insertion point on the bone.
2. Do short, cross-fiber strokes across the tendon.

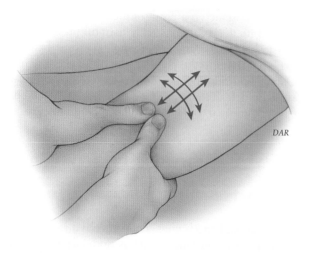

FIGURE 4-16 Hand position for spreading techniques.

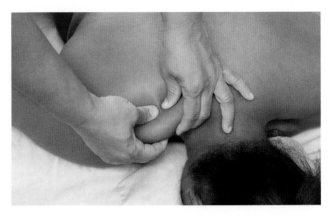

FIGURE 4-19 Sifting technique.

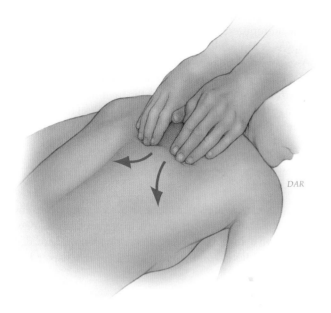

FIGURE 4-17 Fanning stroke.

3. Hold static compression where the tendon attaches to the bone.
4. The thumbs, elbow, fingers, or knuckles may be used (Fig. 4-20).

To Separate Muscles

Stroke along the borders of muscles to separate them from each other. Use elongation strokes with the thumb, elbow, or knuckles (Fig. 4-21).

Client Response

Signs of muscle relaxation are varied. As a muscle relaxes, it feels like it is able to spread more easily and has a softer tone when pressure is applied to it. Contracted fibers may visibly jump, as they are relaxing. Sometimes, a pulsation runs through the entire length of the muscle. Stringy, taut fibers become less pronounced as tone is decreased, and local circulation is restored.

Clients sometimes experience intense sensations during this work. Unhealthy conditions in muscle tissue are usually tender when touched. Trigger points, scar tissue, bands of taut fibers, and spasms can be painful. When these conditions are encountered, the therapist can explain the cause of the painful reaction. This kind of education about their experience may calm feelings of apprehension, and this often

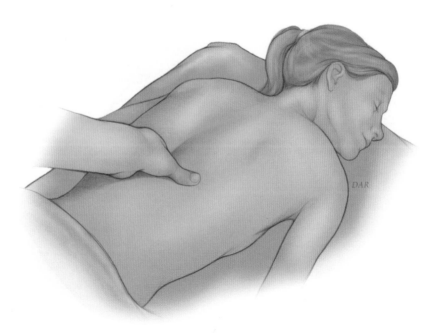

FIGURE 4-18 Static compression using the thumb.

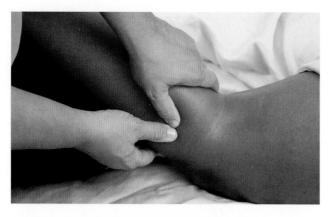

FIGURE 4-20 Hand position for treating a tendon.

lessens the subjective sensation of pain. The therapist must always have the client's input and permission to ensure that the threshold of uncomfortable pain sensations is not crossed.

Evaluation of the Work

During the deep tissue session, the therapist must frequently pause to assess the progress of the work. These pauses also allow the client to assimilate the experience more fully. Softly palpating the massaged muscles enables the therapist to assess the degree of relaxation that has been produced. It is important to ask the client for feedback about his or her reactions to the work done thus far. To enhance the self-sensing

and assimilation process, a gentle hold or polarity contact may be administered to an area of the body after deep tissue therapy is completed.

Assessment of change may include the client's report of pain or relief, range of motion stretches, and a comparison of muscle tone from before and after the treatment. Additional effleurage strokes performed along the length of the muscles may help the client to assimilate a new state of relaxation.

▶ NEUROMUSCULAR THERAPY

The purpose of neuromuscular therapy is to seek out and treat any trigger points, which may be causing pain or muscular weakness. A description of trigger points and their formation was provided in the introduction to neuromuscular therapy in Chapter 1.

Finding Trigger Points

Trigger points are located in one of two ways. First, they may be encountered while performing deep tissue strokes on a muscle. A trigger point is always found within a taut band of muscle fibers that are tender to the touch. An indication that a band of fibers houses a single trigger point, or a group of trigger points, is that the fibers will twitch and elicit a pain response when the therapist's finger strums across them. Once the taut band of fibers is located, the therapist carefully seeks out the point within the fibers that delivers the most concentrated sensation when compressed.

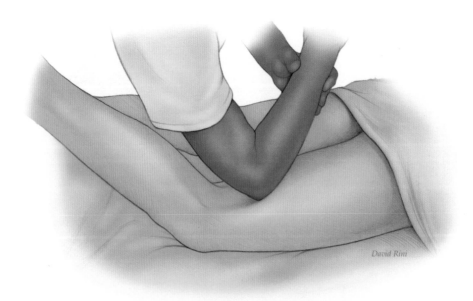

FIGURE 4-21 Deep tissue elongation stroke between muscle bellies.

If active, the trigger point may also elicit pain signals from a predictable remote site, known as a referred pain zone. A trigger point found in a specific location will always refer sensations to the same distant site. The predictability of trigger point referral patterns provides the key to the second method of locating trigger points.

During the interview that takes place before the integrated deep tissue session, the client may describe areas that commonly cause pain and discomfort. This pain may be active, or most pronounced after certain physical activities, or when the person's stress level is high. The client may be describing referred pain sites that are activated by trigger points. If the therapist can pinpoint the exact location and dimension of the pain zone, he or she can be more effective in treatment. A practical way to accomplish this is by the therapist tracing the perimeter of the pain zone on the client's body, with permission, while the client describes it. The therapist can also draw the area of pain on a piece of paper containing a blank figure of the human body. Once the location and size of the referred pain pattern are known, the associated trigger point can be found with the use of a trigger point chart.

A collection of the trigger point maps referred to in this text is included in Appendix B.

Deactivating Trigger Points

The procedure for treating trigger points is simple. Once the location of the trigger point is pinpointed, the therapist presses on it directly, using the thumb, finger, or elbow (Fig. 4-22). Many therapists report the best response with gentle pulsing, rhythmic pressure, as compared to static compression. The degree of pressure should elicit only a mild pain response at the site of the trigger point and at the referral zone. After explaining this to the client, the therapist may incorporate a simple pressure-determining scale graded from 1 to 3 (1 signifying too little pressure, 2 signifying appropriate, satisfying pressure, and 3 signifying too much pressure). By using this scale with the client, the therapist can always gauge his or her pressure perfectly to the client's reaction. This scale can also be used when performing deep tissue strokes to determine the proper amount of pressure.

Active trigger points are painful when pressed or irritated, but they are not usually noticeable otherwise—unless they refer pain to another location. The pain produced by a trigger point may be perceived as coming from the referral site, not necessarily from the location of the trigger point itself. For instance, a person could have a tension-type headache that they feel up over the scalp, but the trigger points behind that pain may be in the sternocleidomastoid muscles. Treatment applied solely at the referral site may offer temporary relief, but it does not solve the underlying problem.

Trigger points are treated with static or rhythmic compression for approximately 8 to 12 seconds. That is usually enough time to interrupt their pain messages. During a treatment, the client should have a significant drop in his or her level of pain. This is a way to check whether treatment is effective: a simple verbal scale can be used to gain information about the level of pain sensation. Every few seconds, as the therapist continues to press, the client is asked if the degree of pain is more, the same, or less. If the treatment is successful, the client should report a continual lessening of the pain, and the constricted area should feel softer, looser, and more moveable.

Immediately after deactivating the trigger point, it is a good idea to stretch the affected muscle, and then return it to its natural resting length. Trigger points cause chronic contractions of groups of muscle fibers. The more regularly a muscle is stretched, the less likely it is to develop trigger points. The client may be taught stretches and exercises (if that is within the therapist's scope of practice) to perform between treatments to maintain healthy muscles.

Charting Trigger Points

Mapping and treating trigger points can be complex, especially if the trigger points have been active for a long time and the client has several overlapping areas of chronic pain. Trigger points can also develop at multiple levels of depth, so deep muscles may have these irritations in addition to superficial muscles. In these clients, each trigger point needs to be addressed in succession, from the superficial muscles to the deeper layers. Several trigger points may cluster around each other within the same muscle, and they may have the same or different referral zones connected to them.

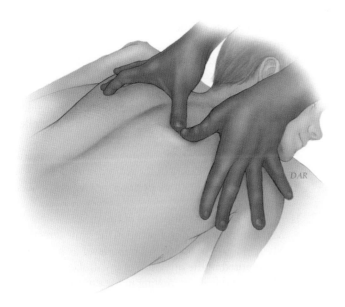

FIGURE 4-22 Hand position for trigger point reduction.

If left untreated, trigger point activity can gradually spread throughout the body. The therapist must carefully map each pain zone and track down the trigger point or points that are causing it to fire. Maintaining a body map for each client that charts each pain zone and the associated trigger points is very helpful in dealing with cases of chronic pain. See Appendix B for a trigger point map that covers the trigger points discussed in this text.

Evaluation of Treatment

The length of time that pain relief from trigger point treatment lasts varies. Among other factors, it depends on the activities and lifestyle of the client. Postural habits and job-related, repetitive movements that aggravate trigger points may have to be relearned or curtailed. Stress management techniques may be incorporated to reduce excessive stimulation within the nervous system. Regular exercise, including slow, sustained stretching, should be practiced on a regular basis. If the necessary steps are taken, relief from trigger point pain may last anywhere from several days to forever.

At the client's next deep tissue therapy session, the therapist would do well to ask about how long local and referred trigger point pain was lessened. If necessary, trigger points can be retreated. If the client has no relief, it is a good idea to suggest a consultation with a physician to examine other possible causes of pain.

Body Mechanics

Of all the essential skills necessary to become a competent integrated deep tissue therapist, one of the most important is learning to use good body mechanics. Correct body alignment and movement allow the efficient execution of the strokes, with minimal effort and wear and tear on the therapist. Straining to perform these techniques not only is detrimental to the therapist's body, it also interferes with the qualities of relaxation and openness that we strive to transmit to the client through our effortless, confident touch.

The study of body mechanics is largely based on learning how to transfer weight through the body structure without creating strain in the muscles. Almost all massage strokes require the transmission of weight from the therapist's body, moving from the feet and legs to the spine, then passing from the shoulder girdle through the arms and hands to the recipient. We create pressure for the strokes when we transfer force into the client's body in a controlled way.

In addition to contending with the force of gravity, the therapist's body must distribute many extra pounds of pressure generated by the compressive movements of the strokes. When the body is not properly positioned, or when the table is not at a proper height, inefficient shearing force around joints like the thumbs and wrists can lead to tissue breakdown and, eventually, disability and a shortened career.

The basic principles of alignment that apply when standing upright are also utilized in performing massage. The best way to understand correct alignment is to become familiar with the proper position of the skeleton to minimize structural stress. When we consciously develop postural and movement patterns that take advantage of good skeletal alignment, these patterns can become ingrained and automatic.

The complex, precise coordinating actions are carried out almost entirely at an unconscious level. Any attempt to consciously control the muscles may inhibit the nervous system's ability to orchestrate smooth muscle function. Using this principle in mastering massage techniques requires learning the correct position of the body for delivering each stroke, and developing the kinesthetic awareness to sense when the body deviates from this position.

The major principles of good body mechanics have been divided into five questions the therapist can easily memorize and recall when performing massage to quickly assess if he or she is using the body properly.

▶ THE FIVE-QUESTION CHECKLIST

1. Are the centers of my joints aligned?
   - My thumb is comfortably extended, not flexed or hyperextended.
   - My spine is straight, not twisted, from the sacrum to the atlas.
   - When my knee is flexed, it lines up over the second toe of the foot.
   - When my leg is straight, the knee is not hyperextended.
   - The tips of my elbows are pointed outward, not rolled inward.
   - My scapulae are relaxed and dropped, and the humerus is resting comfortably in the shoulder joint.
   - My wrists are in a neutral position, not hyperextended or hyperflexed.
2. Is my body facing the direction of my stroke?
   - My shoulders and hips line up in the same direction.
   - My hands are at about the same level as my navel, and pointed in the direction of my stroke.
   - My legs and feet are moving in the same direction as my upper body.
   - My legs are approximating a parallel position, with my feet at least hip-width apart (imagine standing on skis).

3. Am I moving with my whole body?
   - At the beginning of the stroke, most of my weight is on my back foot.
   - My weight shifts forward as I apply pressure and/or as the stroke travels forward.
   - The force needed to perform the stroke flows upward, from my feet to my hands.
   - The more relaxed I am, the more easily strength can flow through my body.
   - Body movement is fluid and continuous; I am never *locked* in a position.
4. Am I lengthening as I apply pressure?
   - For every action, there is a reaction:
     - As I reach my back foot into the floor, my body lengthens upward.
     - As I reach forward, I lengthen backward.

- My joints feel properly aligned and not compressed.
- My body expands and softens as I apply pressure.
- My shoulders are relaxed, my shoulder girdle wide, and my spine long.
- My muscles feel loose and long, not contracted and tense.
5. Am I breathing from my center?
   - The rhythm for each stroke comes from my breathing pattern.
   - I allow myself to relax and fall forward as I exhale into the stroke.
   - My lower body and upper body come into balance at my pelvis.
   - I breathe all tension out of my body as I work.
   - I yield rather than force.

Therapist Self-Care

Massage therapy is a demanding profession. It requires intense mental concentration and regular physical conditioning. As with any care-giving job, burnout is likely to occur if the therapist does not invest in adequate self-care. People who are constantly giving to others often neglect to take the necessary time to replenish themselves. A few simple practices, if done on a regular basis, will assure that the therapist remains healthy and able to sustain a full-time massage practice:

1. *Exercise Daily.* Daily exercise is a requisite for taking care of the body adequately. Practicing proper body mechanics minimizes stress to the therapist's body, but it is not enough to counteract the compressive forces generated by performing massage therapy. The therapist's muscles and joints need to be lengthened and stretched regularly.

   Tai chi and yoga are both excellent practices that maintain a person's flexibility and strength while reducing the build-up of stress. These systems also encourage deep breathing, which is extremely important for rejuvenating the body and the mind. The self-awareness and mental control that tai chi and yoga foster help the massage therapist to increase his or her capacity to empathize with and stay focused on the client throughout the entire deep tissue therapy process.

2. *Take Time for Daily Reflection.* Daily reflection helps the therapist to remain centered, enthusiastic, and committed while caring for others. There are many different ways to clear the internal clutter that accumulates from intense work involving constant interaction with other people. Activities like walking, gardening, reading, and meditating all have the capacity to provide an outlet for the therapist to unwind and relieve potentially toxic mental and emotional build-up.

3. *Eat Real Food and Drink Water.* Massage therapy is intensive work. It involves constant physical activity, moment-to-moment decision making, and unwavering vitality. In short, being a massage therapist calls on all of one's resources. The body must have adequate reserves of energy through intake of nutritious food and clean water to sustain the level of activity required for this work. Maintaining a well-balanced diet is one of the cornerstones of healthy living.

4. *Receive Bodywork Yourself.* Along with the activities mentioned above, the experience of receiving regular massage therapy keeps the body operating at peak performance levels. It also reminds the therapist what the experience of being a massage recipient is like—and what a profound impact we have on clients when we share our integrated deep tissue therapy skills.

REVIEW QUESTIONS

Level 1

Receive and Respond

1. What is the correct order for the three major steps in designing an integrated deep tissue therapy session?
   a. Implement a plan of action; observe changes; plan the next session
   b. Observe patterns; create a plan of action; implement the plan
   c. Observe patterns; implement a plan of action; assess responses
   d. Observe patterns in tension; observe patterns in fascia; observe patterns in posture

2. Muscles that are used mainly for posture are sometimes called ____ muscles.
   a. tonic
   b. clonic
   c. phasic
   d. aphasic

3. Muscles that are used mainly for movement are sometimes called ___ muscles.
   a. tonic
   b. clonic
   c. phasic
   d. aphasic

4. "Swimming," "thumb gliding," and "shingles" are all varieties of. . .
   a. petrissage.
   b. friction.
   c. vibration.
   d. effleurage.

Level 2

Apply Concepts

1. Which is likely to be the most effective order of events during an integrated deep tissue therapy session?
   a. Stretching, followed by Swedish and cross-fiber techniques, followed by accessory work
   b. Polarity and shiatsu, followed by stretching, followed by deep tissue and neuromuscular therapy
   c. Swedish and cross-fiber techniques, followed by reflexology and polarity, followed by deep tissue and neuromuscular therapy
   d. Connective tissue therapy, followed by deep tissue and neuromuscular therapy, followed by stretching

2. In muscle relationships, tonic muscles often become shortened while associated phasic muscles become stretched and weak. A good example of this relationship is. . .
   a. hamstrings vs. rectus abdominus.
   b. biceps vs. triceps.
   c. pectoralis minor vs. rhomboids.
   d. trapezius vs. erector spinae.

3. The neuromuscular therapy portion of an integrated deep tissue massage session is designed to address. . .
   a. fascial adhesions.
   b. imbalances between short and long muscles.
   c. postsession assessment.
   d. myofascial trigger points and referral areas.

4. This text describes deep tissue massage as. . .
   a. therapy that affects tissues close to the core.
   b. therapy that has a deep impact.
   c. therapy that accesses deeply held emotions.
   d. therapy that affects any tissue deeper than the skin.

Level 3

Problem Solving: Discussion Points

1. During your next bodywork session, apply the five-question checklist to your body mechanics. Describe three areas where you could improve. Discuss these with a classmate, and make a plan for how each of you will focus on those areas, and how you will track progress with each other.

2. Consider the recommendations for therapist self-care that are listed in this chapter. Choose one recommendation that you do not currently follow, and analyze why not: what are the obstacles between you and this particular kind of self-care? Are there things you could do to move closer to following this recommendation? Are you willing to try it for a given length of time? Being as specific as possible, discuss your thoughts with a classmate.

REFERENCES

1. Chek P. *Postural and phasic muscles*. WikiEducator. http://wikieducator .org/Postural_Analysis/Postural_and_phasic_muscles. 2005.
2. Schliep R. *Phasic/tonic muscles*. http://www.somatics.de/artikel /for-professionals/2-article/32-phasic-tonic-muscles

Connective Tissue

Role of Fascia

Connective tissues provide shape, support, strength, and continuity to all the structures contained within the human form. In a sense, it is the connective tissues that hold the body together. They include the bones, cartilage, ligaments, tendons, and fascia. Taken as a whole, the body has more connective tissue than any other type of tissue.

Much of our connective tissue is in the form of fascia. Fascia has many forms and locations. It is often a sheet-like membrane that wraps and interweaves all the muscles in the body, from the individual myofibers (endomysium) to collections of fibers (fascicles) to whole muscles (perimysium) and even muscle groups (epimysium), that are then wrapped in superficial fascia (Fig. 5-1).

Fascia can be thought of as a multilayered, three-dimensional net that encases, permeates, and connects all the soft tissue structures, from just below the skin all the way down to the bones. It even wraps and supports internal organs.

The language to describe fascia is in a state of flux, as research reveals that it is far more complex than previously thought. Most scientists now refer to fascia by its qualities or locations: it can be superficial or deep, organized or disorganized, dense or loose. New technologies in imaging have allowed us to see that even within single fascial structures, multiple layers slide over each other during movement. The discovery of a rich supply of mechanoreceptors in fascia that appear to influence nearby muscle tone has added to our knowledge of how massage therapy and bodywork might achieve results. And the discovery that some fibroblasts can become contractile under certain circumstances (often related to injury) has led

to many more exciting questions about the function of this pervasive tissue. (For a truly life-changing view of connective tissue with collagen fibers, view Dr. Jean-Claude Gimberteau's "Strolling Under the Skin," available on You Tube, here: https://www.youtube.com/watch?v=eW0lvOVKDxE.) Fascia blends so seamlessly into all the types of connective tissue, that anatomists now support speaking of the muscle–fascial interface as a single entity instead of a collection of parts. It is anatomically not possible to separate a muscle sheath from a tendon, or a tendon from the periosteum; they are inextricably linked by way of our three-dimensional fascial web.

Massage therapists often claim to affect muscles, but we cannot think about altering the quality of muscle tissue without also addressing the fascial layers that wrap and permeate it. Muscle fibers actively shorten, or contract, to move bony attachments closer together; they lengthen when their antagonists contract in the opposite direction. Deep tissue massage techniques are designed to reduce the tone in chronically shortened muscle fibers through manual compression and slow stretching. However, a muscle cannot regain its resting length, even when contracted fibers are relaxed, if the surrounding fascial membranes bind it up tight. A constricted fascial casing prevents the muscle fibers from lengthening, and so the muscle, even when relaxed, cannot stretch to its capacity. Techniques that address the unique characteristics of fascia must be applied to fully address the whole myofascial component.

Fascia is composed of three primary constituents: two proteins (**collagen** and **elastin**), a liquid medium, and the

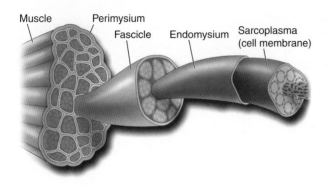

FIGURE 5-1 Every layer of a muscle is surrounded by fascia, from the surface down to the cellular level.

living cells that produce this liquid and fibrous ground substance: fibroblasts. Each of these components contributes a specialized property that gives fascia its diverse characteristics of fluidity, strength, and elasticity.

The liquid medium that suspends the cells and protein fibers is classified as a **mucopolysaccharide**. This medium is a gel, which means it has the capability of moving between a more fluid and a more solid state. The degree of viscosity of this gel is largely dependent on local temperature, movement, and hydration. When the body is in motion it generates heat, which promotes a more fluid state in the fascial medium. Greater fluidity within the fascia promotes freer range of motion, and freer muscle tissue, at least during movement. Exercise helps the body to remain supple, partly as a result of this effect. Lack of movement causes the liquid medium to thicken, which may then inhibit muscular freedom. Possibly because of this phenomenon, the body feels stiffer when a person has been sitting or lying still for long periods. The elements of heat-producing friction, pressure, and stretching used in fascial release techniques replicate natural muscle movements and help to return the fascial medium to a fluid state during treatment sessions.

Within the liquid medium of fascia lie mesh-like layers of collagen, a protein that is composed of long, ropy strands. Collagen can be produced in many versions. "Reticular fibers" are sometimes identified in fascia; these are a subtype of collagen fibers. Other types of collagen are numbered; over 20 different types have been identified so far.

The prevailing collagen fibers found in most healthy fascia are type I fibers. These are extremely strong, with great **tensile** capacity, but very poor rebound: they are strong but not elastic. Adjacent molecular chains of collagen readily link together because of the strong bonding capability of hydrogen, one of collagen's primary components. This creates an extremely durable webbing that can resist stretching even

better than steel wire can.[1] Ligaments and tendons contain a high concentration of dense, linearly arranged collagen, making them very effective in holding the skeleton and muscles together.

Elastin is another protein found within the fascial mesh. Unlike collagen, elastin has great extensibility and rebound capacity, but poor tensile strength. Fascia that is highly invested with elastin is able to stretch, and then return to its original form.

Fascia that wraps around and within skeletal muscle has to be able to stretch, glide, and contain the muscle cells. In some areas—for instance around many superficial muscles—fascia may be loose and stretchy. In other areas, like the lumbodorsal fascia or the compartments of the lower leg, fascia is dense, multilayered, and capable of adding external support to the muscles as they do their work.

Collagen fibers give fascia strength, but they also have a tendency to form chemical bonds with other collagen fibers. When this happens between adjacent surfaces that should move freely, it is called an adhesion. Adhesions can lead to movement and postural problems. In some situations, the external fascial layers of adjacent muscles may adhere to each other, causing the muscles to lose their differentiation of tasks: one cannot move without pulling the other along. As muscles stick together, the body's range of motion is diminished, the risk for injury is increased, and the structure begins to degenerate. Other adhesions can develop between the endomysium wrappings around individual muscle fibers, or in areas where injury or scarring has led to an over-production of sticky collagen.

When connective tissue is healthy and functional, the continuity of the fascial membranes throughout the body provides a medium to absorb and distribute the impact from everyday movements such as walking or jumping, or even from minor trauma like falls, much like the role of shock absorbers in a car. The rich supply of mechanoreceptors that pick up information about gravity, compression, and movement create a powerful feedback loop to maintain optimal muscle tone. For this reason, the quality of a person's fascia and connective tissue in general may be a determining factor in overall health and resilience.

Fascial planes thicken in areas of the body that are under stress as a result of postural misalignment, poor movement mechanics, or injury; this thickening may develop to provide additional bracing. These denser layers or deposits of scar tissue interrupt the flow of mechanical force through the structure, resulting in areas of weakness at the points of discontinuity. The weakened tissues are vulnerable to breakdown, causing degeneration and injury. Re-establishing effective lines of force that flow through the fascia adds immeasurably to the body's overall state of health and vitality by minimizing wear and tear on all tissues.

SESSION IMPRESSION

CONNECTIVE TISSUE CHANGES

The client is a 36-year-old woman named Margaret, who works in sales. She views her job as fairly high stress. She is constantly dealing with people, either in person or on the telephone. Although she exercises regularly, doing stretching and aerobics at least three times a week, she feels unable to relax fully. At times, it is difficult to take a deep breath, because her chest cavity feels muscularly tight and constricted. Her blood pressure is borderline high. Her goal in seeking massage therapy is to be able to relax and reduce the feelings of muscular tension that build up on a daily basis.

On observation, her muscles appear to be well toned. She was athletic in high school, having been on the swimming team, and her body still has an athletic quality. The musculature in her upper trunk and shoulders appears constricted. Her shoulders are medially rotated, with a slight degree of kyphosis in the upper back, and her sternum is depressed, causing her chest to appear somewhat sunken. Her head projects forward, causing the T1 vertebra to be prominent. There is a build-up of connective tissue around the upper thoracic vertebrae. Her pelvis is posteriorly rotated, and she stands with her knees slightly flexed. This postural stance points to short hamstring muscles. Overall, she appears vertically compressed when standing, as if she were carrying a heavy load on her shoulders.

The plan for the initial session was to help relieve the feelings of muscular constriction caused by built-up stress and to open the chest and shoulder region so that she can experience fuller breathing. Future sessions will deal with lengthening the spinal column and bringing the head and pelvis into a better relationship with each other.

Soon after the session began, it became apparent that the client was unable to accept deep, direct pressure to the muscles. The muscles were tight. When moderate pressure was applied, the client reported feeling uncomfortable pain, and her upper body retreated further into its medially rotated stance. The therapist decided that a connective tissue approach was the preferred treatment for this client. The fascial compartments needed to be stretched so that her muscles could lengthen. The client was uncomfortable with firm pressure and did not like sustained pressure to specific areas of soft tissue, even when the contact was light.

Myofascial mobilization and spreading techniques were applied to the pectoralis major, pectoralis minor, and serratus anterior to help expand the chest region and widen space across the shoulder girdle. The fanning stroke was also used in the upper thoracic region to help lift the sternum. Long Swedish strokes, combined with connective tissue spreading, were used on the rest of the body to promote feelings of length and relaxation. Overhead stretching of the arms was used at the end of the session to stretch the chest.

The client reported feeling much lighter at the end of the session. Her breathing felt much fuller without forcing it. Her comment was, "I feel like a burden has been lifted off of me."

Topics for Discussion

1. What are some indications that a connective tissue approach should be the primary course of treatment for a particular client?
2. Explain the reasons for performing connective tissue strokes slowly.
3. What kind of self-care treatment would be most beneficial for a client receiving connective tissue massage?
4. How would you explain to a client why connective tissue strokes feel different from other massage techniques that he or she may have received?
5. Why is connective tissue therapy a useful addition to any other form of massage treatment?

Working with Fascia

Different areas of the body have different capacities for movement and stretch. Part of this depends on a history of injury, patterns of muscle holding, and postural habits, but much of it is related to the density of the fascial structure, and the ratio of collagen to elastin fibers. When the condition of fascia is not optimal, the integrated deep tissue therapist works to restore whatever capacity for freedom of movement might be possible. Working to improve the quality of the fascia requires

BOX 5-1 | Fascial "Release": What Does the Science Say?

What really happens when we sense that fascia softens or releases? This is an interesting question, and it is difficult to answer.

The traditional thinking has suggested that the heat and movement associated with massage or other manual therapies may influence the fluid medium that suspends the cells and protein fibers of fascia to become looser (a thixotropic effect), but research shows that this result only lasts as long as the tissue is directly heated; the fluid medium in connective tissue returns to a gel state almost immediately when heat is removed.[1]

Another possibility is that the mechanical distortion of the fascia stimulates the many proprioceptors located there. Among these are Ruffini receptors, which are especially sensitive to sustained shearing pressure. The response to these mechanoreceptors may cause local capillary dilation, increased passage of fluid into the local area, and a nearby reduction in muscle tone as some motor units stop firing.[2] However, Ruffini nerve endings comprise only a small portion of the many mechanoreceptors located in fascia, so it is probable that the much smaller and more numerous "interstitial" receptors are also involved in any reflex arc activity that impacts CNS signals to motor units. However, this has not yet been demonstrated, so it is only a theory at this point.

Noting that collagen behaves like "liquid crystal", some researchers wondered whether the changes seen in fascia might be due to the production of an electrical charge when fascia is deformed (piezoelectricity).[3] However, this theory has never been rigorously tested, and the significance of any fascial electrical change has never been demonstrated.

Finally, we must consider whether some sense of "release" comes from the reduction of adhesions between fascial layers. Again this is difficult to demonstrate scientifically, so we would not really know until we have imaging technology to show us. Research shows that massage can resolve interperitoneal adhesions after surgery in rats,[4] but human studies have not shown such a clear result. It is safe to say that massage therapy can have a profound effect on certain kinds of scars,[5–7] but whether we are manually separating layers of fascia between or within muscles is difficult to determine.

The power of manual therapy to affect the palpable quality of fascia is clear, but the mechanisms are still being explored. For this reason, we have to be very careful about the language we use: "release of the fascia" may turn out to be an incorrect description of what really happens. As we learn more through research, we gain the tools to become increasingly effective for our clients. This is why it is so important to stay informed about what the science says about muscles, fascia, and massage therapy.

---

sensitivity to the limits of a particular area: tissue is taken to its stretch point, and then patiently held until a sense of softening or lengthening is perceived. Tissue is never forced beyond its capacity to yield.

Because contractile muscle fibers and their fascial membranes are so intricately intertwined, it is physically impossible to touch one without affecting the other. The therapist's intention while manipulating tissues is the key to distinguishing which component of the myofascial unit is being emphasized. Helpful images for sensing softening when working with fascia can include visions of an ice cube slowly melting on a sidewalk, or a flower opening, or butter melting in a frying pan.

As the therapist's hands are placed on the body, pressure is applied only to the point at which resistance is first felt in the muscle tissue. This might be registered as a slight recoil or a feeling of the tissue thickening. The therapist then waits for a softening of the resistance, which allows his or her hands to continue to glide through the tissue until further resistance is encountered. This slow, methodical sensing of the tissue's reaction to the therapist's manipulation assures that the state of the fascia is being affected (see Box 5-1).

Connective Tissue Routine

This description of the connective tissue procedures in this chapter does not include the specific muscles being addressed, because the goal of these strokes is to stretch the fascial membranes that wrap all of the muscles. The therapist's focus

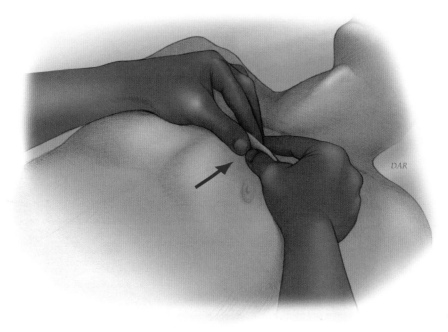

FIGURE 5-2 Lifting and rolling the superficial fascia of the upper chest.

while performing these strokes is on sensing the softening and stretching of the tissues in response to the slow movements of the hands.

The techniques described here are meant to be incorporated into the lessons of the following chapters in the "connective tissue" sections of the protocols. This will allow therapists to provide the benefit of both fascial and muscular softening for their clients.

The body regions are presented here in the same order as they appear in Chapters 6 to 10.

▶ CHEST

Position

- The client is lying supine.
- The therapist is standing at the side of the table.
  1. *Fascial Lift and Roll Technique.* Grasp the skin of the upper chest lightly between your thumb and fingers. Slowly, roll it superiorly toward the clavicle (Fig. 5-2). Cover as much of the chest as you can. When working with female clients, avoid the breast tissue.
  2. *Fanning Strokes on the Upper Chest.* Place the fingers of both hands on the sternum. Sink into the tissues, and spread slowly outward from the midline with a fanning stroke (Fig. 5-3). Repeat the stroke several times, moving in a superior direction toward the clavicles. ▶
  3. *Myofascial Mobilization of the Tissues Over the Ribs.* For female clients, drape the breast area for this section. Beginning at the lower portion of the rib cage, place

your fingers on the lowest ribs, and slide the tissues up and down over the rib (Fig. 5-4). Feel for areas where the tissue either does not move or feels like it is sticking to the rib. Work to free all the tissue. Progress up the rib cage, working over each rib until you reach the clavicle. Repeat on the other side of the chest.
  4. *Compress and Spread the Chest Tissues.* Holding the wrist, abduct the client's arm 90°, and flex it at the elbow. Move the arm into various stretched positions while you compress and spread the stretched myofascial tissues of the chest with the heel of your other hand (Fig. 5-5).

▶ BACK

Position

- The client is lying prone.
- The therapist is standing at the head of the table.
  1. *Myofascial Mobilization of the Back.* With your fingertips or palms, sink into the tissues enough to be able to move the skin without sliding over it. Using a short up-and-down and side-to-side motion, move the skin over the underlying tissues (Fig. 5-6). Work in small sections, and cover the entire back. This procedure can also be performed with a rolled-up towel to move the skin.
  2. *Myofascial Spreading of the Back.* Standing at the side of the table, sink into the tissues with your fingers or knuckles. Glide through the tissues with a spreading

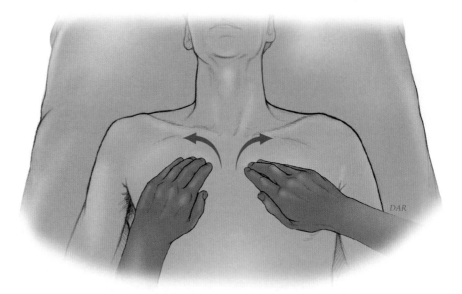

FIGURE 5-3 Fanning stroke on the chest.

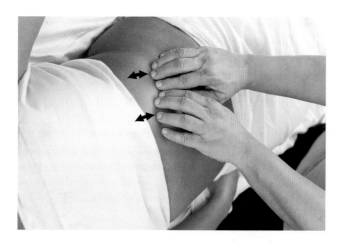

FIGURE 5-4 Myofascial mobilization of the tissues over the ribs.

motion, moving as the fascia softens and pausing at resistance. Begin the stroke at the spine, and move outward in horizontal motions across the back (Fig. 5-7). If using the fingers, work on the opposite side of the client's back from the side of the table where you are standing, and stroke from the spine away from yourself. When using the knuckles, work on the same side of the back, and stroke from the spine toward yourself.

3. *Myofascial Release of the Tissues Over the Bones.* Using a circular friction motion, roll the myofascial tissue over the bones. In the upper back, roll the tissues over the ribs and scapulae. In the lower back, roll against the 12th rib, the lumbar spine, and the iliac crest.

4. *Back Stretch.* Have the client lift up onto his or her hands and knees while under the sheet and then sit back on the heels, resting the chest on the thighs and the forehead on the table in front of the knees to stretch the muscles of the back (Fig. 5-8).

ARM

Position

- The client is lying supine.
- The therapist is standing at the side of the table, next to the client's hand.
  1. *Myofascial Spreading of the Palm.* The client's palm is facing away from the therapist. Using both hands, curve your fingers under the client's hand, pressing your fingertips into the palm. Slowly slide your hands apart, stretching the tissues of the palm (Fig. 5-9). Perform this move very slowly, and pause to allow the fascia to stretch.
  2. *Fascial Lift and Roll Technique.* The client's arm is resting on the table. Place your hands in the skin rolling position, parallel to the muscle fibers, above the client's wrist. Roll and lift the tissues of the forearm, in horizontal strips, from wrist to elbow (Fig. 5-10).
  3. *Myofascial Spreading of the Forearm.* Flex the client's arm at the elbow. Place your hands around the forearm at the wrist, with your fingers sinking into the midline of the palmar side of the forearm using the same hand position as described in move 1. Slowly spread the fingers away from the midline, stretching the tissues

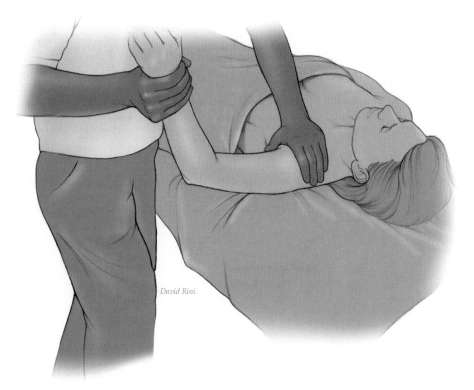

FIGURE 5-5 Compressing and spreading the myofascial tissues of the chest.

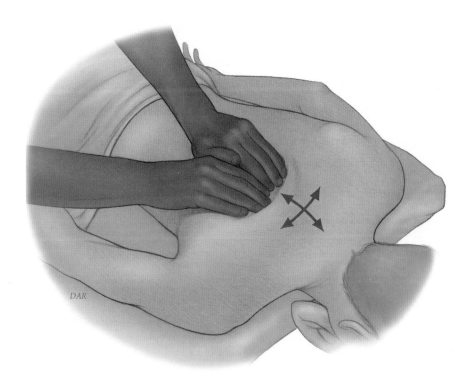

FIGURE 5-6 Myofascial mobilization of the back.

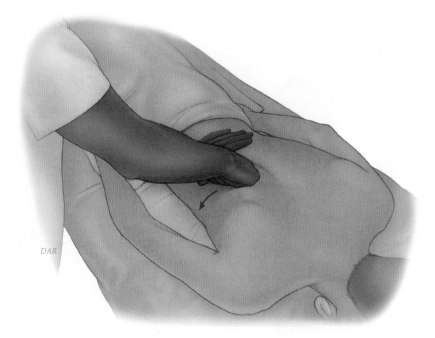

FIGURE 5-7 Myofascial spreading of the back.

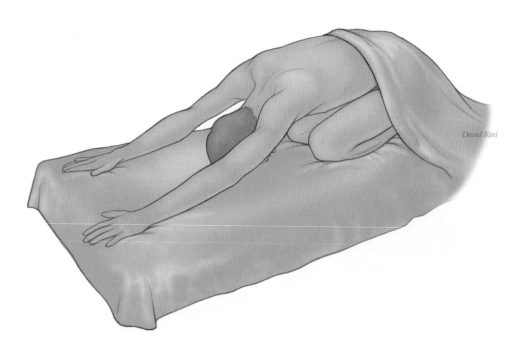

FIGURE 5-8 Back stretch from a kneeling position.

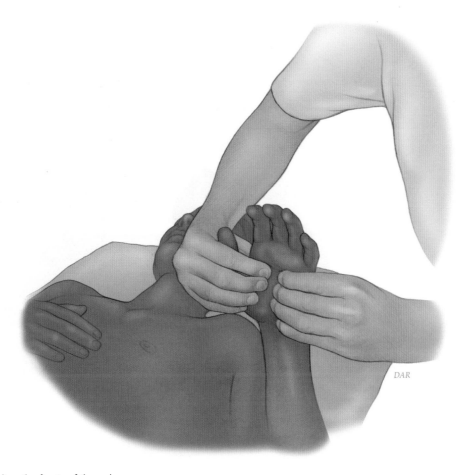

FIGURE 5-9 Spreading the fascia of the palm.

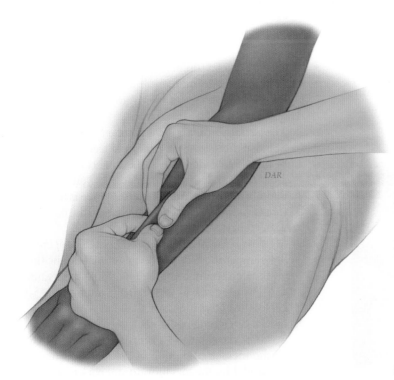

FIGURE 5-10 Lifting and rolling the forearm tissues.

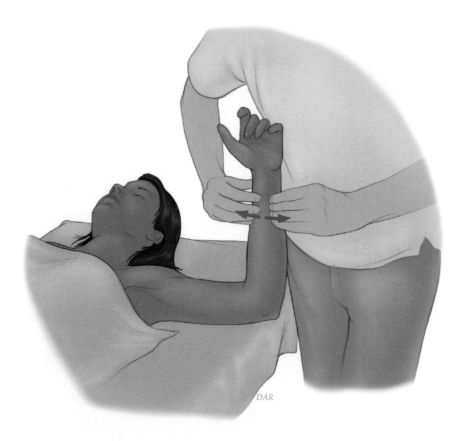

FIGURE 5-11 Myofascial spreading of the forearm.

(Fig. 5-11). Continue, in horizontal strips, to the elbow. Repeat the move on the other side of the forearm. ▶

4. *Myofascial Spreading of the Upper Arm.* The client's arm is lying on the table. Begin the stroke just above the elbow. Using the heels of your hands or the broad side of your thumbs, spread the tissues evenly from the midline out to the edges of the upper arm (Fig. 5-12).

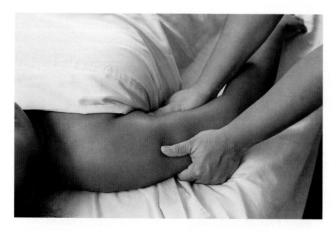

FIGURE 5-12 Myofascial spreading of the upper arm.

▶ FOOT

Position

- The client is lying supine.
- The therapist is standing at the side of the table next to the client's foot and is facing away from the client's head.
  1. *Myofascial Spreading of the Plantar Surface of the Foot.* Stand at the side of the table, and face the dorsal side of the client's foot. Curve the fingers of both hands around the underside of the foot. Sink your fingers into the sole of the foot until mild resistance is felt. Slowly spread your fingers from the midline to the outer edges of the foot (Fig. 5-13).
  2. *Myofascial Mobilization on the Dorsal Side of the Foot.* Standing at the base of the table, place your fingers on the dorsal surface of the foot. Slide the tissues up and down and side to side in small sections (Fig. 5-14). Cover the entire surface of the foot.
  3. Fascial Stretching of the Foot
     a. Grasp the client's toes with one hand while holding the metatarsal portion of the foot with the other hand. Flex the toes forward and back to stretch the foot (Fig. 5-15).

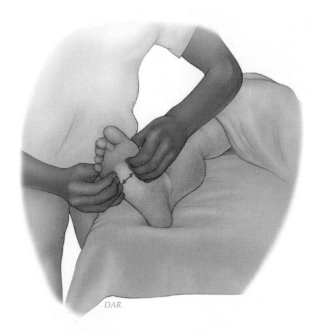

FIGURE 5-13 Myofascial spreading of the plantar surface of the foot.

b. Hold both sides of the client's foot with your hands. Shift the bones of the foot back and forth by alternately moving one hand toward you and the other hand away from you in a continuous motion (Fig. 5-16).

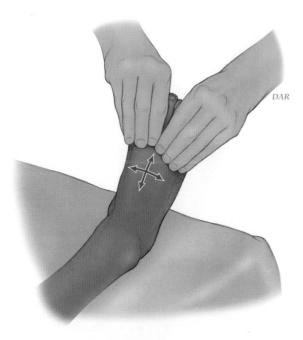

FIGURE 5-14 Myofascial mobilization on the dorsal side of the foot.

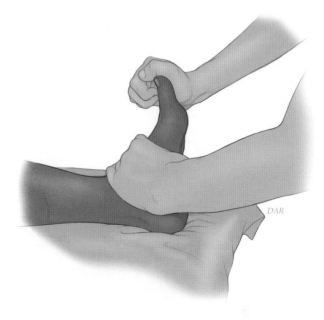

FIGURE 5-15 Fascial stretching of the foot.

▶ LEG

Position

- The client is lying supine.
- The therapist is standing at the side of the table next to the client's ankle.
  1. *Myofascial Spreading of the Leg.* Place the hands around the tibia, with the heels of the hand meeting at the midline of the leg. Slowly spread the hands apart, with pressure against the base of the palms (Fig. 5-17). Begin the sequence at the ankle. Moving in horizontal strips, work your way up the leg to the knee.
  2. *Myofascial Mobilization of the Leg.* Using the fingers or knuckles, roll across the lateral leg muscles until they slide freely over the bone (Fig. 5-18). Begin at the ankle, and work in horizontal strips up to the knee.
  3. *Fascial Stretches for the Leg.* With one hand on the ankle and the other hand on the metatarsal, alternately flex and extend the client's foot. Place one palm on the dorsal surface of the foot and the other palm on the plantar surface of the foot. Invert the foot, and then hold, allowing the myofascial tissues to stretch. Evert the foot, and hold.

▶ CALF

Position

- The client is lying in a prone position.

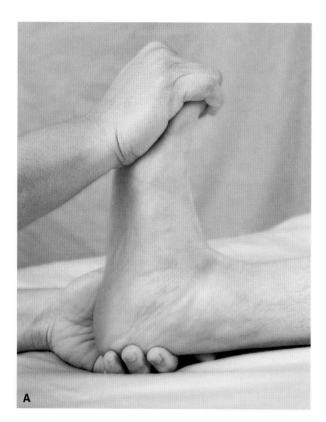

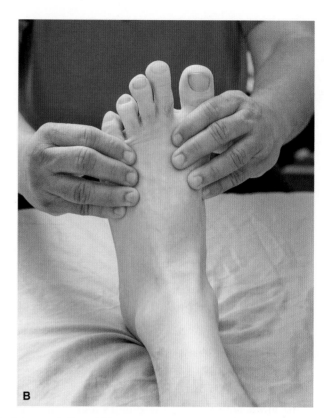

FIGURE 5-16 Position for foot stretch (**A** and **B**).

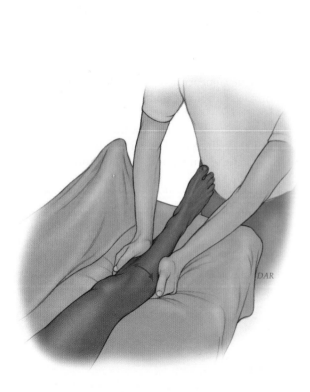

FIGURE 5-17 Myofascial spreading of the leg.

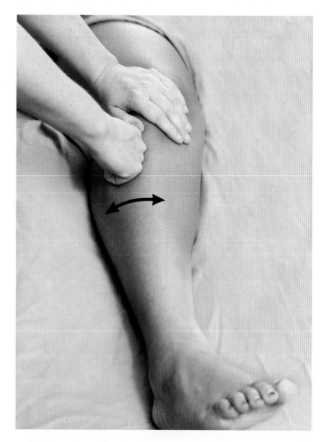

FIGURE 5-18 Myofascial mobilization of the leg.

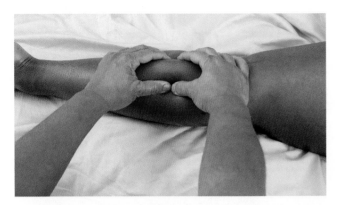

FIGURE 5-19 Lifting and rolling the calf tissues.

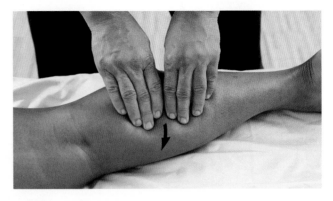

FIGURE 5-20 Myofascial spreading of the calf.

- The therapist is standing at the side of the table next to the client's calf.
  1. *Fascial Lift and Roll Technique.* Lift and roll the skin and muscles of the calf, the gastrocnemius and the soleus, moving in horizontal strips (Fig. 5-19).
  2. *Myofascial Spreading of the Calf.* Placing the heels of the hands on the midline of the calf, spread laterally. Variation—Use the fingertips to spread each side of the calf separately, from the midline laterally (Fig. 5-20).
  3. *Myofascial Mobilization of the Calf.* Using your fingers, roll the muscles against the underlying muscles and bones. Work to release any areas that feel adhered.
  4. *Flex the Knee, Bringing the Leg Perpendicular to the Table.* Dorsiflex the foot, and hold the stretch.

❱ ANTERIOR THIGH

Position

- The client is lying supine.
- The therapist is standing at the side of the table next to the client's knee.
  1. *Fascial Lift and Roll Technique.* Place your hands in the skin rolling position on the thigh, parallel to the muscle fibers. Lift and roll the tissues of the thigh (Fig. 5-21). Move from the knee to the hip, and work in horizontal strips, covering the entire thigh.
  2. *Myofascial Spreading of the Thigh.* Place the hands around the thigh, with the heels of the hand meeting

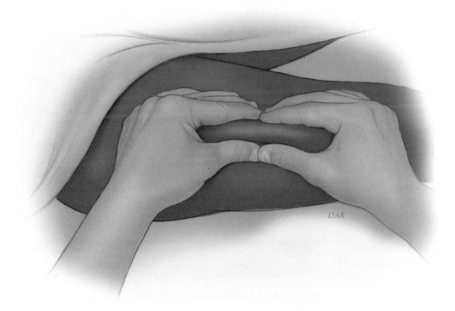

FIGURE 5-21 Lifting and rolling the myofascial tissue of the anterior thigh.

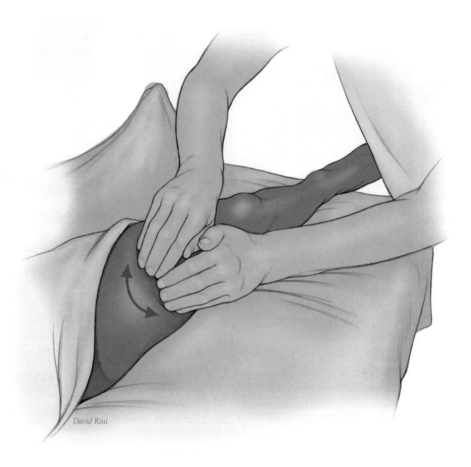

FIGURE 5-22 Myofascial mobilization of the anterior thigh.

David Rini

at the midline. Applying pressure with the base of the palm, slowly slide the hands apart, spreading the tissues of the thigh. Begin the stroke at the knee. Repeat the spreading action in horizontal strips to the hip.

3. *Myofascial Mobilization of the Thigh.* Using the fingers of both hands, roll the muscles of the thigh over the bone until they slide freely (Fig. 5-22).

▶ MEDIAL THIGH

Position

- The client is positioned supine, with the leg to be worked on bent at the knee and turned out, or in side posture, with the top leg flexed 90° and the bottom leg straight. The underneath leg is the one to be massaged.
- The therapist is standing at the side of the table next to the client's knee.
  1. *Myofascial Spreading of the Medial Thigh.* Place the sides of the thumbs next to each other on the midline of the medial thigh. Slowly spread the thumbs apart, stretching the myofascia (Fig. 5-23). Begin the stroke

at the knee. Working in horizontal strips, continue to the groin.

2. *Myofascial Mobilization of the Medial Thigh.* Using your finger pads, roll the muscles against the bones, helping them to slide freely.

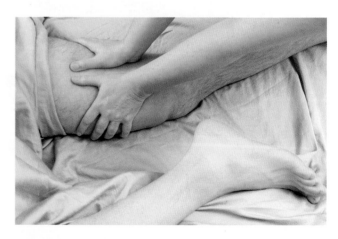

FIGURE 5-23 Myofascial spreading of the medial thigh.

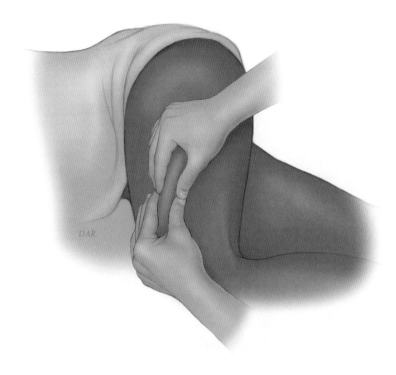

FIGURE 5-24 Lifting and rolling the tissues of the lateral thigh.

▶ LATERAL THIGH

Position

- The client is placed in side posture. The upper leg is flexed, with a bolster under the knee. This is the leg that will be massaged.

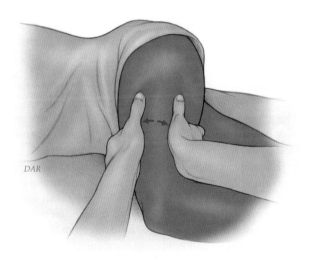

FIGURE 5-25 Myofascial spreading of the lateral thigh.

- The therapist is standing on the front side of the table and is facing the thigh of the client's top leg.
  1. *Fascial Lift and Roll Technique.* Place the hands in the skin rolling position along the lateral thigh, parallel to the muscle fibers. Lift and roll the muscles (Fig. 5-24). Start at the knee, and continue, in horizontal strips, to the hip.
  2. *Myofascial Spreading of the Lateral Thigh.* Place the heels of the hands against the midline of the lateral thigh. Slowly spread the hands apart (Fig. 5-25). Begin the first stroke at the knee. Repeat, in horizontal strips, to the hip.
     Variation—Spread each half of the thigh individually. Place the hands parallel along the midline of the thigh. Using the fingertips, spread from the midline outward. Work in horizontal strips, and continue to the hip. Repeat on the other side.
  3. *Myofascial Mobilization of the Hip.* Standing behind the client, place the forearm across the hip area. Slowly roll the muscles in a back and forward motion (Fig. 5-26). Place the forearm farther back into the gluteal area, and repeat.

▶ POSTERIOR THIGH

Position

- The client is lying prone.
- The therapist is standing at the side of the table next to the client's thigh.

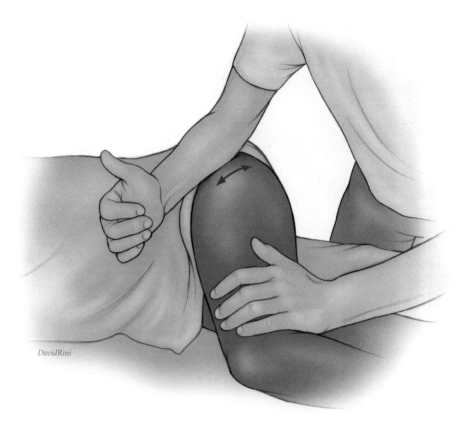

FIGURE 5-26 Myofascial mobilization of the hip.

1. *Fascial Lift and Roll Technique.* Lift and roll the skin and muscles, working parallel to the fibers. Begin the stroke slightly above the knee joint. Move in horizontal strips to the hip.
2. *Myofascial Spreading of the Posterior Thigh.* Use either the heels of the hands or the knuckles. Place your hands on the midline of the thigh, just above the knee. Slowly and evenly spread the hands apart. Move in horizontal strips, from the knee to the hip.

   Variation—Stand at the side of the table, and face the client's thigh. Place the fingertips of both hands on the midline of the thigh. Allow the fingers to sink into the tissues until mild resistance is felt. As the tissues soften, let the fingers slowly slide in a medial direction. Walk around to the other side of the table, and repeat the stroke on the posterior thigh in the opposite direction.
1. *Myofascial Mobilization of the Posterior Thigh.* Using the fingers, roll the muscles of the thigh over each other and against the femur. Work to free the individual muscles from adhering.

▶ POSTERIOR HIP

Position

- The client is lying prone.

- The therapist is standing at the side of the table next to the client's pelvis.
    1. *Fascial Lift and Roll Technique.* Lift and roll the gluteal muscles in a superior direction (Fig. 5-27).
    2. *Myofascial Spreading of the Posterior Thigh.* Using your knuckles or the heels of the hands, spread the tissues from the sacrum to the trochanter (Fig. 5-28).
    3. *Myofascial Mobilization of the Posterior Thigh.* Using your fingers, roll the muscles to re-establish individual action (Fig. 5-29).

▶ ABDOMEN

Position

- The client is lying supine, with a bolster under the knees.
- The therapist is standing at the side of the table and is facing the client's abdomen.
    1. *Fascial Lift and Roll Technique.* Reach across the client's body, and grasp the skin at the waistline between your thumb and fingers. Roll the skin, moving slowly toward the midline (Fig. 5-30). When you encounter tightness or resistance, slowly lift the skin away from the underlying muscle, and hold until a softening is felt. Cover the entire side of the abdomen thoroughly, working in horizontal strips from the side of the trunk to the midline.

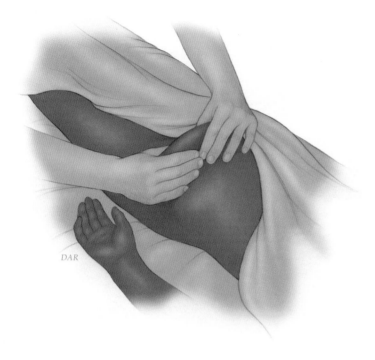

FIGURE 5-27 Lifting and rolling the gluteal tissues.

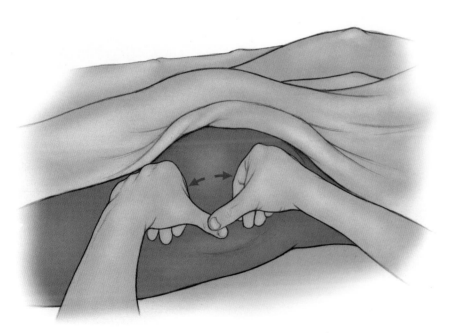

FIGURE 5-28 Myofascial spreading of the gluteal area.

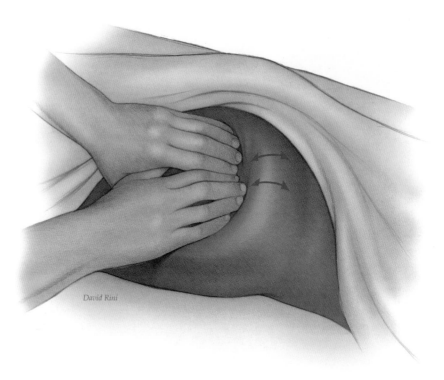

David Rini

FIGURE 5-29 Myofascial mobilization of the gluteal tissues.

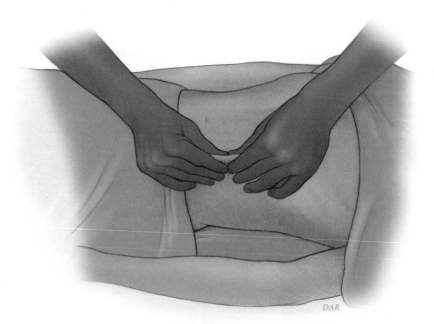

DAR

FIGURE 5-30 Lifting and rolling the abdominal tissue.

Walk around to the other side of the table, and repeat the procedure on the other half of the client's abdomen.

2. *Myofascial Stretch of the Abdomen.* Place the right palm on the abdomen, over the navel area. Place your left palm on top of your right hand. Begin to make a slow, clockwise, spiraling motion, moving the skin over the underlying tissues (Fig. 5-31). Do not glide over the skin. Gradually increase the size of the spiral, stretching the skin and fascia to their maximum degree.

3. *Abdominal Stretch of the Abdomen.* With the client's knees flexed, have him or her stretch both arms overhead and reach fully. Encourage the client to take a deep breath, lifting the chest and pulling the abdomen in while continuing to stretch the arms overhead until a stretch is felt in the abdominal muscles (Fig. 5-32). A useful image to aid this stretch is to tell the client to imagine the navel touching the front of the spine as he or she reaches.

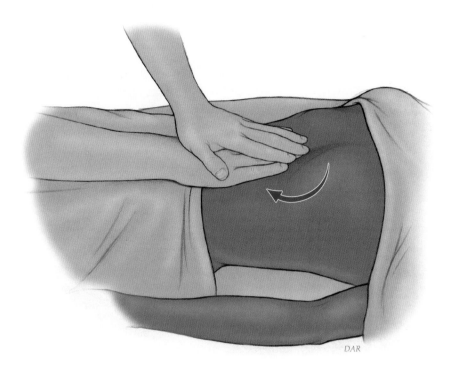

FIGURE 5-31 Myofascial stretching of the abdomen using the palms of the hands.

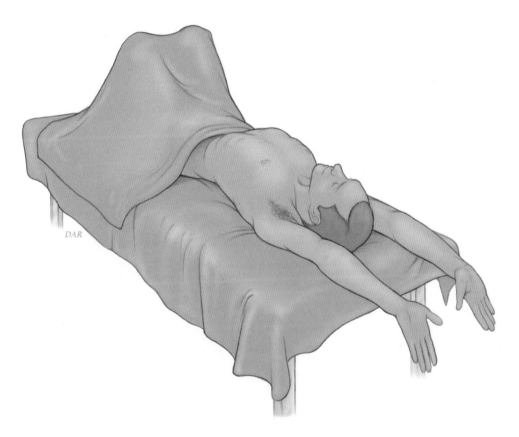

FIGURE 5-32 Abdominal stretch.

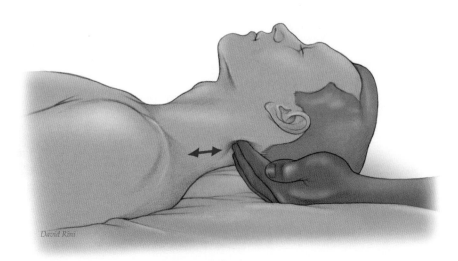

FIGURE 5-33 Longitudinal neck release.

❱ NECK

Position

- The client is lying supine on the table.
- The therapist is sitting at the head of the table.
  1. *Longitudinal Neck Release.* Place the fingers of both hands under the occipital ridge. Allow the fingers to sink into the tissues until a slight resistance is felt.

    Move the tissues of the neck with short up-and-down strokes but without sliding over the skin (Fig. 5-33). Move the fingers down a couple of inches to the next section of the neck, about an inch below the first section, and repeat the up-and-down stroke. Continue with this pattern to the base of the neck.

Return to the occiput, and place the fingers farther away from the midline than on the first pass. Repeat the sequence down the neck.
  2. *Lateral Neck Release.* Place the fingers lengthwise, from underneath, on either side of the spinous processes of the neck. Let the fingers sink into the tissues. Slowly spread them laterally, away from the spine (Fig. 5-34). Slide farther down the neck, and repeat. Continue, spreading in horizontal strips, to the base of the neck.
  3. *Horizontal Neck Release.* Turn the client's head slightly to the side. Using your fingers, sink in along the anterior border of the sternocleidomastoid muscle. Slowly glide the fingers in a posterior direction as far as you can reach (Fig. 5-35). Repeat, in horizontal strips, throughout the length of the neck.

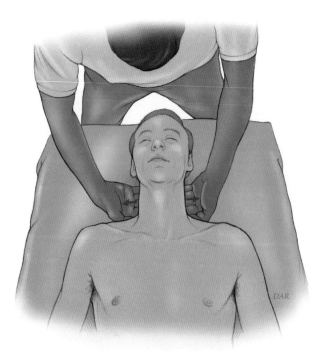

FIGURE 5-34 Lateral neck release.

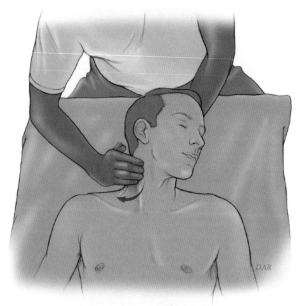

FIGURE 5-35 Horizontal neck release, with the working hand moving posteriorly.

4. *Laterally Flex the Client's Neck.* Place your fingers into the front portion of the trapezius muscle on the flexed side, slightly behind the clavicle. Gradually sink in until mild resistance is felt, and perform the short up-and-down movements with your fingers.
5. Repeat moves 1 through 4 on the other side.

REVIEW QUESTIONS

Level 1

Receive and Respond

1. What is the best description of fascia?
   a. A loose, highly innervated, slightly contractile sheath of tissue that connects the skin to underlying tissues
   b. An interconnected network of connective tissue layers that wraps, supports, separates, and infiltrates tissues throughout the body
   c. A tough, dense membrane that surrounds muscles and muscle groups
   d. An umbrella term for all tissues in the body composed primarily of protein fibers, liquid medium, and invested with few living cells

2. Which statement is most accurate?
   a. Fascia, muscles, and muscle sheaths are inextricably interwoven, and cannot be separated into discrete structures
   b. Fascia is now considered to be a subtype of connective tissue with its own innervation and separate embryologic roots
   c. Fascia is now considered to be an outgrowth of muscle and is no longer discussed as a separate tissue type
   d. Fascia and muscles have been seen to work together to adapt to weight-bearing stress; this means all fascia is contractile material

3. What are the three main constituents of fascia?
   a. Tendons, ligaments, cartilage
   b. Hyaluronic acid, mucopolysaccharides, thixotropic gel
   c. Collagen, elastin, reticular fibers
   d. Protein fibers, liquid matrix, fibroblasts

4. What is an adhesion?
   a. A complication of scar tissue from trauma or overuse
   b. A site of linkage between adjacent collagen fibers
   c. An area where chronic muscle tightness has caused the muscle sheaths to stick together
   d. An area where collagen has overgrown and become sticky

5. Fascia is most heavily invested with what type of sensory neuron?
   a. Thermoreceptors
   b. Mechanoreceptors
   c. Nociceptors
   d. Proprioceptors

Level 2

Apply Concepts

1. Collagen has good tensile strength, but poor elasticity. What does this mean?
   a. Fibers resist stretching and have excellent rebound capacity
   b. Fibers can withstand stress, but they do not rebound well
   c. Fibers are good for wrapping and shock absorption, but not for pulling or stretching
   d. Fibers can rebound well, but they tear easily

2. Fascia is sometimes referred to as a three-dimensional web. How might this concept be applied to a client with persistent knee pain?
   a. His knee pain is a result of dura mater restrictions within the central nervous system
   b. His knee pain will lead to back and hip problems if it is not addressed quickly
   c. His knee pain might be a sign of a history of trauma relating to running away from something frightening
   d. His knee pain may be related to distant fascial restrictions that lead to movement inefficiencies

3. Most of the connective tissue routines described in Chapter 5 follow which sequence?
   a. Fascial lift and roll; joint mobilization; myofascial mobilization
   b. Myofascial spreading; fascial lift and roll; myofascial mobilization
   c. Myofascial mobilization; fascial lift and roll; joint mobilization
   d. Joint mobilization; fascial lift and roll; myofascial release

4. A fascial lift and roll technique is intended to address. . ..
   a. periosteum.
   b. muscle sheaths.
   c. superficial fascia.
   d. epimysium.

5. Myofascial spreading on an extremity is typically done. . .
   a. from proximal to distal.
   b. from lateral to medial.
   c. from medial to lateral.
   d. from inferior to superior.

Level 3

Problem Solving: Discussion Points

1. Read Box 5-1 "Fascial 'Release': What Does the Science Say?" Working with a partner, explain what "fascial release" means to you. What has been your experience of this phenomenon? What is an appropriate way to describe it?

2. Working with a partner, practice the stroke, "myofascial spreading of the plantar surface of the foot." How much pressure do you need to reach the sense of mild resistance? What changes as your fingers move laterally? Analyze these sensations and try to describe them to your partner.

REFERENCES

1. Schleip R. Fascial plasticity—a new neurobiological explanation. *J Bodyw Mov Ther.* 2003;7(1):11–19.
2. Schleip R. Fascial mechanoreceptors and their potential role in deep tissue manipulation. Excerpted from Schleip R 2003: Fascial plasticity—a new neurobiological explanation. *J Bodyw Mov Ther.* 2003;7(1):11–19 and 7(2):104–116. http://www.fasciaresearch.com/images/PDF/Innervation Excerpt.pdf
3. Oschman JL. *Excerpts from publications by James L. Oschman, Ph.D. Readings on the scientific basis of bodywork and movement therapies.* http://www.somatics.de/artikel/for-professionals/2-article/24-excerpts-from-publications-by-james-l-oschman-ph-d
4. Bove GM, Chapelle SL. Visceral mobilization can lyse and prevent peritoneal adhesions in a rat model. *J Bodyw Mov Ther.* 2012;16(1):76–82.
5. McKay E. Assessing the effectiveness of massage therapy for bilateral cleft lip reconstruction scars. *Int J Ther Massage Bodyw.* 2014; 7(2):3–9.
6. Wilk I, Kurpas D, Mroczek B, et al. Application of tensegrity massage to relieve complications after mastectomy—Case Report. *Rehabil Nurs J.* 2015;40(5):294–304.
7. Cho YS, Jeon JH, Hong A, et al. The effect of burn rehabilitation on massage therapy on hypertrophic scar after burn: a random trial. *Burns.* 2014;40(8):1513–1520.

The Lessons

The Fundamentals—Breath and Support

The Chest

▶ GENERAL CONCEPTS

The integrated deep tissue therapy series begins with the chest. Because the overall goal of deep tissue therapy is to bring a person's body to a condition of better balance and function, the logical place to begin is with the breathing mechanism. It is through the breath that the body receives the oxygen that is necessary to carry out its vital processes. The first breath we take marks our entry into this world, and the last breath signals our departure. How we manage all the breaths in between has much to do with determining the quality of the lives we lead.

The movement of the breath in and out establishes a primary rhythm through the body. It represents our general ability to take in and assimilate, and to give out and let go. The smooth flow of breath is also crucial to the bodywork process. During an integrated deep tissue therapy session, the recipient is called on to accept challenges in stretching and pressure, to process change, and to let go of stored tension. If the breath is restricted, this sequence of events is less effective, and the person cannot derive the full benefits of the therapy.

Tension in the muscles of the chest inhibits the movement of the lungs, diminishing the amount of oxygen that is taken into the body. Decreased access to oxygen affects metabolism all the way to the cellular level. With less oxygen available, the body's connective tissues become thickened: a barrier to both cellular-level metabolism, and to larger-level muscular action. Over time, the fascia may constrict our musculature in a way that limits our interaction with our surrounding environment. Through observation and palpation, the integrated deep tissue therapist evaluates the patterns of myofascial constriction that limit full breathing capacity, and then focuses on reducing or eliminating them to allow the unhindered movement of breath.

The benefits of open, full breathing are many. Contributors to guarded breathing and muscle resistance often have to do with the perception of threat. When a person can relinquish patterns of muscle resistance, overall levels of tension in the body may subside. At the same time, reducing muscular resistance in breathing allows more access to oxygen, and more capacity for activity: effort goes down, and energy levels and endurance may be substantially increased.

Free, effortless movement of the breath allows the body to shed carbon dioxide efficiently, and helps to keep the blood pressure normalized. The medulla oblongata, a structure in the brainstem, oversees the size and tone of the blood vessels. If carbon dioxide is high, the medulla elevates blood pressure (perhaps with the intended outcome that blood will be delivered to the lungs more efficiently for the necessary O_2–CO_2 exchange).

The movement of breath presents a clear picture of how mood may be reflected in the physical body, and vice-versa, how a person's physical state can influence mood or perception of threat. The sense of stress or physical threat raises our muscle tone, including in the thoracic cavity. Although we are designed to breathe more deeply when we are under short-term threat (the better to run away from danger), long-term, low-grade stress appears to have the opposite effect as the intercostals become locked, and diaphragm moves more shallowly, and the scalenes must do more work to raise the top ribs. This pattern can become ingrained as proprioceptors interpret it as a normal level of tension. Breathing shallowly and with resistance then reinforces any sensation of fear or threat, and the cycle becomes self-fulfilling, even to the point of hyperventilation and involuntary muscle contractions to consume dangerously high levels of oxygen in the blood.

By contrast, if a person can drop some of that unnecessary tension and mindfully expand the thoracic cavity from the floor (diaphragm), walls (intercostals), and roof (scalenes), the movement of air in and out becomes more effortless. In this situation, instead of reinforcing a sense of dread, breathing can help to create a sense of equilibrium. For this reason, deep breathing techniques are an important aspect of treatment for people with anxiety disorders, chronic pain conditions, and for those with conditions that exacerbate breathing disturbances, like asthma, chronic bronchitis, and emphysema.

▶ MUSCULOSKELETAL ANATOMY AND FUNCTION

The chest, or thoracic cage, is one of the three major weight segments supported by the spine. It consists of 12 pairs of ribs, the 12 thoracic vertebrae, the costal cartilage, and the sternum (Essential Anatomy Box 6-1 and Fig. 6-1). The thoracic portion of the spine is its least moveable segment, providing a stable attachment for the ribs in the back of the body. The ribs join the sternum on the anterior side by means of the costal cartilage. The cylindrical, cage-like design of the chest forms a protective housing for the heart and lungs. Refer to Figure 6-1C for an illustration of the bones of the thorax.

The *pectoralis major* muscle is made up of three overlapping sections that fan across the anterior chest cavity. All three sections attach on the lateral side of the upper humerus, on the lateral side of the bicipital groove. The upper section originates on the medial half of the clavicle and is the most superficial of the three sections. The middle section attaches along the sternum. The lower section, which is also the deepest, attaches to the costal cartilages. The broad, fan-like arrangement of the pectoralis major fibers allows it to act on the arm from numerous angles. This design also distributes force coming from the arm over the entire anterior rib cage, minimizing impact stress to the thorax.

All three sections of pectoralis major contribute to horizontal flexion and internal rotation of the arm. In these actions, it is opposed by the latissimus dorsi, which powerfully extends the arm. Both muscles work together to adduct the arm, internally rotate at the shoulder, and to lift the thorax toward the arm in pull-ups. Chronically contracted pectoralis major muscles are characterized posturally by a collapsed chest, with the arms drawn forward and rolled inward when hanging at the sides of the body. The *subclavius* muscle lies deep to the clavicular section of the pectoralis major. It attaches on the first rib and to a groove on the underside of the clavicle. It fixes the clavicle to the chest wall and depresses it.

Although 46 muscles are involved in the breathing process, the primary breathing muscle is the *diaphragm.* This dome-shaped muscle is connected to the lower ribs, sternum, and lumbar spine in a rim around the body. The bases of the lungs attach to the superior surface of the diaphragm. The diaphragm forms the floor of the chest cavity and the roof of the abdominal cavity. The movement of the diaphragm lowers the floor of the thoracic cavity while other muscles expand the walls and raise the roof. This causes a vacuum, and air rushes in to fill the low-pressure area.

BOX 6-1 ESSENTIAL ANATOMY | **The Chest Routine**

MUSCLES
Pectoralis major
Subclavius
Intercostals
Diaphragm
Serratus posterior superior
Serratus posterior inferior

BONES AND LANDMARKS
Ribs
Sternum
Manubrium
Xiphoid process
Sulcus intertubercularis
Locations of vertebrae T1–T3, T11–L2
Clavicle

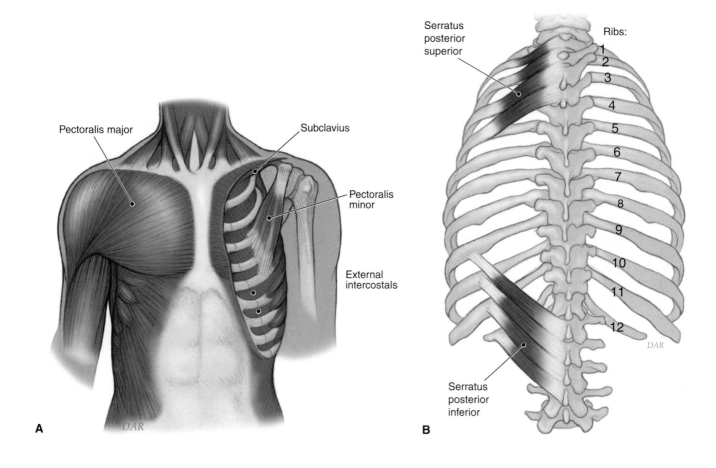

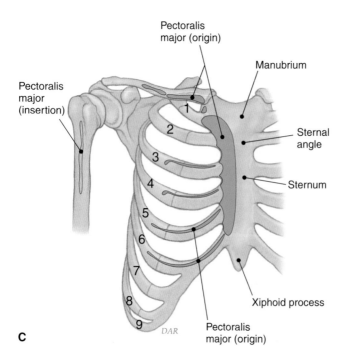

FIGURE 6-1 A. Muscles of the chest. **B.** Posterior breathing muscles. **C.** Muscle attachments on the thorax. **D.** The diaphragm.

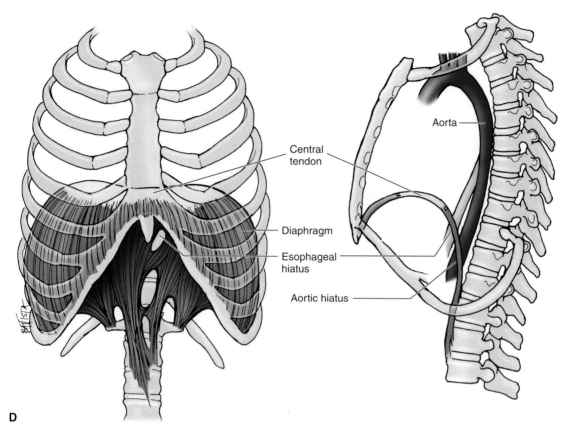

Central
tendon

Aorta

Diaphragm

Esophageal
hiatus

Aortic hiatus

D

FIGURE 6-1 (continued)

The diaphragm has two main portions (Fig. 6-1D). The central tendon, which is noncontractile connective tissue, forms the central roof of the dome and blends with the pericardium. The central tendon helps the diaphragm to maintain its shape parachute-like shape.

Surrounding the central tendon are muscular fibers that are arranged in a radial design like spokes on a wheel. This muscular portion of the diaphragm consists of two sections, the crural part and the costal part. The crural portion forms a muscular extension of the diaphragm that runs in two sections down the anterior surface of the lumbar spine, attaching on the vertebral bodies and discs of L1–L3 and on the aponeurotic arcuate ligament. The crura blend with superior fibers from the psoas, and form a connection for the breathing apparatus between the upper and lower spine.

When the diaphragm contracts during the inhalation phase of breathing, the fibers pull the central tendon downward toward the crura. As the diaphragm descends, the abdominal contents are pushed downward and outward; the phrase, "breathe into your belly" refers to this sense of distension.

The *external intercostal* muscles also contract during inhalation, elevating the ribs—the walls of the thoracic cavity—and causing the lower portion of the rib cage to lift and expand laterally. The intercostal muscles attach to adjacent ribs all the way around the circumference of the rib cage. They are extensions of the abdominal oblique muscles into the chest cavity. The fibers of the external intercostals angle obliquely downward and inward, in the same direction as the external abdominal oblique muscles.

The *serratus posterior superior* works with the external intercostals to expand the ribcage during inhalation. It lies deep to the rhomboids in the upper back. Serratus posterior superior connects the C7–T3 vertebrae and ribs 2–5 at a 45° downward angle. When the serratus posterior superior contracts, it lifts the upper ribs, also expanding the walls of the chest. This muscle can be strained when a person engages in too much forceful, high chest breathing without incorporating the abdominal muscles.

The *scalenes* are the final contributors to inhalation: they pull up on the top ribs, raising the "roof" of the thoracic cavity. They are relatively minor contributors to healthy breathing, however, and they will be addressed in Chapter 10, *Balancing the Upper Pole.*

When inhalation has reached its peak and comes to a pause, those muscles relax and the elastin in the lungs pulls the thoracic cavity back to its original shape. The lungs are compressed, and air rushes out. To take exhalation even further than the normal passive process, the *internal intercostals*

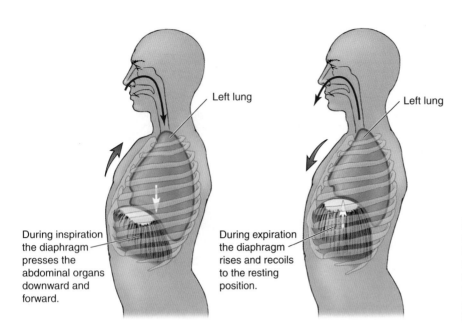

Left lung

Left lung

During inspiration the diaphragm presses the abdominal organs downward and forward.

During expiration the diaphragm rises and recoils to the resting position.

FIGURE 6-2 Mechanics of normal breathing: during inhalation the diaphragm pushes the abdominal contents downward, while the external intercostals, serratus posterior superior, and scalenes lift and expand the ribcage. During exhalation, the diaphragm relaxes and rises, while the ribcage returns to its original shape.

contract, causing the ribs to move downward and inward and assisting in diminishing the size of the lungs. Refer to Figure 6-2 for a visual representation of the breathing process (see Box 6-2 The Mechanics of Breathing).

The *serratus posterior inferior* muscle attaches to the T11 and T12 and the L1 and L2 vertebrae. Its fibers angle upward at about a 45° angle, mirroring the serratus posterior superior, to attach to ribs 8–12. It stabilizes the lower ribs, and it assists in exhalation. Serratus posterior inferior can be strained during lifting, twisting, and reaching actions, such as stretching to grasp an item located on a high shelf. Figure 6-1A and B illustrates the muscles of the chest.

As mentioned previously, many other muscles are involved in the breathing process, assisting in the essential movements and stabilizing muscles and bones. Full, unrestricted breathing is a full-body phenomenon. The breath is experienced as a pressure wave moving throughout the entire body. Watching a small baby breathe demonstrates this effect beautifully. The deep tissue massage therapist should be aware of how the client's body is moving as he or she breathes, and where the breath is inhibited. The restoration of full-body breathing is an important goal of integrated deep tissue therapy.

▶ CHEST ENDANGERMENT SITES

- The xyphoid process is a bony prominence at the inferior end of the sternum. It overhangs the liver, and any sharp, downward pressure at this site may cause a bone fracture and liver damage.
- The floating ribs are not connected to the rest of the rib cage by way of costal cartilage. Careless massage may

create an uncomfortable sensation by pinning soft tissues on the points of the floating ribs (see Fig. 6-3).

BOX 6-2 | **The Mechanics of Breathing**

Breathing is a vital and complex activity that involves not only all the bones and muscles of the chest area but also accessory muscles in the abdomen, shoulder girdle, and neck. These muscles must be free to do the coordinated actions necessary to achieve full breathing with minimal resistance.

The act of inhalation is carried out primarily by the diaphragm, the external intercostal muscles with the serratus posterior superior, and the scalenes. The act of exhalation is mostly a function of the elastin fibers that permeate the lungs: when the inhalation pauses, they recoil and bring the lungs (and the attached walls of the thoracic cavity) back into their original size. Extra exhalation, beyond this passive recoiling mechanism, is a function of the internal intercostals, transversus abdominus and serratus posterior inferior.

The breathing mechanism is so efficient that a healthy person at rest invests only 5% of his or her energy into the act of providing enough oxygen for the needs of every cell in the body. But when we develop resistance in the system through disease or inefficient muscular patterns, then the act of breathing claims a much larger portion of our resting energy.

▶ CONDITIONS

1. *Asthma* is a respiratory disorder that is characterized by episodes of difficulty in breathing accompanied by coughing and a build-up of mucus secretion. Asthma involves permanent inflammation of the bronchial tubes and excess mucus production, and transient attacks are triggered by allergens, strenuous exertion, a sudden change in temperature, or emotional factors. Massage may be beneficial if the client is comfortable; be sure to use hypoallergenic lubricant and avoid any scents or perfumes in the treatment room. Massage therapy may help to expel excess mucus (with tapotement on the thorax), reduce tension in the chest muscles, and reduce stresses that may contribute to attacks.

2. *Chronic obstructive pulmonary disease (COPD)* is a condition in which the lungs are damaged due to genetic predisposition, or long-term exposure to irritants. This condition is often, but not always, related to smoking. COPD has two main components: chronic bronchitis and emphysema. In chronic bronchitis the tiny bronchioles that lead into the alveoli are irritated and filled with mucus. In emphysema, the alveoli are over-inflated. They may fuse together into larger bubbles, called bullae. Emphysema interferes with breathing because these bullae reduce surface area in the lungs, so less

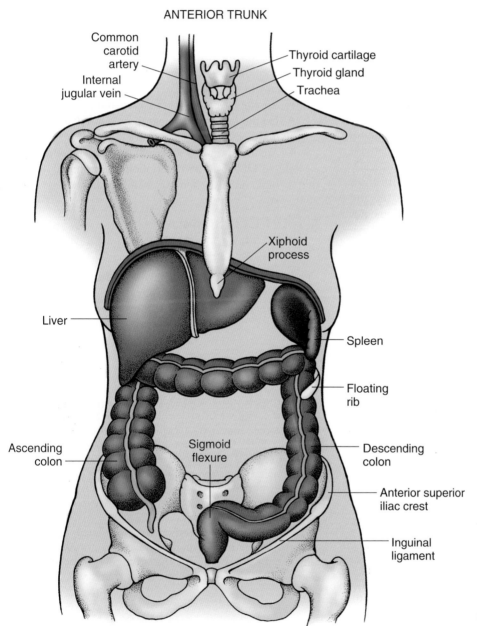

ANTERIOR TRUNK

Common carotid artery
Internal jugular vein
Thyroid cartilage
Thyroid gland
Trachea
Xiphoid process
Liver
Spleen
Floating rib
Ascending colon
Sigmoid flexure
Descending colon
Anterior superior iliac crest
Inguinal ligament

FIGURE 6-3 Endangerment sites of the chest.

oxygen can enter the blood, and less carbon dioxide can leave. Breathing exercises and massage that focuses on reducing resistance in the breathing muscles may be helpful for people with COPD, if the condition is not too advanced.

3. *Acute bronchitis* is an inflammation of the tubes leading from the trachea to the lungs in the upper respiratory tract. It is usually a bacterial infection that arises as a complication of cold or flu. It is typically short in duration, but can be severe. It is accompanied by coughing and heavy mucus production, along with a low-grade fever and constriction behind the sternum. Because it is an infection, it contraindicates massage until the symptoms subside and the patient starts to expel built-up mucus.

4. *Pneumonia* is any infection of the lungs. It can be caused by viruses, bacteria, or other agents. Pneumonia can be contagious, and in some cases it can be life-threatening: it is the leading cause of death by infection in the United States. It contraindicates massage therapy until the patient is in recovery, at which point they may benefit from any work that helps to restore strength and vitality.

5. *Pleurisy* is inflammation of the pleurae, the membranes covering the lungs. It causes the visceral and parietal layers of the pleurae to stick together, which drastically limits movement within the thoracic cavity. It causes difficulty in breathing and sharp pain under the ribs and extending into the abdomen. Pleurisy contraindicates massage therapy until the contributing factors have been resolved.

6. *Rib fractures* are broken bones, and best left alone until the bones have healed. They usually heal easily, but taping is sometimes required.

See Appendix A for more information on these conditions.

POSTURAL EVALUATION

1. Describe the general shape of the chest (see Fig. 6-4A–C).
   - Do the right and left halves match?
   - Are the upper and lower portions symmetric?
2. Check the position of the sternum.
   - Is it lifted?
   - Is it depressed?
3. Observe the position of the ribs.
   - Where do the ribs appear to be squeezed together?
   - Where are the spaces between the ribs expanded?
4. Observe the breathing pattern.
   - Which phase of breath (inhalation or exhalation) is favored, if any?
   - Which portions of the chest appear to move easily with the breath?
   - Which portions of the chest appear to be rigid and not moving with the breath?
5. Look at the region of the diaphragm, at the level of the lower ribs.
   - Are the lower ribs spread apart and pulled up?
   - Do the lower ribs appear to be relaxed and hanging downward?
   - Are the lower ribs squeezed or drawn together?

Refer to Table 6-1 for a description of common distortions of the chest and possible muscles involved.

EXERCISES AND SELF-TREATMENT

1. *Stretch for the Pectoralis Major Muscles.* Stand in a doorway with your arms spread apart and your hands or forearms resting against the sides of the door frame

HOLISTIC VIEW

"I need to get something off my chest"

The chest serves as a container for the heart, and we identify the heart with feeling, especially with our capacity to experience and radiate love. Love is considered to be a warm emotion. It is often associated with fire. We feel the fires of passion burning, or the warm glow of a smoldering ember in our chest when we are in love. When the chest is open, our feeling expands outward to others and is returned to nourish our heart center.

A chest that is tight, closed, and shut off squeezes the heart, and reduces its capacity to produce warm, loving emotions. The fire has died, and we are left with the experience of cold-heartedness: the absence of both happiness and sadness.

When we let go of chronic tightness in the muscles of the chest cavity, we often feel an energizing of the heart-felt emotions. Tears may accompany the reconnection to the capacity for joy, sadness, affection, and intimacy.

The outward, expansive movement of the body that accompanies inhalation represents our capacity to give outwardly of ourselves, to share. The inward, contractive movement of expiration denotes our ability to receive, to surrender, to take in.

Balance of the mind/body system is reflected in a full, integrated breathing rhythm that allows us to shift easily between these two phases. The rib cage and abdomen are mobile, with the ability to change shape and size easily. ■

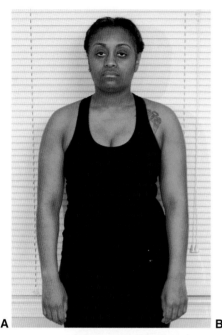 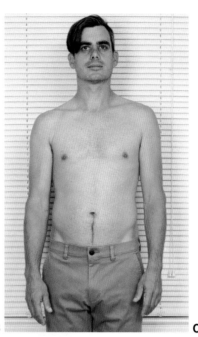 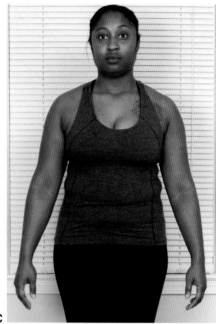

FIGURE 6-4 Postural evaluation: anterior chest.

TABLE 6-1 | Body Reading for the Chest

Postural Patterns	Muscles That May Be Shortened
Overexpanded chest—the sternum is lifted, ribs are expanded, shoulders drawn back	Scalenes External intercostals Rhomboids
Hollow chest—the sternum is depressed, upper ribs are compressed, shoulders are pulled forward	Pectoralis major Pectoralis minor Subclavius Internal intercostals Anterior deltoid Diaphragm Rectus abdominus

(Fig. 6-5). Shifting your weight forward from your pelvis, allow the back to arch slightly and the chest to lift and stretch. Breathe deeply. Positioning the arms higher or lower along the sides of the door frame will alter the muscle fibers being stretched.

2. *Stretch for the Chest and Abdomen.* Lie on your back across a bed with your midthoracic spine on the side edge of the mattress so that your upper body can hang down toward the floor, with the arms extended. Take deep breaths. Alternative surfaces are an exercise ball (Fig. 6-6), the arm of a large couch, or several blankets rolled up tightly into the shape of a cylinder at least 18 inches in diameter and fastened with belts or rope.

3. *Self-Massage for the Contracted Diaphragm and Serratus Posterior Muscles.* Lie on your back on the floor. Place

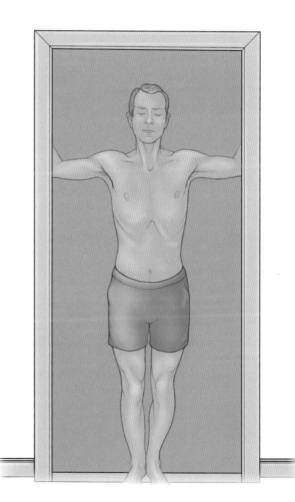

FIGURE 6-5 Using a door frame to stretch the pectoral muscles.

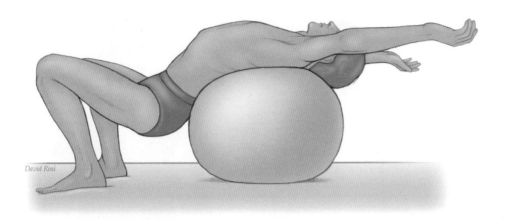

David Rini

FIGURE 6-6 Stretching the chest and abdominal muscles.

two tennis balls on either side of the low back, at the level of the 12th rib. Slowly allow your weight to sink into the balls as you relax, and breathe fully.

❱ CHEST ROUTINE

Objectives

- To restore the chest cavity to its full volume
- To resolve inhibiting factors in the breathing muscles
- To integrate effective breathing patterns
- To realign the shoulders and ribs

Energy

POSITION

- The client is lying supine on the table, with a bolster under the knees.
- The therapist is standing at the side of the table next to the client's chest.

POLARITY

The left palm is placed over the manubrium, and the right palm slides under the back and is positioned between the shoulder blades. Envisioning the smooth, pump-like motion of the lungs, the therapist's hands move in accordance with the rising and sinking of the client's thorax with each breath. The position is held for at least 1 minute, allowing the client time to relax and focus on the breath.

SHIATSU

Moving to the head of the table, the therapist presses the finger pads into the intercostal spaces on both sides of the upper chest simultaneously to stimulate points on the lung, stomach, and kidney channels (Fig. 6-7). The fingers move to different spaces, covering the upper chest

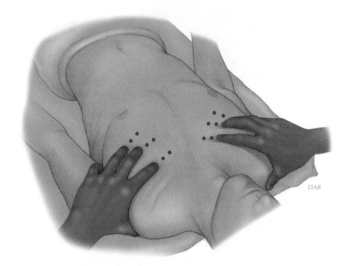

DAR

FIGURE 6-7 Fingertip compressions of the intercostal spaces.

area thoroughly. Each set of fingertip compressions is held for the length of the client's exhalation and is released as the client inhales.

Swedish/Cross-Fiber Massage

1. *Shingles Stroke on the Pectoralis Major Muscles.* The therapist stands on the side of the table at the client's shoulder level. One hand is placed on the opposite side of the upper chest from the side on which the therapist is standing, with the heel of the hand against the sternum and the fingers facing the client's shoulder. Perform short, alternate strokes with the palms across the chest to the client's shoulder. Repeat several times.
2. *Petrissage Strokes on the Pectoralis Major Muscles.* Each side of the chest may be worked individually, or both sides may be worked simultaneously.
3. *Fingertip Raking Across the Upper Chest Muscles.* Slide the fingers in both directions perpendicular to the direction

of the pectoralis major muscle. Avoid the breast tissue when working on a woman.

Connective Tissue Therapy

Perform the fanning stroke on the upper portion of the chest. Begin with the sides of the thumbs touching each other. The tips of the fingers of both hands may be used as an alternative to the thumbs. Slowly spread them apart, stretching the tissues. Keep the strokes small, spreading the thumbs or fingers 2 or 3 inches apart with each stroke.

Start at the midline of the chest over the sternum, just above the level of the breasts. The fanning strokes move upward toward the clavicles. Repeat the stroke a number of times, covering the entire upper segment of the chest. The intention is to free the fascia of the upper thorax, creating a sense of lift in the chest.

Deep Tissue/Neuromuscular Therapy

SEQUENCE

1. Pectoralis major (attachments and belly)
2. Subclavius
3. Intercostal muscles (from supine and side position) ▶
4. Diaphragm ▶
5. Back muscles (serratus posterior superior and inferior)

⊙ It is likely that the chest muscles will be restricted in many areas, because the breathing mechanism is compromised in the majority of the adult population as a result of stress and the lack of encouragement of full expression of feeling and sensation. The reductions of trigger points not only assist in opening up the breathing but also are instrumental in rebalancing the shoulder girdle and freeing the ribs.

SESSION IMPRESSION

THE CHEST

The client is a 10-year-old boy named Joey, who has asthma. He has been picked on in school because of his small stature, and because he cannot participate fully in sports activities. His mother wants him to receive integrated deep tissue therapy to help alleviate the condition and possibly boost his self-esteem.

Postural evaluation of Joey reveals that his chest area is severely constricted. There are noticeable hollow areas under the clavicles and along the borders of the anterior deltoids, indicating that the pectoralis minor muscles are extremely contracted. The central sternal region of the chest is lifted, but in a strained manner. This position of the chest may also partly be a consequence of struggling to breathe during asthma attacks.

The focus of the session was to relieve tension in the chest and ease restrictions in the breathing muscles. Because Joey was a minor, his mother sat in on the session. Based on observation and the information gathered about his asthmatic condition, the areas chosen to focus on included the pectoralis major and minor, subclavius, scalenes, intercostals, and diaphragm. A connective tissue approach to these muscles was mandated because of the child's sensitivity to touch in the chest area.

Joey responded well to the front to back polarity contact on his sternum and upper back. He visibly relaxed, and his breath deepened. Swedish massage strokes were used to warm up the muscles thoroughly before the deep tissue/connective tissue strokes were applied. The integrated deep tissue protocol was followed, but with full attention given to sensing a melting of the tissues before applying any further pressure or moving through the muscle fibers.

The chest muscles were addressed in layers, from superficial to deep. Many trigger points were encountered in the intercostal muscles. As a trigger point was pressed, Joey was encouraged to breathe deeply and imagine the point melting. He enjoyed participating in the process and felt a sense of accomplishment when the uncomfortable feelings generated by the trigger points dissolved. The diaphragm was contacted and massaged very carefully.

The session was concluded with long, Swedish strokes along the erector spinae and with fingertip raking into the intercostal spaces between the ribs in the back to balance the work performed on the front of the chest cavity. After the session, Joey's mood was much lighter. He was thrilled to be able to take fuller breaths without struggling, and he commented to his mother how much broader his chest and shoulders felt. He was extremely proud of himself. Joey was shown the door frame stretches for the chest muscles, and it was suggested that he practice them every day to maintain the newfound length in his pectoralis major and minor muscles. ∎

Topics for Discussion

1. Give at least three reasons for beginning a series of deep tissue sessions with chest work.
2. Describe several possible manifestations of chest constriction along with the muscles involved.
3. What precautions should be taken when performing deep tissue therapy on the diaphragm muscle?
4. How might restricted breathing patterns be revealed by observing a client's thorax?
5. Where are the most likely areas for trigger points to form in the thoracic region, and why?

Pectoralis Major (Attachments and Belly)

Origin:
 Clavicular—medial half of the clavicle.
 Sternal—sternum to the seventh rib, cartilages of upper six ribs.
Insertion: Lateral lip of the bicipital groove of the humerus.
Action: Adduction of shoulder. Medial rotation of shoulder.
 Clavicular—shoulder flexion, medial rotation of shoulder, horizontal adduction of humerus.
 Sternal—adduction of humerus diagonally downward, anterior shoulder stabilizer.

Pectoralis Major (Origin)

Strokes

- Elongation stroke on the sternum, just lateral to the midline, from the xiphoid process to the manubrium, using the fingers or the thumb (Fig. 6-8).
- Elongation stroke along the inferior border of the medial half of the clavicle, using the fingers or the thumb. Move medial to lateral. Feel for small knots and stringy fibers. If they are tender or refer pain, work on them with cross-fiber strokes and direct compression.

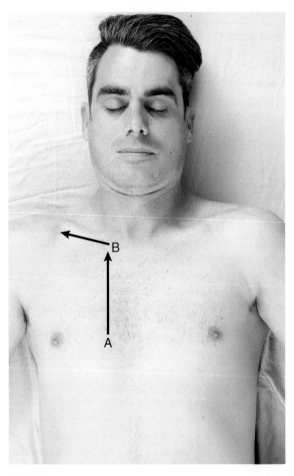

FIGURE 6-8 Directions of elongation strokes on the sternal and clavicular attachments of the pectoralis major.

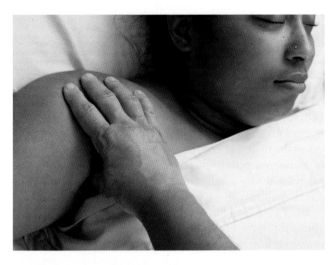

FIGURE 6-9 Contacting the attachment of the pectoralis major on the lateral lip of the bicipital groove of the humerus.

- Insertion of the pectoralis major. Perform the side-to-side stroke and static compression with the fingers on the lateral lip of the bicipital groove of the humerus (Fig. 6-9). To locate it, take the client's arm to an abducted position. Slide your fingers along the border of the pectoralis major and the anterior deltoid to reach the point of attachment on the humerus. It is superior to the deltoid tuberosity on the lateral lip of the bicipital groove. Check for trigger points. If any are found, pause there for several seconds while checking with the client about the level of pain reduction.

Pectoralis Major (Belly)

The pectoralis major muscle has three major segments. They are named after their sites of origin: clavicular, sternal, and costal. Trigger points in the upper or clavicular portion may be found along the lateral border, underneath the edge of the anterior deltoid muscle. They refer pain throughout the anterior deltoid and into the area of the pectoralis major near the trigger point.

Trigger points in the sternal section tend to accumulate in the medial and lateral portions between ribs 3, 4, and 5, near the insertion points of pectoralis minor. Check along the inferior border of the costal section of the muscle for trigger points. The pain pattern is into the front of the chest and down the arm.

Trigger points in the lower section of the muscle tend to form along the lateral border. They refer pain into the breast and nipple.

Heavy lifting, prolonged holding of the arms in an abducted position, and postural changes related to emotional stress may all contribute to the formation of trigger points in this muscle.

Strokes
- The client's arm is still in the abducted position. Using your knuckles, perform the elongation stroke from the sternum to the insertion on the humerus in several strips (Fig. 6-10). Begin the first strip just inferior to the clavicle. Begin the last strip across the muscle at the xiphoid process.
- With a female client, the knuckle stroke should only be done on the upper chest, superior to the breast tissue. At the level of the breast, stroke outward, using the fingers or thumb, from the sternum to the medial border of the breast.

Subclavius (Fig. 6-11)

Origin: Upper border of the first rib.
Insertion: Groove on the inferior surface of the clavicle.
Action: Depresses and moves the clavicle forward. Stabilizes the clavicle during shoulder movements.

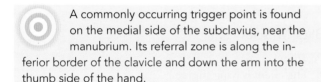 A commonly occurring trigger point is found on the medial side of the subclavius, near the manubrium. Its referral zone is along the inferior border of the clavicle and down the arm into the thumb side of the hand.

Strokes
- Stand at the side of the table, and face the inferior border of the client's clavicle. The client's arm is flexed at 90°. Hold it slightly inferior to the elbow. Drawing the clavicle slightly away from the chest wall for easier access to the subclavius muscle, traction the arm toward the ceiling.
- Using the pads of the index and middle fingers or the pad of the thumb, stroke under the inferior border of the clavicle from the medial to the lateral end.

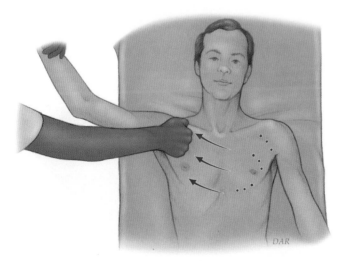

FIGURE 6-10 Elongation stroke on the clavicular, sternal, and costal sections of the pectoralis major.

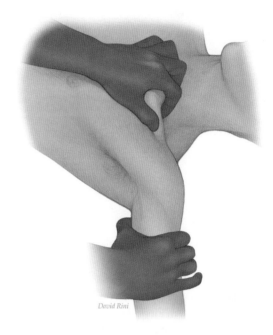

David Rini

FIGURE 6-11 Accessing the subclavius.

Intercostal Muscles

Origin:
   External—from the lower border of each of the upper 11 ribs.
   Internal—from the cartilages to the angles of the upper 11 ribs.
Insertion:
   External—superior border of the rib below the origin.
   Internal—superior border of the rib below the origin.
Action:
   External—elevation of ribs during inspiration.
   Internal—depression of ribs during exhalation.

Intercostals (Supine Position)

Trigger points are likely to be found in concentration along the borders of the ribs where the intercostal muscles attach. Contracted muscles related to inhibited breathing are the probable cause of their formation.

Strokes
- Begin at the base of the rib cage, in the rib space between the 10th and 9th ribs. Place your fingers between the two ribs. Allow the fingers to sink into the tissues until resistance is met (Fig. 6-12).
- Perform a short, side-to-side stroke, feeling for deviations in the tissues (i.e., stringy fibers, tiny knots). Hold with static compression on tender points until pain diminishes. The thumbs may be used instead of the fingers if more pressure is required.
- Continue with this procedure, working between each pair of ribs, to the clavicle. Be thorough.

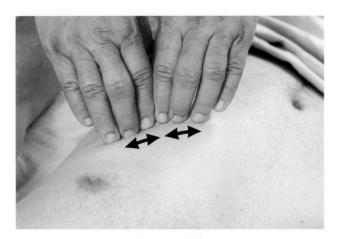

FIGURE 6-12 Working with the intercostals.

Intercostals (Side Posture)

Position

- The client is put in side posture, with the knees flexed and a pillow placed between them. The top arm is positioned in front of the client, allowing access to the side of the chest. A pillow may be placed under the side of the head for comfort.
- The therapist stands behind the client.

Strokes

- Perform fanning strokes with the fingers or heels of the hand in a superior direction on the side of the chest, from the base of the rib cage to the axilla, to soften the superficial fascia and prepare the tissues for deeper work.
- Find the space between ribs 10 and 9 (Fig. 6-13). Sink the fingers into the tissues until resistance is met, and begin short, side-to-side strokes, working the intercostals in sections. Continue, working in each rib space, to the top of the axilla to reach the spaces between the upper ribs.

Diaphragm

Origin:
  Sternal part—inner surface of the xiphoid process. Costal part—inner surfaces of the cartilages of ribs 7–12.
  Lumbar part—L1–L3 vertebrae.
Insertion: Central tendon.
Action: Increases volume of the thoracic cavity during inhalation by drawing the central tendon down.

> ◎ An active trigger point along the diaphragm attachment on the underside of the costal cartilage may be found approximately 1-inch lateral to the xiphoid process.

Position

- The client is placed back in a supine position with a bolster under the knees.
- The therapist is standing at the side of the table facing the client's rib cage.

Strokes

- With the palm supinated, slide your fingers under the border of the costal cartilage of ribs 7–10, just lateral to the xiphoid process. The finger pads must stay in contact with the underside of the costal cartilage to avoid pressing into the underlying organs. Take time to let the fingers sink into the tissues (Fig. 6-14).

> ⚠ Avoid pressing directly on the xyphoid process, because it is not well supported.

- Do short, side-to-side motions with your fingers, feeling for tightness and trigger point activity. Move laterally along the border. Place the palm of your nonworking hand over the lower ribs to give additional support to the upward pressure of your working hand.
- Work with the client's breath. On the exhalation, sink into the tissues with your fingers until resistance is felt. On the inhalation, allow the client's abdomen to push your fingers out from under the ribs.

Back Muscles

Position

- The client is lying supine.
- The therapist is standing or sitting at the side of the table.

Serratus Posterior Superior

Origin: Spinous processes of the C7 and the T1–T3 vertebrae. Ligamentum nuchae.
Insertion: Upper borders of ribs 2–5, just lateral to their angles.
Action: Elevates upper ribs. Possible assistance in inspiration.

> ◎ This muscle may house a trigger point just medial to the superior angle of the scapula. It is a common cause of shoulder pain. The pain is felt deep, under the upper portion of the scapula. It can also extend over the posterior deltoid and down the triceps.

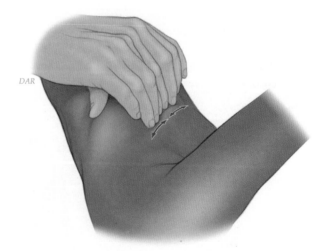

FIGURE 6-13 Working with the intercostals from side-lying position.

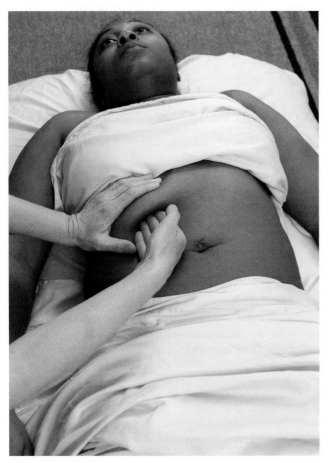

FIGURE 6-14 Working with the diaphragm.

Strokes

- Slide your hands under the client's back at the level of the upper thoracic spine (T1–T3). Beginning at the spinous processes, perform short back and forth motions with your finger pads moving toward the vertebral border of the scapula.
- Hold static compression over sensitive points as the client breathes deeply.
- As an alternative move, use the knuckles instead of the fingers.

Serratus Posterior Inferior

Origin: Spinous processes of T11–T12 and L1–L2 vertebrae.

Insertion: Inferior borders of ribs 9–12, lateral to their angles.

Action: Depresses lower ribs and moves them dorsally. Possible assistance in expiration.

> To locate trigger points, examine the serratus posterior inferior's attachments along the inferior borders of ribs 9–12. The pain pattern is throughout the muscle itself and over the lower ribs.

Strokes

- Slide your hands under the client's back at the level of the lower thoracic and upper lumbar vertebrae (T11–T12 and L1–L2). (If the client is too large or heavy to slide your hands under his or her trunk effectively, you may position the client in side posture to address the serratus posterior superior and inferior muscles.) Beginning at the spinous processes, perform short back and forth motions with your finger pads in a diagonally upward direction, toward the muscle's insertion on the inferior borders of ribs 9–12 (Fig. 6-15).

> ⚠ When performing the strokes on ribs 11 and 12, be careful to contact only the inferior edge of the ribs. Do not press down on the body of the ribs, because they have little support underneath them.

- Hold with static compression over sensitive points as the client breathes deeply.
- As an alternative procedure, use the knuckles instead of the fingers.

STRETCH

1. The therapist stands at the head of the table. The client extends his or her arms overhead toward the therapist. Take hold of the client's arms slightly superior to the elbow joints. Pull the arms toward you and slightly downward while the client takes full breaths, focusing on expanding the chest (Fig. 6-16).

2. The client turns onto his or her side, with the knees flexed. The client's straightened superior arm reaches behind him. The therapist stands behind the client's

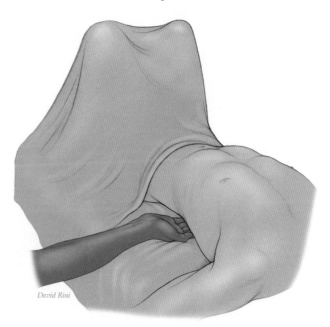

David Rini

FIGURE 6-15 Accessing the serratus posterior inferior along ribs 9-12.

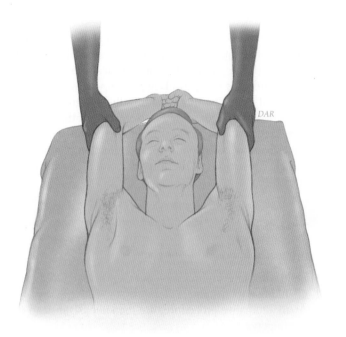

FIGURE 6-16 Thoracic stretch with the client supine.

shoulder. Hold the extended arm, and slowly increase the stretch while your fist is placed against the client's scapula to prevent the client from rolling backward too far (Fig. 6-17). This position stretches the pectoralis major muscle.

ACCESSORY WORK

1. Perform an elongation stroke on the erector spinae and paraspinal muscles. Using the forearm, begin the stroke between the scapula and spinous processes on one side of the back. The forearm is parallel to the spine until you clear the inferior angle of the scapula. Then, it is rotated perpendicular to the spine to make contact with a broader section of the back. Continue the stroke to the iliac crest of the pelvis (Fig. 6-18). Repeat on the other side of the back. Press points along the inferior border of the 12th rib, which is near the attachment of the diaphragm muscle (Fig. 6-19). Both sides may be palpated simultaneously. Begin with the thumbs on either side of T12, and move them apart laterally.

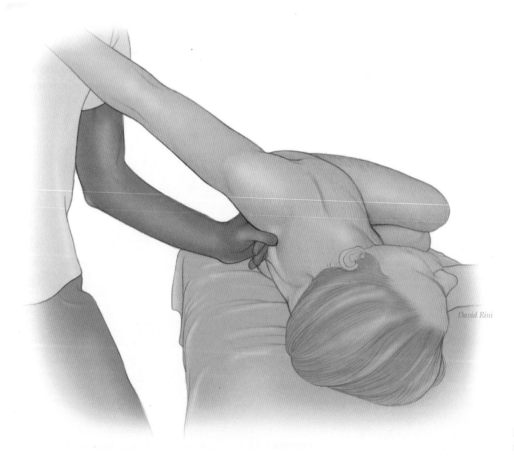

FIGURE 6-17 Pectoralis major stretch from side-lying position.

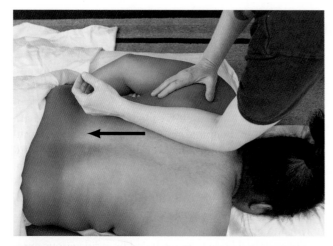

FIGURE 6-18 Elongation stroke for the erector spinae muscles.

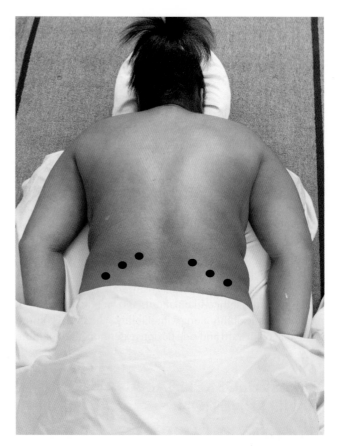

FIGURE 6-19 Pressure points for the diaphragm.

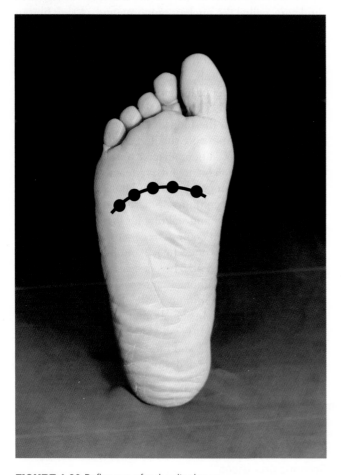

FIGURE 6-20 Reflex zone for the diaphragm.

2. Concentrate on diaphragm reflex points on the foot (Fig. 6-20). Press points along the diaphragm line on the plantar surface of the foot, moving medial to lateral. The line is located slightly inferior to the metatarsal bones, and it runs all the way across the surface of the foot. It is easy to distinguish, because the color of the skin is darker above the diaphragm line and lighter below it.

CLOSING

Sitting at the foot of the table, lightly hold the heels of the client's feet in your hands for 30 to 60 seconds. Remove your hands slowly.

The Back and Spine

▶ GENERAL CONCEPTS

The spine acts as the primary support structure for the entire body. Functional alignment of the spine is essential so that it can carry the three major weights that are connected to it (the head, rib cage, and pelvis) without adding unnecessary stress in the muscles of the trunk. A poised, balanced spine results in the effortless elongation of the trunk that is associated with healthy posture. The muscles attached to the spine must be free of restrictions so they can achieve the equalization of forces along the spinal column that allows a balanced relationship between its components. This is the next goal in the integrated deep tissue series.

The spine is constructed so that many muscles and ligaments attach to it in a lattice-like pattern, allowing a great deal of mobility and flexibility along with stability. The spinal column is capable of forward and side flexion, extension, and rotation.

▶ MUSCULOSKELETAL ANATOMY AND FUNCTION

Spinal Column

The spinal column consists of 33 bones: 7 cervical vertebrae, 12 thoracic vertebrae, 5 lumbar vertebrae, and at birth, 5 modified sacral vertebrae and 4 small vertebral remnants forming the coccyx. The bones of both the sacrum and the coccyx fuse later in life, leaving 24 functional vertebrae in the adult. Twenty-three intervertebral discs are sandwiched between the vertebral bones (Essential Anatomy Box 6-3 and Fig. 6-21).

All vertebrae except C1 are composed of two parts: a rounded body on the anterior side, and a posterior segment, called the vertebral arch. The vertebral arch is a complex structure with several landmarks. The spinous and transverse processes are on the vertebral arch; these provide attachment sites for many muscles and ligaments. The opening between the vertebral body and arch is called the vertebral foramen. Lined up within the spinal column, the foramen form a tunnel, called the vertebral canal, within which the spinal cord is located. See Figure 6-21A for an illustration of a vertebra.

Stacked vertebrae also create bilateral holes on the horizontal plane. These are called the intervertebral foramina, and they allow the spinal nerves to exit the central nervous system and become part of the peripheral nervous system.

The vertebral bodies are separated by cartilaginous discs. The two components of the disc are a central, compressed fluid core, called the nucleus pulposus, and a tough fibrous covering, called the annulus fibrosus. The discs act as cushions, helping to transfer weight evenly between the vertebrae, and absorbing the shock of the vertical and shearing pressures that occur when we walk, run, bounce, and twist. The discs in the lumbar and cervical segments of the spine are thicker in relation to the height of the vertebrae, allowing greater movement between the individual vertebrae, but the discs in the thoracic segment are smaller, decreasing the amount of possible motion. When adjacent vertebrae are properly aligned, compression on the intervertebral disc is distributed evenly, allowing a smooth downward transfer of weight.

One of the spinal column's primary functions is to provide an anchor of support and stability for the cranium, thorax, and pelvis. The spinal column has a series of four opposing curves that offset the uneven size and placement of these three weights (Fig. 6-22). The cervical and lumbar curves are concave, while the thoracic and sacral curves are convex. This design creates continuity of weight transfer and shock absorption throughout the spinal column. The vertebral joints where the curves change (C7–T1, T12–L1, and L5–S1) bear the greatest weight load, and must be in best alignment for the spine to be an integrated, stress-free unit.

BOX 6-3 ESSENTIAL ANATOMY | **The Back/Spinal Column Routine**

MUSCLES	BONES AND LANDMARKS
Trapezius	Vertebral column
Latissimus dorsi	Spinous processes
Erector spinae	Transverse processes
Rhomboid minor	Lamina groove
Rhomboid major	Scapula
Intercostals	Ribs
Quadratus lumborum	Iliac crest
Sacral ligaments	Sacrum
	Coccyx

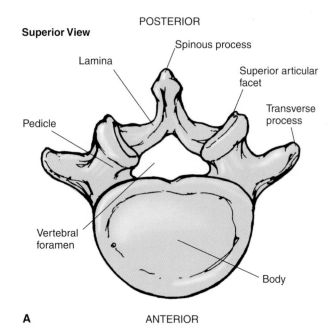

Superior View

POSTERIOR

Spinous process

Lamina

Superior articular facet

Pedicle

Transverse process

Vertebral foramen

Body

A

ANTERIOR

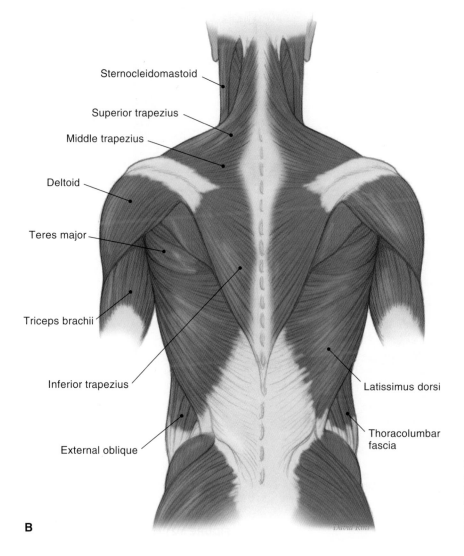

Sternocleidomastoid

Superior trapezius

Middle trapezius

Deltoid

Teres major

Triceps brachii

Inferior trapezius

External oblique

Latissimus dorsi

Thoracolumbar fascia

B

FIGURE 6-21 A. Superior view of lumbar vertebra. **B.** Superficial muscles of the back with areas of possible trigger point formation. **C.** Middle layer of back muscles. **D.** Deep layer of back muscles. **E.** Sacral ligaments.

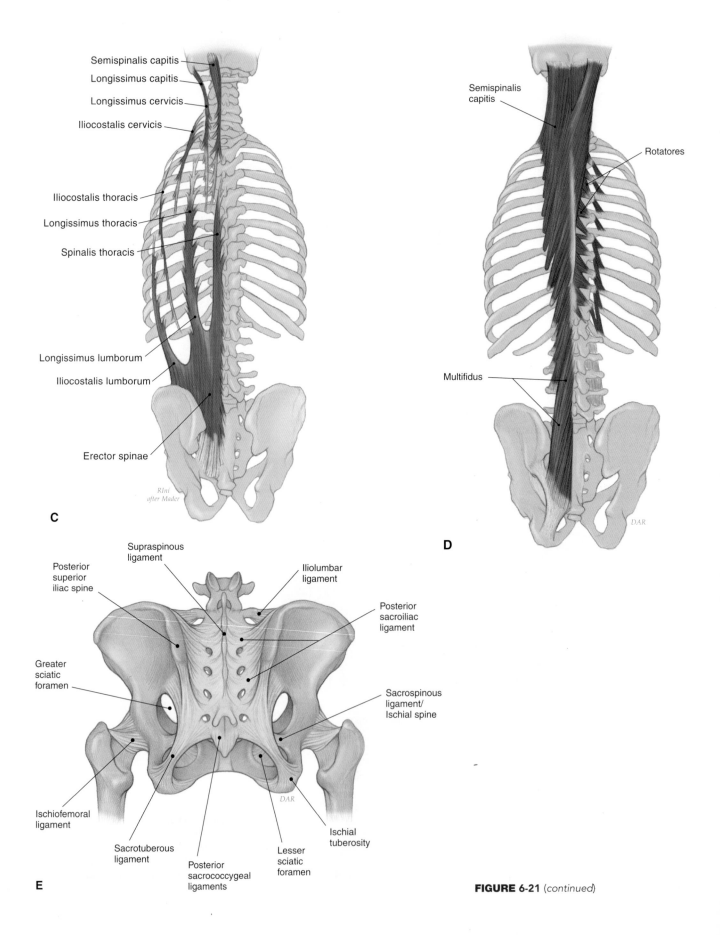

C

- Semispinalis capitis
- Longissimus capitis
- Longissimus cervicis
- Iliocostalis cervicis
- Iliocostalis thoracis
- Longissimus thoracis
- Spinalis thoracis
- Longissimus lumborum
- Iliocostalis lumborum
- Erector spinae

RIni after Mader

D

- Semispinalis capitis
- Rotatores
- Multifidus

DAR

E

- Supraspinous ligament
- Posterior superior iliac spine
- Iliolumbar ligament
- Posterior sacroiliac ligament
- Greater sciatic foramen
- Sacrospinous ligament/ Ischial spine
- Ischiofemoral ligament
- Sacrotuberous ligament
- Posterior sacrococcygeal ligaments
- Lesser sciatic foramen
- Ischial tuberosity

DAR

FIGURE 6-21 (*continued*)

ligaments, which constantly transfer and redistribute forces to maintain postural equilibrium.

The concept of tensegrity provides useful description of the relationship between the bones and soft tissues of the back. In a tensegrity structure, weight is transferred through the tension members (these are represented by muscles, tendons, and ligaments), rather than through the compression members (as represented by bones) (see Fig. 6-23). The compression members act as spacers and points of attachment for the tension components to maintain the necessary shape and distribution of force in the structure.

In the back, the spine, ribs, cranium, and pelvis act as spacers, maintaining the proper lengths for the muscles and other tissues that are attached to them. Thus, the bones are suspended in a web of soft tissue support. When the muscles become chronically shortened and dysfunctional, they are unable to distribute weight effectively, and the spine begins to act more like a compression-style column, setting the stage for breakdown and injury.

Chronic compression of the spine is the cause of many back difficulties. The ligaments and the intervertebral discs take over the job of transferring weight, which should be done by the muscles. The ligaments may become inflamed and even tear, because they have to reinforce and carry weight beyond load they were designed to support. The discs become chronically compressed, losing their springiness and ability to cushion the vertebrae. In this process, the discs can become

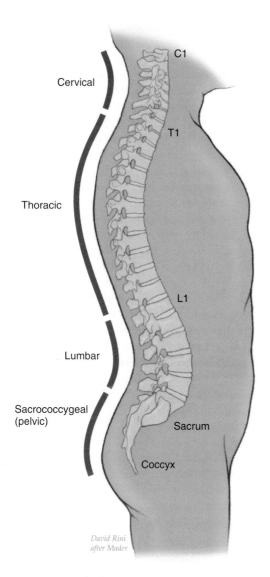

David Rini
after Mader

FIGURE 6-22 The four counterbalancing spinal curves.

Mechanically speaking, all the bony weights of the trunk should be placed as close to the central axis of the body and as close to each other as possible to minimize stress on the weight-bearing spine. This is an important factor in determining correct posture and movement. For this balance to occur, the soft tissues of the back must be able to contract and lengthen freely to accommodate all the shifts of weight and movements that are necessary to maintain this dynamic equilibrium.

The spine is often referred to as a column, but this is not a completely accurate description. A column transfers weight vertically through its central axis by internal compression of its structural components. It does not rely on outside forces to distribute weight. The spine does not function this way. Because of its curved design, it is not rigidly in line with the body's central axis and cannot maintain balance on its own. It must rely on the aid of the attached muscles, tendons, and

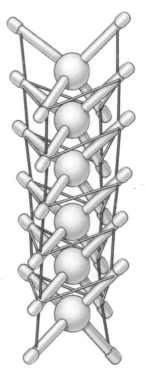

FIGURE 6-23 The relationship between the bones, ligaments, and muscles can be represented in a tensegrity structure.

damaged in a way that puts pressure on nearby nerve tissues, causing substantial pain and disability.

Spinal Muscles

The muscles that move the spine consist of two groups, the superficial and the deep paraspinal muscles. The superficial group is called the *erector spinae* (Fig. 6-21C). It is made up of three muscles, the *iliocostalis*, *longissimus*, and *spinalis*. Depending on their location along the spine, these muscles are subdivided into segments called the *cervicis*, *thoracis*, and *lumborum*. They span the entire length of the back with iliocostalis lumborum, extending all the way down to the sacrum.

The longissimus and iliocostalis muscles are the strongest of the group as well as the most likely to be injured and to develop trigger points. The spinalis is a smaller and weaker muscle. It is the most medially placed, attaching to the spinous processes of the L2–T2 vertebrae. Collectively, the erector spinae muscles extend the vertebral column. The iliocostalis and longissimus are also responsible for lateral flexion of the spinal column.

The deep paraspinal muscles, also known as the *transversospinalis muscles*, connect the transverse processes of the vertebrae to the spinous processes in a layered, upwardly angled pattern. From the most superficial to the deepest-lying, they are the *semispinalis, multifidi,* ▶ and *rotatores* (Fig. 6-21D).

The semispinalis segments span five to six vertebrae. The multifidi segments span three vertebrae, and the rotatores connect adjacent vertebrae. All three muscles extend, laterally flex, and rotate the vertebrae. They also serve to elongate the spinal column. These muscles are active most of the time, because they are responsible for maintaining the alignment of the spinal column as the body shifts its position, even when lying down.

An important purpose of integrated deep tissue therapy on the back is to relieve compression and other stresses along the spine by re-establishing effective muscle function. Massage therapy, along with exercise and proper spinal mechanics, can help to relieve many back problems.

▶ SOURCES OF BACK PROBLEMS

Back pain is a complicated and multifactorial condition. One contributor to back pain is instability of the spinal joints. The discs and ligaments alone provide minimal support for the amount of force exerted on the vertebral joints in everyday movements. Adjacent spinal vertebrae are constantly adapting to the body's many movements through minute amounts of sliding and tilting motions in relation to each other. Too much play between vertebrae disrupts the integrity of the facet joints, resulting in tissue damage, arthritis, and potential nerve impingement.

Broad, strenuous and percussive movements may put hundreds of pounds of force through the spine. The support

required to brace the spinal joints against this kind of stress is provided primarily by the ligaments and deep paraspinal muscles, which connect the vertebrae as described above, along with other stabilizing muscles of the trunk. If those ligaments or muscles are injured or strained, back pain will almost certainly develop.

Age, long-term poor alignment, trauma and other factors may lead to damage of the intervertebral discs. The nucleus pulposus may bulge or even rupture, or the annulus can crack. A prolonged and extreme inflammatory response often accompanies such an injury. Disc damage is especially painful if anything puts pressure on the spinal cord, or on a spinal nerve root as it exits through the intervertebral foramen.

Besides providing support, one of the major functions of the discs and ligaments is to sense the positions of the vertebrae through a proprioceptive feedback connection with the nervous system. When stress is placed on a spinal joint and the vertebrae are close to moving beyond a safe proximity to each other, messages from the nervous system activate stabilizing muscles to support the areas of the spine that are under duress. The most important stabilizing muscles of the spine are the multifidi, transverse abdominus, quadratus lumborum, and psoas.

Trauma to the spine, as well as the normal wear and tear of age, can damage discs and ligaments, interfering with their ability to send position-sensing information to the nervous system. When this occurs, the stabilizing muscles are less effective, creating spinal instability and its related problems. Lack of support from the stabilizing muscles causes the outer layer muscles that control large movements of the spinal column (the erector spinae muscles) to forcibly contract, resulting in a protective splinting action to prevent further damage to the weakened area. This phenomenon is commonly known as a muscle spasm.

Chronic low back pain is a common and expensive disorder, affecting millions of adults every year. The most successful therapies for back pain often include a combination of modalities, including soft tissue manipulation, chiropractic or osteopathic care, physical therapy, exercise, and stretching. Surgery for back pain is typically avoided unless every other avenue has been pursued.

The integrated deep tissue therapy system specifically addresses the multifidi on the posterior aspect, and the transversus abdominus on the anterior side as an effective strategy for many cases of back pain. Programs that target awareness and control of the stabilizing muscles as well as provide educational information about proper spinal mechanics have been very effective in providing long-term relief from back pain for many clients.

Possible Contributors to Back Pain

- Improper standing and sitting postures contribute to strain in the soft tissues around the spine. Many people wear shoes with high heels, which throw the body forward of the line of gravity. To remain upright, the upper back is brought backward, causing an increased lumbar curve with resulting compression in the soft tissues.

- Sitting in a slumped position with the low back rounded is a common habit. This position eliminates the proper lumbar curve. In this position the vertebrae are no longer aligned, placing stress on the surrounding ligaments and muscles. Unfortunately, most furniture is not designed to position the spine properly, and many people with desk jobs find themselves slumping as the day wears on.
- Lack of variation in position or activity can contribute to back pain and other problems; this may be even more important than postural issues.
- Incorrect lifting techniques are a major cause of back injury. The spine should always maintain its integrity as a unit during any kind of lifting activity. The most current guidelines on correct lifting emphasize the importance of starting with the heavy item close to the lifter, and they also suggest to lift, whenever possible, in the "power zone," between the mid-thigh and mid-chest. It is also important to avoid twisting, reaching, or other awkward positions while lifting.
- The abdominal muscles help to support the low back. When they are weak, they may not be sufficient to counteract low back strain. If the psoas muscle is tight, it will also cause tightness and compression in the low back. Short, restricted hamstring muscles pull the pelvis downward, which reduces the lumbar curve and places stress on the ligaments of the low back.
- A sudden, unexpected movement or force, such as slipping on a wet floor or even sneezing (particularly if the back is already in a weakened condition), can result in muscle spasms and tears.

SPINAL ENDANGERMENT SITES

- The kidneys are fist-sized organs located just lateral to the spine. They are partly protected by the 12th ribs. The right kidney is slightly lower than the left. Deep pressure in this area may cause the paraspinal muscles to tighten in response (Fig. 6-24).

CONDITIONS

1. *Postural deviations* are a collection of distortions of the alignment of the spine. Functional deviations typically involve soft tissues, while structural deviations may suggest bony deformation. Postural deviations include hyperkyphosis, hyperlordosis, scoliosis, and rotoscoliosis.
2. *Disc disruptions* refer to any deterioration of the material of the disc that may lead to mechanical pressure on the spinal cord or nerve roots. These problems may include degenerative disc disease, herniated disc, or internal disc disruption. More on disc injuries can be found in Chapter 10.
3. *Muscle spasms* are a protective reaction to, rather than a cause of, damage in the back, but they can become a persistent source of pain and limitation.

See Appendix A for more information on these conditions.

POSTURAL EVALUATION

The client is standing and facing away from the therapist so that the back may be observed.

1. Imagine a vertical line running down the spine, or have the person's spine lined up to a plumb line, dividing the back into left and right segments (see Fig. 6-25A–C).
   - Check for balance of the musculature on the right and left sides.
   - Observe underdevelopment and/or overdevelopment of muscles.
2. Check for exaggeration or underdevelopment of the spinal curves (see Fig. 6-26A–C).
   - Sacral

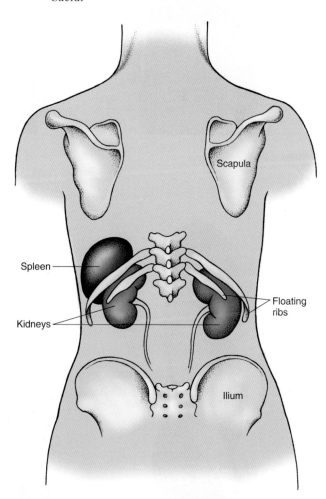

FIGURE 6-24 Endangerment sites of the trunk.

- Lumbar
- Thoracic
- Cervical
3. Note if any vertebrae are protruding or sunken. This is determined by observing or palpating the spinous processes.
4. Check for evenness in the height of the iliac crests.
5. Look for scoliosis. Lack of symmetry in the musculature on the left and right sides may be an indication of this

condition. To confirm this, run your fingers down the back, over the spinous processes, and check for lateral deviations.

Refer to Table 6-2 for a description of abnormal spinal curvatures and muscles that are possibly involved.

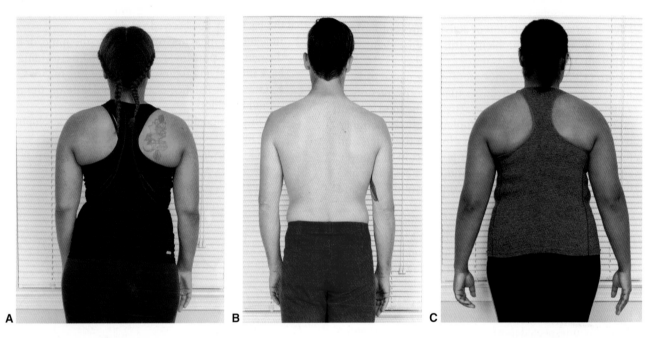

A   **B**   **C**

FIGURE 6-25 Posterior view.

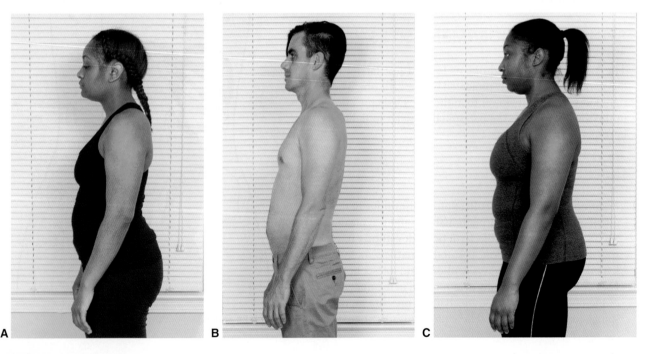

A   **B**   **C**

FIGURE 6-26 Lateral view.

TABLE 6-2 | **Body Reading for the Back**

Postural Patterns	Muscles That May Be Shortened

Scoliosis	Muscles on concave sides of the spinal curves:
	    Erector spinae
	    Paraspinal muscles
	Check for lateral imbalances in:
	    Iliopsoas
	    Quadratus lumborum
	    Biceps femoris

Hyperkyphosis	Head extensors Neck extensors Pectoralis minor Anterior deltoid
Hyperlordosis	Iliacus Psoas major Rectus femoris Quadratus lumborum

HOLISTIC VIEW

"There's nothing like millions of years of really frustrating trial and error to give a species moral fiber and, in some cases, a backbone." (T. Pratchett)

The spine is the major support structure of the body. Strength of character is often judged by the degree of strength exhibited by our posture. We speak of a courageous, forthright person as "having a strong backbone." Someone who is considered to be weak or cowardly is labeled as "spineless."

A baby's spine is extremely flexible, because the muscles around it have not yet developed the strength to support it and the balancing spinal curves have not yet formed.

Newborn infants are almost completely helpless. They cannot sit up or hold the weight of the head and thorax through the spine. Children's early movements of kicking and squirming are necessary to develop the musculature of the pelvis and low back. By exploring and exerting themselves through movement, infants gradually develop the core strength of support. Even the actions of crying and screaming are important in building up the muscles that will stabilize the necessary lumbar curve so that the child can hold the head up and, eventually, be able to sit and stand without aid.

When lying on the abdomen, a very young baby cannot lift his or her head off the floor. It is a great accomplishment when infants can finally pull the trunk up. As they survey the world around them, they are beginning the first stages of asserting themselves as individuals.

Contractions of the extensor muscles control the lift and arching motion of the spine. The Feldenkrais approach associates the stance of opening the chest and stretching the arms back is with joy, expansion, and self-expression. In this context the extensor muscles are the "happy muscles," because their use tends to elicit a happy response in individuals throughout life.

When the trunk is open and lifted, we show that we are available to receive and interact with the world around us. On the other hand, contraction of the flexor muscles causes the trunk to be pulled forward and the spine to flex. This position may reflect feelings of withdrawal, fear, and lack of initiative.

Integrated deep tissue therapy can open the tight muscles in the chest and create a sense of expansion and lift. The recipient then has the freedom to explore this posture, and the sense of confidence, energy and power that go along with it.

Dr. Ida Rolf referred to the spine and its intrinsic support muscles as the inner core of the body. This core represents our sense of security and our will. If the spine and its associated muscles are weak, there may be a feeling of not being able to stand up for one's self or a lack of trust that one has the inner resources to handle all the conflicts or problems that may arise in life. By contrast, if the spine and supporting muscles are supple and strong, we may experience a sense of independence and self-reliance.

The low back provides a bridge between two solid bony structures, the pelvis and the thorax. In an emotional interpretation, the low back is responsible for mediating feelings between these two areas. Having no bony protection around it, the lumbar spine is mobile, but vulnerable. Pain and tightness in this area may reflect areas of vulnerability within a person. When weakness and degeneration in the lumbar spine are present, it may be beneficial to look at areas in one's life where security and support are not present. This could relate to a person's finances, job, home life, or relationships.

The upper back has a direct structural relationship to the shoulders. Feelings of anger or even rage can lodge in this segment. We tend to "hold back" aggressive actions of the arms, like punching, with the upper back muscles; we also associate strength and rigidity here with a military stance. The thoracic curve corresponds to the heart center. It is usually when the heart center is shut down that hostile and resentful feelings arise. ■

▶ EXERCISES AND SELF-TREATMENT

Deep Breathing on All Fours

This exercise emphasizes the stabilizing action of the transverse abdominis and multifidus muscles. It may be incorporated during the exercises on the ball described below.

Position—Kneel on your hands and knees, with the spine in a neutral position parallel to the floor (Fig. 6-27).

Execution—Inhale deeply, allowing the chest to expand and the abdomen to relax. Exhale, lifting the navel toward the spine and allowing the abdominal wall to partially contract. Do not alter the position of the spinal column. Maintain this lift of the navel for 5 to 10 breaths. If low back pain is present, focus on contracting the multifidus muscles attaching to the vertebrae at the level of the injury. Try to keep the other multifidus muscles relaxed. This precise muscular isolation is difficult to achieve but with practice can be accomplished.

Exercises Using a Ball

Incorporating a fitness ball into a back training program is beneficial because the act of maintaining the ball in a stable position during the exercises engages the primary stabilizing muscles that support the spine.

- *One-leg raise* (Fig. 6-28)

Position—Sit on top of the ball with both feet planted on the ground. Imagine the crown of your head being pulled up toward the ceiling by a thread. Allow your arms to hang at your sides with the hands resting against the ball.

Execution—Inhale deeply, maintaining an elongated spine. Exhale, raising the right leg several inches off the floor while the navel pulls toward the front of the spine. Inhale, lowering the right foot back to the floor. Repeat the lift with the left leg. Perform 5 to 10 sets.

- *Rear leg lift* (Fig. 6-29)

Position—Lie prone on top of the ball with both hands touching the floor in front and both legs extended in back with the toes tucked under, making contact with the floor.

Execution—Exhale, raising the right leg straight off of the floor with the toes pointed. Inhale, lower the right leg back to the starting position. Repeat the lift with the left leg. Perform 5 to 10 sets.

- *Side stretch for the abdominal muscles and quadratus lumborum* (Fig. 6-30)

Position—Sit on top of the ball with your arms at your sides and the palms of the hands against the ball.

Execution—Inhaling, raise the right arm overhead. Exhaling, shift your hips to the right as you extend your right arm toward the left, bringing your navel toward the front of the spine. Use your left hand to brace yourself from sliding off the ball. Hold the stretch for several breaths. To let go of the stretch, bring the right arm back to your side as you center your pelvis back on top of the ball. Repeat the stretch on the left side.

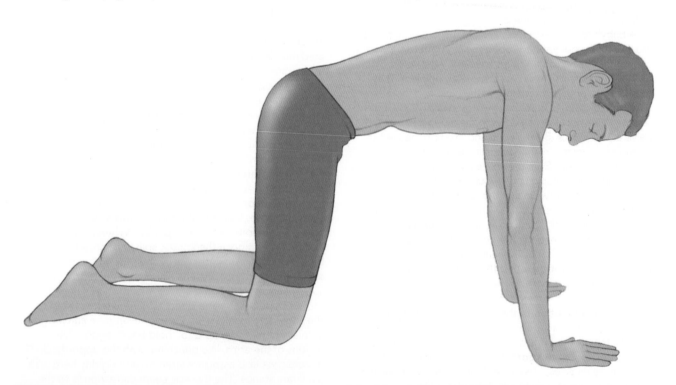

FIGURE 6-27 Exhaling in the all-fours position, isolating the transverse abdominis and affected multifidus muscles.

- *Spinal lift* (Fig. 6-31)

  Position—Lying on your back with your arms on the floor at your sides, place your feet on the ball.

  Execution—Inhale, pressing your palms against the floor. Exhale, raise your pelvis several inches off the floor as you press into the ball with your feet. Pull your navel in toward the front of the spine. Inhaling, lower your hips back down to the floor. Repeat the pelvic lift several times.

- *Forward bend* (Fig. 6-32)

  Position—Sit on the floor with your legs extended in front of you and the ball placed in between them. Place the palms of both hands on the ball.

  Execution—Inhale, elongating the spine toward the ceiling. Exhale, rolling the ball forward with your hands as you flex the torso forward over your extended legs. Draw the navel in toward the front of your spine. Remain in the stretch for several breaths as you visualize extending the crown of the head forward toward the ball.

Self-Massage for the Back Muscles

Place two tennis balls under your back, one on either side of the spine, beginning between the shoulder blades. Take deep breaths, allowing the muscles to sink into the balls and visualizing the tension melting. Reposition the balls farther down the spine, and repeat the procedure. Continue, down to the sacrum.

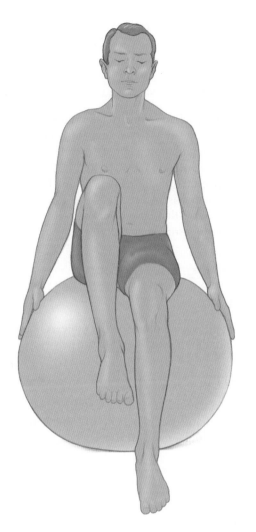

FIGURE 6-28 Single leg raise.

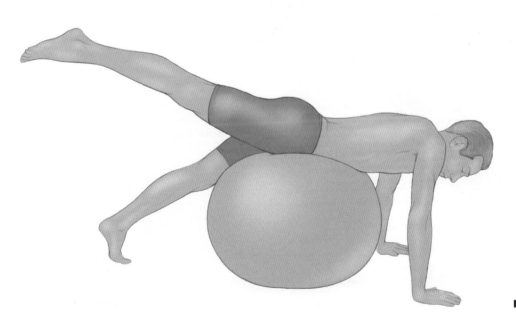

FIGURE 6-29 Rear leg lift.

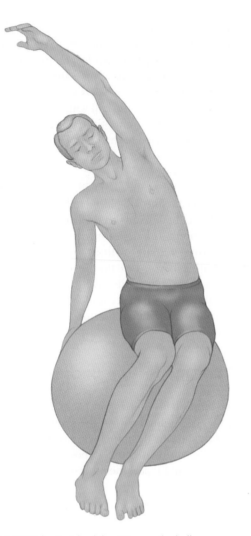

FIGURE 6-30 Side stretch while sitting on the ball.

▶ BACK AND SPINAL COLUMN ROUTINE

Objectives

- To relax the back area, which tends to hold excessive tension
- To lengthen the spine by releasing the muscles that control the position and movement of the vertebrae
- To reduce tension in the posterior breathing muscles
- To balance the weight segments along the spine (head, thorax, and pelvis)
- To treat tissues that have been strained by back injuries and/or poor postural habits

Addressing Energy Flow

POSITION

- The client is lying prone on the table. A bolster may be placed under the ankles and/or the pelvis.

POLARITY

Contact the sacrum and occiput with the palms of your hands. Imagine the spine decompressing and lengthening between your hands. Hold for at least 30 seconds.

SHIATSU

Cat's Paws

With your hands placed on either side of the spine at the level of the upper back, alternately press your palms down the back, as if

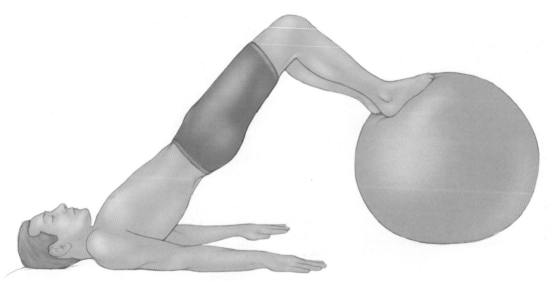

FIGURE 6-31 Spinal lift.

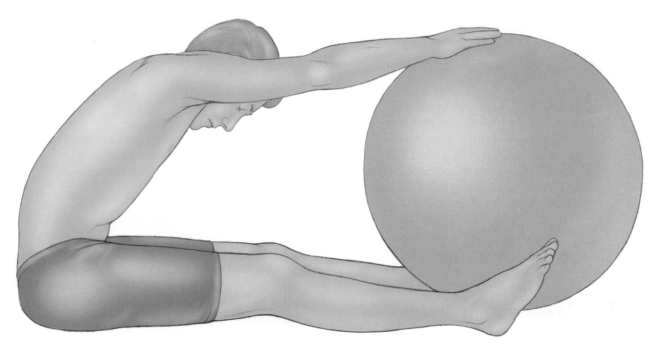

FIGURE 6-32 Forward bend.

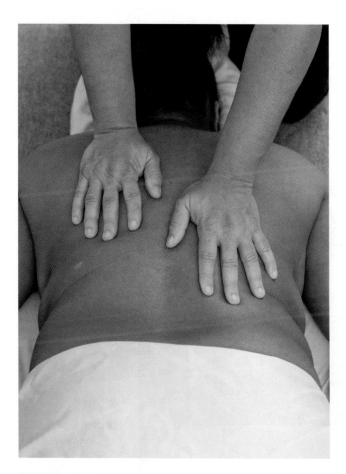

FIGURE 6-33 Cat's paws.

walking on your hands. When you reach the iliac crests, bring your hands back to the shoulders, and perform the sequence again, only this time with the hands wider apart (Fig. 6-33).

Swedish/Cross Fiber

1. Perform basic effleurage strokes on the musculature of the back.
2. Stand at the side of the table, and face the client's back. Perform the swim stroke by rolling and spreading your forearms across the back muscles, avoiding pressure on the spinous processes.
3. Apply cross-fiber strokes to the erector spinae muscles with the heel of the hand or the knuckles.

Connective Tissue

MYOFASCIAL MOBILIZATION TECHNIQUE

Using the fingers or the palms, roll the muscles of the back over the underlying ribs and vertebrae. Use the myofascial spreading technique on areas of tissue that do not easily slide over the bones.

Deep Tissue/Neuromuscular Therapy

SEQUENCE

1. Erector spinae group

2. Deep paraspinal muscles (the lamina groove) ▶
3. Iliac crest
4. Sacral ligaments
5. Intercostals

◎ Trigger points may be located in any of the musculature of the back, particularly where injuries have occurred and tissues have been damaged. Observe the client's posture and movement patterns. Note where bending and reaching are initiated along the spine. These are stress points and likely candidates for trigger point formation and connective tissue thickening.

Erector Spinae Group (Spinalis, Longissimus, Iliocostalis)

Origin:
    Iliocostalis lumborum—external lip of the iliac crest, posterior surface of the sacrum.
    Iliocostalis thoracis—upper borders of ribs 12–7.
    Longissimus thoracis—transverse processes of L1–L5 vertebrae.
    Spinalis thoracis—spinous processes of T11–T12 and L1–L2 vertebrae.

Insertion:
    Iliocostalis lumborum—angles of ribs 6–12.
    Iliocostalis thoracis—transverse process of C7, angles of ribs 1–6.

Longissimus thoracis—accessory processes of L1–L3 vertebrae, transverse processes of T1–T12 vertebrae, between the tubercles and angles of ribs 2–12.
Spinalis thoracis—spinous processes of T1–T4 vertebrae.

Action:
Iliocostalis lumborum and thoracis;
longissimus thoracis—extension and lateral flexion of the vertebral column, depression of the ribs.
Spinalis thoracis—extension and rotation of the vertebral column.

◎ The longissimus and iliocostalis muscles are the most likely sites for trigger point activity. Trigger points in the iliocostalis thoracis at its upper level tend to refer along the scapular border and between the shoulder blades. In the lower portion of the muscles, pain may be referred downward, into the lumbar and hip region and into the abdomen.

Strokes
- Perform elongating strokes down the back and parallel to the spine, beginning at the level of T1 and ending at the iliac crest. Use the base of the palm, forearm, or knuckles (Fig. 6-34). Cover each of the three erector spinae muscles.
- Using the elbow or thumbs, stroke along the borders of the muscles. Begin at the level of T1, and end at the iliac crest.

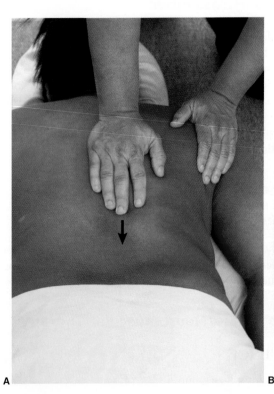

A

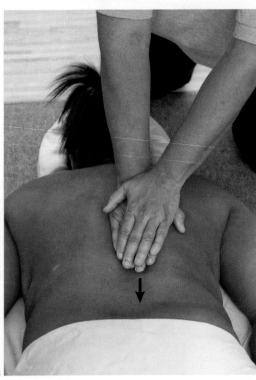

B

FIGURE 6-34
Elongation stroke for the erector spinae muscles using the base of the palm.

Deep Paraspinal Muscles (Semispinalis, Multifidi, Rotatores)

Origin:

Semispinalis thoracis—transverse processes of T6–T10 vertebrae.

Semispinalis cervicis—transverse processes of T1–T5 vertebrae.

Semispinalis capitis—transverse processes of C4–C7 and T1–T6 vertebrae.

Multifidi—sacrum to S4 foramen, erector spinae aponeurosis, posterior superior iliac spine, posterior sacroiliac ligaments, mammillary and transverse processes of T1–T12 vertebrae, articular processes of C4–C7 vertebrae.

Rotatores—transverse process of all vertebrae.

Insertion:

Semispinalis thoracis—spinous processes of C6–C7 and T1–T4 vertebrae.

Semispinalis cervicis—spinous processes of C2–C5 vertebrae.

Semispinalis capitis—occiput, between superior and inferior nuchal lines.

Multifidi—spinous process of two to four vertebrae above origin.

Rotatores—base of spinous process of next highest vertebra.

Action: Extend and rotate vertebral column.

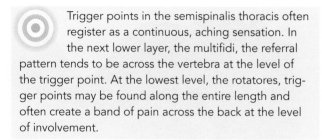

Trigger points in the semispinalis thoracis often register as a continuous, aching sensation. In the next lower layer, the multifidi, the referral pattern tends to be across the vertebra at the level of the trigger point. At the lowest level, the rotatores, trigger points may be found along the entire length and often create a band of pain across the back at the level of involvement.

Strokes

- Perform elongating strokes down the spine in the space between the spinous processes and the transverse processes of the vertebrae, from T1 to the sacrum (Fig. 6-35). Use the thumbs or the elbow.
- Use static compression and/or short spreading techniques in muscular areas that feel dense, fibrous, or unyielding.
- Place the thumbs end to end at C7 (Fig. 6-36). Do an elongating stroke along the lamina groove of the cervical spine to the occiput. Repeat, using the side-to-side strokes, along the muscle fibers.

Iliac Crest, Iliolumbar Ligament

Position

- Place a pillow under the client's pelvis for the next three sections (iliac crest, iliolumbar ligament, sacral ligaments).

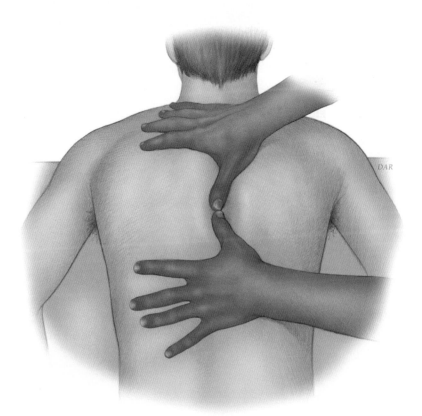

FIGURE 6-35 Placement of the thumbs next to the spinous processes to access the deep paraspinal muscles.

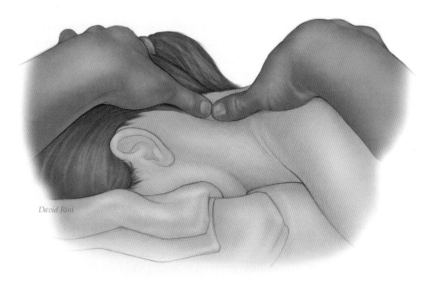

FIGURE 6-36 Hand placement to access the cervical paraspinal muscles.

Superior Border of the Iliac Crest

Strokes

- Trace the edge of the iliac crest using the thumbs or the elbow. Feel for congested areas of tissue and/or tender spots.
- Use static compression on tender spots. Do the side-to-side spreading technique across the congested tissues to reduce tension in them.

Thoracolumbar Fascia

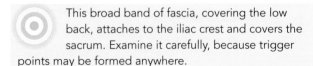 This broad band of fascia, covering the low back, attaches to the iliac crest and covers the sacrum. Examine it carefully, because trigger points may be formed anywhere.

Iliolumbar Ligament

Strokes

- Find the junction formed by the lumbar spine and the pelvis. Place your elbow into it, pressing inward and downward, at approximately a 45° angle toward the iliac crest (Fig. 6-37).
- Hold, with static compression. Perform short, cross-fiber strokes.

Sacral Ligaments

Strokes

- Warm up the sacral area by applying fingertip friction over the entire sacrum.
- Using the thumbs or fingers, do all the deep tissue spreading techniques over the sacrum (up-down, side-side, and combination) (Fig. 6-38).

Intercostals

Strokes

- Stand on the opposite side of the table from the section of ribs on which you are working. Place your fingers just

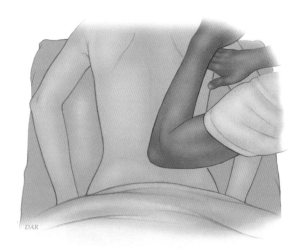

FIGURE 6-37 Elbow position for contacting the iliolumbar ligament.

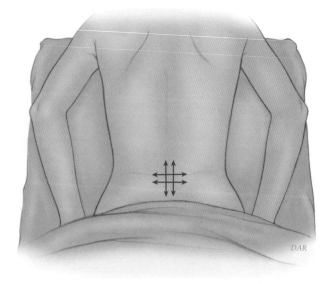

FIGURE 6-38 Direction of strokes on the sacrum.

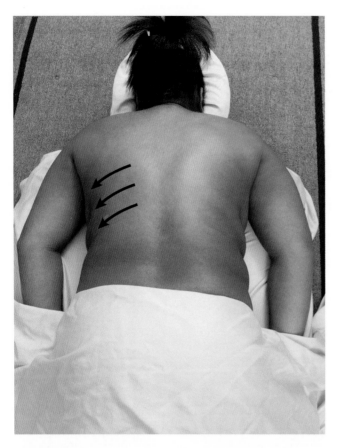

FIGURE 6-39 Direction of strokes on the intercostal muscles.

below the inferior angle of the scapula. Moving your fingers back and forth and up and down, feel for the spaces between the ribs.

- Using short back and forth motions, feel for restricted areas in the soft tissues between the ribs (i.e., knots, strings, lumps) (Fig. 6-39). Check for trigger point activity. The thumbs or a knuckle may be used in the intercostal spaces, where more pressure is required.
- Continue to the 12th rib.

STRETCH

1. Bring the client's knees to his or her chest. Either holding the client's knees with your hands or by pressing your forearm against them, slowly lean forward, flexing the thighs to the chest (Fig. 6-40). This stretches the client's low back muscles.

2. Reaching across the table, press down on the client's shoulder to stabilize it against the table. With your other hand, slowly pull the client's knees toward you and down toward the table, creating a twist for the spine and back muscles (Fig. 6-41).

3. Have the client hold the knees to the chest. Standing at the head of the table, hold the client's head in your hands. Traction the neck very slightly by drawing the head toward you, then by lifting the head off the table and bringing the forehead toward the knees. This stretches the upper back muscles.

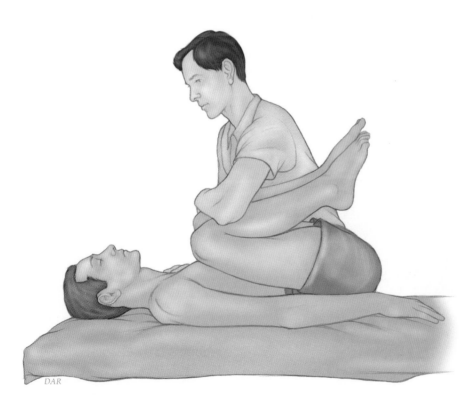

DAR

FIGURE 6-40 Stretching the client's low back.

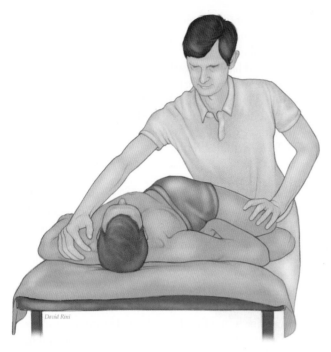

FIGURE 6-41 The spinal twist.

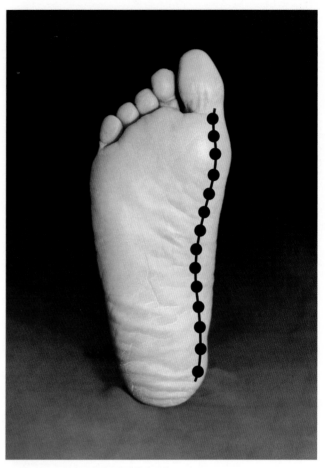

FIGURE 6-43 The spinal reflex zone.

ACCESSORY WORK

1. *Occipital Muscles.* Sitting at the head of the table, slide your fingers under the client's occipital ridge and lift the head slightly (Fig. 6-42). Wait for the muscles to soften and for the sensation of an even pulse on both sides of the occiput.

2. *Spinal Reflex Points on the Foot.* With your thumb, press points along the medial border of the foot, beginning at the big toe and working down to the heel. The curves of the instep correspond to the curves of the spine (Fig. 6-43). Hold sensitive spots for 8 to 12 seconds.

CLOSING

Sitting at the foot of the table, lightly hold the heels of the client's feet in your hands for 30 to 60 seconds. Remove your hands slowly.

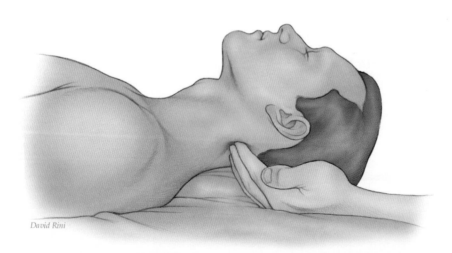

FIGURE 6-42 Hand position to access the occipital muscles.

SESSION IMPRESSIONS

THE BACK

The client is a 29-year-old man named Clint, who works in real estate. He has received massage treatments from different therapists on an irregular basis over several years. His goal is to relax and relieve tension in tight neck, shoulder, and back muscles. Clint is tall and muscular. He used to lift weights but quit 4 years ago because he strained his low back and found that weight lifting put stress on his neck muscles. Recently, he has felt the need to return to exercising and has just begun to work out again. He is in good health. His only physical problem is residual tightness in low back muscles from the weight-lifting injury 4 years ago.

Clint's upper body is more developed than his lower body. His shoulders and arms carry more bulk, relatively speaking, than his hip and thigh muscles do. He exhibits a small degree of posterior pelvic tilt. His erector spinae muscles are very pronounced, particularly on the right side. He used to play baseball regularly and exhibits the right side–left side muscular imbalance that one-handed sports generate. His neck appears short as a result of contracted trapezius muscles as well as other shortened head and neck extensors. The focus of this session will be to elongate the spinal column by reducing tension in the erector spinae and deep paraspinal muscles.

During the session, initial work on the back revealed that the superficial musculature was fairly relaxed. However, the deep muscles along the spine were extremely contracted. The client requested very deep pressure on these muscles. He barely felt any sensation in the deep paraspinal muscles regardless of the depth of pressure. These muscles seemed to be numb. Deep pressure applied with the elbow did not cause the contractions in the muscles to yield. The lack of feeling and response from these muscles seemed to suggest that maybe the tension was psychologically based. In other words, the client may be armoring himself on a subconscious level, to prevent certain feelings from arising to conscious awareness.

Although the client wanted very deep pressure applied to these muscles so that he could feel something there other than numbness, the tissues were guarding against the invasion by contracting further. It was explained to the client that this deep, invasive pressure was counterproductive, so the pressure was decreased. Although the client could not feel anything in the deep muscles, these muscles relaxed to a small degree when the pressure was lessened.

The session continued with deep tissue strokes applied to the muscles along the entire spinal column. Then, the client turned supine so that balancing work could be applied to the anterior neck and chest areas. Shiatsu compression moves were performed on the legs, and the session was completed with massage of the spinal reflex points on the feet.

After the session, the client described himself as high strung and unable to relax. This description matched the assessment of the condition of the soft tissues of the back. It was suggested that, if interested, he could participate in a yoga class, where he could learn slow, sustained stretching movements along with coordinated deep breathing to begin to relieve some of the deep-seated stress in his intrinsic muscles. Regular yoga practice, along with deep tissue therapy sessions, would help to uncover and reduce the tightly held tension that had accumulated along his spinal column. The client appreciated the suggestion and added that he had wanted to start taking yoga and this session had been a good incentive for him to follow through on it. ■

Topics for Discussion

1. Describe a viable course of treatment for a client experiencing low back pain, assuming that pain is muscular in origin.
2. What other areas of the body should be included in a session focusing on the spine to achieve an even distribution of forces along the vertebral column?
3. How would you approach a client who cannot feel any response in his back muscles, no matter how much pressure you apply?
4. What self-care suggestions might you give to a client who is experiencing back strain?
5. What are some visual indications of exaggerated curvatures of the spine (kyphotic, scoliotic, or lordotic) in a client who is lying in a prone position?

REVIEW QUESTIONS

Level 1

Receive and Respond

1. Which muscles are most involved in healthy breathing?
   a. Diaphragm, psoas
   b. Intercostals, diaphragm
   c. Pectoralis minor, scalenes
   d. Scalenes, pectoralis major

2. The diaphragm is shaped like a. . .
   a. dome.
   b. fish.
   c. triangle.
   d. diamond.

3. Which of the following is an endangerment site of the anterior chest?
   a. Zygomatic arch
   b. Xyphoid process
   c. Linea alba
   d. Umbilicus

4. The term "tensegrity structure" is sometimes used in the context of the spine. What does this mean?
   a. Strength is supported through vertical stacking
   b. Forces are conveyed through compression and leverage
   c. Strength is supported through weight-bearing stress
   d. Forces are conveyed through tension lines

Level 2

Apply Concepts

1. If a client has a chest that seems expanded and round, with shoulders that are retracted and a lifted sternum, what are some muscles that may be shortened?
   a. Latissimus dorsi, pectoralis major, anterior deltoid
   b. Diaphragm, internal intercostals, obliques
   c. External intercostals, scalenes, rhomboids
   d. Scalenes, pectoralis minor, pectoralis major

2. Your client has demonstrably shortened pectoralis minor muscles that cause his chest to be rounded. What is a simple activity he can do to help create more freedom of movement in this area?
   a. Resisted lateral rotation of the humerus
   b. Resisted internal rotation of the humerus
   c. Doorway stretch
   d. Breathing deeply while on all fours

3. An integrated deep tissue therapy approach for client who has back pain is most likely to include addressing the. . .
   a. trapezius and pectoralis major.
   b. diaphragm and psoas.
   c. latissimus dorsi and teres major.
   d. multifidi and transversus abdominus.

4. What is the recommended sequence for neuromuscular therapy to the anterior chest?
   a. Diaphragm, followed by serratus anterior, followed by pectoralis minor, followed by scalenes
   b. Pectoralis major, followed by intercostals, followed by diaphragm, followed by serratus posterior and inferior
   c. Pectoralis major, followed by pectoralis minor, followed by subclavius, followed by scalenes
   d. Intercostals, followed by diaphragm, followed by iliopsoas, followed by intestinal work

5. What is the most likely contributor to back pain?
   a. Trauma
   b. Poor posture
   c. Genetic predisposition
   d. Sedentariness and lack of movement

Level 3

Problem Solving: Discussion Points

1. Read the *Session Impressions* piece for the client named Clint. Assuming this client comes back for another session, how would you design his next treatment? Be specific about what structures you plan to address and why. Discuss this with a classmate who has a different plan.

2. Your client is a middle-aged woman who has a chronic low-grade cough, but no diagnosed disease or infection. Today she has a painful area in her midback on the right side. It is so tender that she can't breathe deeply, bend, reach, or do many of her typical daily activities without pain. Using elements of integrated deep tissue therapy, describe your plan for today's session with her.

CHAPTER 7

Aligning the Upper Extremity

LEARNING OBJECTIVES

Having completed the reading, classroom instruction, and assigned homework related to Chapter 7 of *The Balanced Body*, the learner is expected to be able to. . .

- Apply key terms and concepts related to integrated deep tissue therapy as related to the arm, shoulder, and hand
- Identify anatomical features of the relevant areas, including
  - Bony landmarks
  - Muscular and fascial structures
  - Endangerments or cautionary sites
- Identify common postural or movement patterns associated with pain or impaired function of the arm, shoulder, and hand
- Use positioning and bolstering strategies that provide safety and comfort for clients to receive integrated deep tissue therapy to the arm, shoulder, and hand

- Generate within-scope recommendations for client self-care relevant to the arm, shoulder, and hand
- Safely and effectively perform the integrated deep tissue therapy routines as described
- Organize a single session to address the arm, shoulder, and hand, using the integrated deep tissue therapy approach, customized to individual clients
- Plan a series of sessions to address whole-body incorporation using the integrated deep tissue therapy approach, customized to individual clients

The Shoulder, Arm, and Hand

▶ GENERAL CONCEPTS

The shoulder, arm, forearm, and hand form the upper extremity. This is an extremely important area, because it is largely through the shoulder–arm complex that we express ourselves bodily and make contact with the world. The way in which people hold and use their shoulders and arms conveys a lot about attitudes and self-expression.

Functionally, the pectoral girdle forms a base of support for the arms that allows almost unlimited range of motion. Structurally, the pectoral girdle (also called the shoulder girdle) includes the scapula and clavicle. These bones provide a base for the humerus.

The pectoral girdle and pelvic girdle share a similar function: They both support and anchor the limbs. The major difference between them is that the pelvis is a more rigid structure. Unlike the pectoral girdle, the pelvic bones are fused together, limiting its movement. The shoulder girdle is open in the back, because the scapulae do not connect to each other. This design allows the arms much greater freedom of individual motion at the shoulder joints than the legs are capable of at the hip joints.

The pectoral girdle and pelvis need to be aligned with each other for optimal balance and function of the body. The muscles of the pectoral girdle and arms should be free to adjust to weight shifts that occur from movements in the lower body. The pectoral girdle acts like a yoke suspended over the rib cage by muscles attaching to the neck and head. The arms should hang loosely from the shoulder joints, with freedom to swing. Tension in the muscles of the shoulders produces rigidity in the upper back and neck that contributes to imbalance and stress throughout the body.

When the muscles of the upper extremity work in a coordinated fashion, the centers of the shoulder joints are directly at the sides of the body, creating maximum width in the upper torso.

Function of the pectoral girdle is of particular relevance to massage therapists, because when all the joints of the upper extremity are balanced, a force applied through the fingers and hand will pass through the wrist, up the forearm and humerus, and through the scapula to the trunk. From there, the force will pass down the vertebrae to the sacrum and flare out across the ilium to the hip joints. Then, it will pass down the bones of the legs to the ankles and across the

111

feet. In this way, forces are transferred smoothly through the body, eliminating strains caused by soft tissues having to brace uneven twisting, pulling and pushing around misaligned joints.

Integrated deep tissue therapy on the shoulder girdle, arms, and hands helps to remove uneven pulls on the scapula and clavicle and balances the humerus in the shoulder joint. Soft tissue reorganization at the shoulder girdle improves movement of the arms, increases breathing capacity, and reduces the risk of injury to the area.

▶ MUSCULOSKELETAL ANATOMY AND FUNCTION

See Essential Anatomy Box 7-1 for a summary of musculo-skeletal anatomy and function.

The Shoulder

The shoulder girdle consists of the clavicles and the scapulae. It is mostly held in place by soft tissues; its only connection to axial skeleton is where the medial ends of the clavicles attach to the sternum. The clavicles support the shoulder joints and keep the scapulae away from the chest wall so that they may move freely and independently. In maintaining this distance from the thorax, the clavicle prevents the shoulder girdle from interfering with the important functions of circulation and respiration, and it protects the brachial plexus nerves as they pass under the coracoid process and out to the axilla. The clavicle also absorbs shocks coming through the shoulder and arm, protecting the sternum and ribs from the force of direct impact.

The humerus and scapula are joined via a ball-and-socket type joint. The rounded head of the humerus fits into a concave depression on the side of the scapula, called the glenoid fossa. This fossa is shallow, and it does not fit around the humerus as deeply as the acetabulum houses the femur. The humerus is held in the joint by a ligamentous capsule and the work of the rotator cuff muscles. The glenohumeral joint has much less bony and ligamentous support than most joints. This allows a great range of motion, but at the cost of stability and protection: the shoulder joint can be vulnerable to injury.

The motions of the arms are controlled by a series of muscles attached around the shoulder joint and along the humerus (Fig. 7-1A). These muscles form a wheel-like design, fanning out from the shoulder joint to connect to the skeleton over a broad area, all the way to the sacrum and ilium. Thus, the strength and action of the arms rely partly on support and coordinated action from the trunk and legs. Isolated movement of the arms, without support of the rest of the body, creates strain that can lead to injury.

The muscles that control the movements of the arm include those that must also stabilize the scapula. It is important that the scapula is free to move in combination with all movements of the humerus, but it must also remain anchored to the body wall through muscular action to provide leverage for the head of the humerus.

In the back, the ***trapezius*** and rhomboids help to support the scapulae (Fig. 7-1A). The upper trapezius, with assistance from the lower trapezius, elevates the shoulders.

A trigger point that frequently develops near the attachment point of the ***levator scapula*** muscle on the superior angle of the scapula is often attributed to holding the shoulders in an elevated position. More likely, however, this soreness is caused by a chronic forward head position. When the head is held forward, the levator scapulae are constantly active, drawing the neck posterior to bring the head back toward the vertical axis of gravity. The scapulae must be held steady to stabilize the pulling action of the muscles, causing the

---

BOX 7-1 ESSENTIAL ANATOMY | **The Shoulder and Arm Routines**

MUSCLES	BONES AND LANDMARKS
Trapezius	Scapula
Supraspinatus	Spine of scapula
Infraspinatus	Acromion process
Teres minor	Humerus
Teres major	Olecranon process
Latissimus dorsi	Olecranon fossa
Deltoid	Deltoid tuberosity
Biceps brachii	Lateral epicondyle
Triceps brachii	Medial epicondyle
Brachialis	Ulna
Forearm extensors and flexors	Radius
Hand muscles	Carpals and metacarpals
	Phalanges

scapular attachments of the levator scapulae to become strained. The stress on these muscles is relieved by properly positioning the head on the neck, thus reducing the pulling action by the levator scapulae.

The *rhomboids*, which retract the scapulae, are opposed by the *serratus anterior* muscles, which protract them. When the musculature controlling the placement of the scapulae is balanced, the rhomboids lie on the horizontal plane along with the clavicles. When the rhomboids are weak, they cannot fix the vertebral borders of the scapulae to the body wall, and the lower portion of the scapulae will lift away from the back, or wing.

Several large muscles emanating from the spine, sternum, and ribs contribute to arm movements. These muscles include the trapezius, latissimus dorsi, and pectoralis major. This arrangement is advantageous, because it distributes forces generated from the arms throughout the length of the spine, helping to stabilize the spine against large, peripheral motions.

The ligamentous capsule surrounding the head of the humerus is quite loose, allowing increased range of motion for the arm. Because of this laxity of the capsule, it cannot maintain the head of the humerus in the joint. Instead, this support is accomplished by the tendons of four muscles positioned around the shoulder joint, known as the rotator cuff. The muscles that comprise the rotator cuff are the *supraspinatus, infraspinatus, teres minor*, and *subscapularis*. They are joined in their function of reinforcement by the tendon of the long head of the *biceps brachii* on the top of the joint and the long head of the *triceps brachii* on the underside of the joint. The balance of all these muscles is crucial to proper positioning of the humerus in the shoulder joint.

The primary abductors of the humerus are the *deltoids*. Because of their position at the superior end of the humerus, however, they lack the leverage to initiate abduction when the arm is against the side of the body. Instead, the supraspinatus muscle

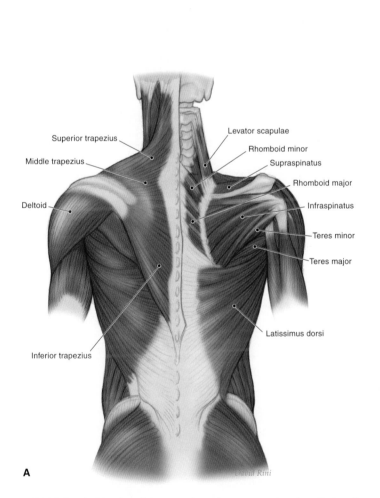

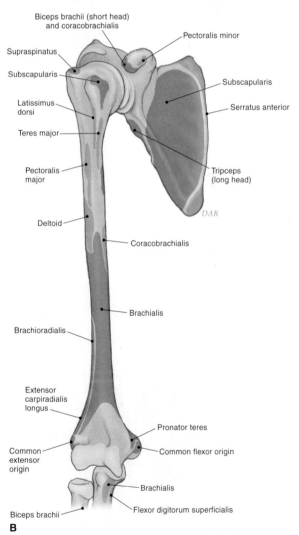

FIGURE 7-1 A. Muscles of the scapula and arm, posterior view. **B.** Attachment sites of the muscles of the scapula and arm, anterior view. **C.** Attachment sites of the posterior muscles of the scapula and arm. **D.** Attachment sites of the anterior muscles of the forearm and hand. **E.** Muscles of the hand, anterior view.

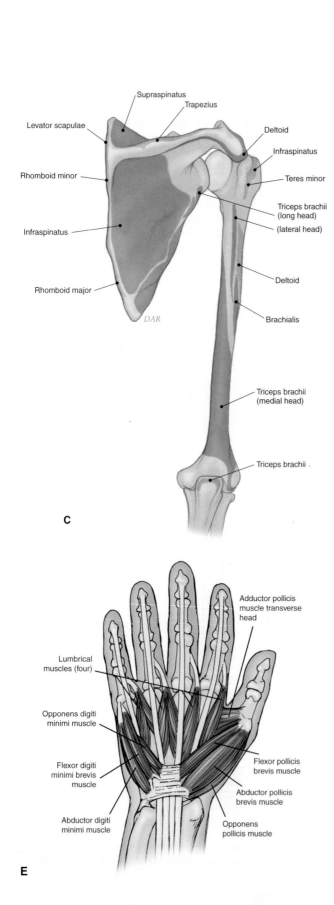

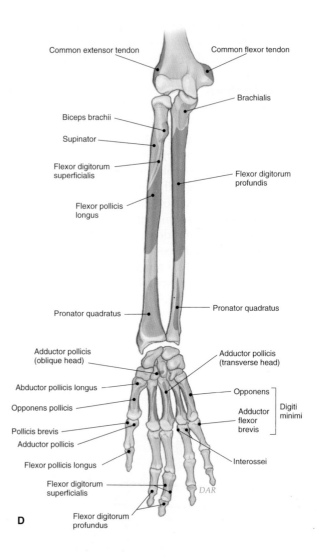

FIGURE 7-1 (continued)

initiates abduction, which is taken over by the deltoids when the arm is abducted about 12 inches from the side of the body.

The infraspinatus muscle is responsible for external rotation of the humerus. It is opposed by the subscapularis, which internally rotates the arm. Both muscles help to stabilize the humerus in the glenoid fossa, and they are easily strained by swinging the arm forward or backward from a horizontal position.

The teres minor assists the infraspinatus in external rotation and stabilization of the head of the humerus against the scapula. The ***teres major*** assists the ***latissimus dorsi*** in internal rotation and extension of a flexed arm. The teres major and latissimus dorsi muscles form the posterior axillary fold, which is the back of the armpit.

The ***pectoralis minor*** ▶ connects the scapula to the anterior side of the rib cage. It brings the scapula forward, downward, and medial. Shortened pectoralis minor muscles are characterized by rounded or stooped shoulders. The lateral bundle of nerves of the ***brachial plexus*** and the axillary artery pass underneath the pectoralis minor. When this muscle is chronically contracted, it may impinge blood flow and nerve supply to the arm when that arm is abducted and externally rotated. In this position, the pectoralis minor is unable to lengthen, and it presses against these structures.

The Forearm and Hand

The forearm consists of two bones, the ulna and the radius (Fig. 7-1D). The radius is capable of rotation around the ulna at its proximal end via a ligamentous ring that joins the two bones. This ring also prevents the radius from being pulled away from the ulna by the biceps muscle as it supinates the forearm and hand and flexes the elbow. The radius and ulna are tied together by an interweaving interosseus membrane. This gives additional strength to the forearm while keeping it much lighter than if it were composed of one large bone.

The ***brachialis*** is deep to the biceps, and of the two, it is the stronger flexor of the forearm. Both muscles are opposed by the triceps, which extends the forearm. The triceps is usually much weaker than the biceps and brachialis, and it is prone to overuse injuries from actions that require repetitive flexing and straightening of the forearm (e.g., hammering). It often requires strengthening to balance movement at the elbow joint.

The hand connects to the forearm by the wrist joint, which is formed between the radius and ulna and the eight small carpal bones. The number of small gliding joints that this design creates allows great mobility and flexibility at the wrist. A unique feature of the human hand is that the thumb is opposable, meaning it is capable of touching each of the fingers. This allows for an oppositional type grip and a superior degree of control and refinement of movement.

Most of the muscles that control the hand lie along the forearm. The extensor muscles merge at the ***common extensor tendon***, which attaches on the lateral epicondyle of the humerus. The

flexor muscles merge at the ***common flexor tendon***, which attaches on the medial epicondyle of the humerus.

▶ UPPER EXTREMITY ENDANGERMENT SITES

- Brachial plexus: The brachial plexus emerges from C5-T1, and travels between the anterior and medial scalenes, under the clavicle and coracoid process, out to the axilla. Parts of the brachial plexus are vulnerable at the lateral neck, in the groove between the pectoralis major and deltoid, and in the axilla (Fig. 7-2).
- Other nerve entrapment sites

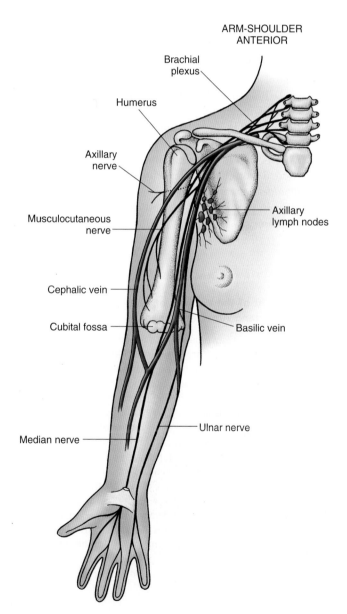

ARM-SHOULDER ANTERIOR

Brachial plexus

Humerus

Axillary nerve

Musculocutaneous nerve

Axillary lymph nodes

Cephalic vein

Cubital fossa

Basilic vein

Median nerve

Ulnar nerve

FIGURE 7-2 Endangerment sites of the upper extremity.

- The radial nerve travels down the posterior side of the arm. It is sometimes vulnerable to pressure and irritation on the back side of the humerus.
- The "funny bone" refers to the sensation of irritation to the ulnar nerve as it passes through the groove between the ulna and medial epicondyle.
- The median nerve is vulnerable in the cubital fossa at the anterior elbow.

▶ CONDITIONS

Shoulder

1. *Bursitis.* This is acute or chronic inflammation of the subacromial bursal sac, which prevents the head of the humerus from hitting the inferior aspect of the acromion process.
2. *Osteoarthritis.* This is a general term covering a broad range of joint inflammations. Osteoarthritis at the shoulder can be brought on by chronic misuse of the arm, trauma, or misalignment in the shoulder girdle.
3. *Rotator Cuff Injuries.* The muscles of the rotator cuff are frequently injured, and they often refer pain in unusual patterns, so it may be difficult for a client to tell exactly where a shoulder injury is originates.
4. *Shoulder Separation.* The source of this injury is usually a tear in the ligament that binds the clavicle and the acromion.

5. *Shoulder Dislocation.* The humerus is held in place at the glenoid fossa, mainly through ligamentous binding. It is fairly easy to knock the humerus out of the socket, which is painful and results in irritation and possible chronic stretching of the ligaments, along with painful spasm of the muscles that cross the shoulder joint.
6. *Nerve Impingement Syndromes.* When any part of the brachial plexus is irritated by mechanical pressure from a tight muscle or fascial entrapment, symptoms may affect that spot, or they may refer to the termination of the nerve. Further, any nerve that is irritated in one zone may develop edema along the entire length of the structure—which puts it at risk for entrapment at other areas as well. Nerve entrapment syndromes include thoracic outlet syndrome, carpal tunnel syndrome, pronator teres syndrome, and multiple crush syndrome.

Forearm and Hand

1. *Tennis Elbow (lateral epicondylitis).* This term describes an injury to the extensor tendon that connects the extensor muscles of the hand in a long attachment along the lateral epicondyle of the humerus.
2. *Golfer's Elbow (medial epicondylitis).* This occurs when the origin of the wrist flexors at the medial epicondyle of the humerus is irritated and possibly inflamed.

See Appendix A for more information on these conditions.

HOLISTIC VIEW

The Weight of the World is on Our Shoulders (and Arms, and Hands)

In the olden days we used yokes, a broad piece of wood with ropes or chains attached at either end for hanging buckets or bundles of some sort, to help carry heavy loads. We carried these on our neck and shoulders. Interestingly, the shape and location of the shoulder girdle is similar to an old-fashioned yoke. Although in the Western world we no longer use yokes to carry heavy loads, the shoulders themselves often continue to serve that function psychologically: In our minds and emotions, we often carry heavy loads across our shoulders.

The muscles of the shoulder girdle often reflect our concerns and worries about our ability to carry all the responsibilities and burdens that accompany us in life. It is not uncommon to see a person literally stooped over, as if weighted down by some tremendous, invisible load.

As explained previously, the position of the shoulders is dependent, perhaps more than any other joint, on muscle action. Because muscles are controlled by the nervous system, which ultimately is controlled by the mind, there is an obvious relationship between the way a person positions the shoulders and his or her beliefs and attitudes in general. An interesting experiment is to stand in front of a mirror and put your shoulders and arms into different poses. Observe how the way you feel and the image you project change based on your body posture.

Our shoulders, arms, and hands reflect how we interact with the world. The shoulders can be set back and open, or closed in and protective. Our arms can be ready to be a barrier, pushing people away, or they can draw people in with an embrace. Closed hands are unreceptive, but open hands give and receive energy in the form of stimulus, awareness, and qi. It is through the medium of the hands that healing therapeutic touch is administered. The Chinese qi gong and Indian yoga systems both refer to the existence of energy centers in the hand.

What do your shoulders, arms, and hands say about you? ■

▶ POSTURAL EVALUATION

See Figure 7-3 A–I
1. Check the position of the clavicles. How close are they to being horizontal?
2. Compare the height of the right and left shoulders. Observe the distance from the shoulder to each ear.
3. Compare the length of both arms. Where do the fingertips reach on the thigh?
4. Make note of any hollow spaces around the clavicles.
5. Have the client raise the arms to the sides. Do the arms move independently of the shoulder girdle? (They should.)
6. Note any areas of restriction or muscle tension around the shoulder girdle.
7. How do the arms hang?
   • Are the arms straight or flexed at the elbow?
   • What direction do the hands face?
   • What is the distance of the arms from the sides of the body? Is it the same on both sides?
8. From a lateral view, observe the alignment of the tip of the shoulder to the ear, hip, knee, and ankle.
9. From the posterior view, check the position of the scapulae. Are they. . .
   • Protracted?
   • Retracted?
   • Depressed?
   • Elevated?
   • Upward or downward rotation?
   • Relaxed and properly positioned?
10. Observe the condition of the musculature affecting the scapulae.

Refer to Table 7-1 for a description of common distortions of the shoulder girdle and possible muscles involved. Table 7-2 lists the muscles responsible for various actions of the upper extremity.

▶ EXERCISES AND SELF-TREATMENT

Shoulders

1. *Stretch for Pectoralis Minor and Clavicular Division of Pectoralis Major.* Standing in a doorway, extend your arms upward, and open them slightly wider than shoulder width. Placing your palms against the top of the door frame, and lean your body forward, leading with the hips and chest, until you feel a stretch in the shoulders. Hold for a few seconds as you breathe deeply into the stretch.
2. *Stretch for Anterior Deltoid and Sternal Division of Pectoralis Major.* Stand in front of a dresser or table, and face away from it. Reach your arms behind you with the elbows flexed, and place your palms on top of the flat surface,

with the fingers facing you. Squeezing your shoulder blades and elbows toward each other, slowly flex your knees, and sink down as if sitting into a chair until you feel a stretch in the shoulder area. Hold as you breathe deeply, and focus on releasing tension in the shoulders.
3. *Exercises from a Seated Position.* The following shoulder exercises may be performed from a seated position:
   • *Strengthen Upper Trapezius.* As you inhale, raise both shoulders toward your ears. Hold for a few seconds. Light weights may be held in the hands to increase resistance.
   • *Stretch for Upper Trapezius.* Exhaling, lower your shoulders slowly, feeling the tension flowing out of the muscles.
   • *Contract Rhomboids.* Inhaling, draw both shoulders back, squeezing the vertebral borders of the scapulae toward each other.
   • *Stretch for Rhomboids.* Exhaling, press the outside edges of the shoulders forward, feeling the space between the scapulae stretching.
   • *Stretch for Rotator Cuff.* Slowly circle the shoulders. Inhale for half of the circle, and exhale for half of the circle. Repeat a few times, and then reverse the direction of the circle.
4. *Stretch for Rotator Cuff Muscles, Pectoralis Major, and Latissimus Dorsi.* Lie on your side with both knees flexed. Your head may rest on the arm closest to the floor. The uppermost arm is straight and placed on the floor in front of your chest, with the palm facing downward. Slowly circle the arm around your body, tracing the circle on the floor with your fingers. As the arm moves overhead, allow it to rotate naturally so that the palm is facing upward. Pause in positions that feel tight or restricted, and imagine breathing into the shoulder. Repeat a few times, and then reverse the direction of the circle. Turn onto your other side, and repeat the entire exercise.

Arms

1. *Strengthen Biceps, Brachialis, and Triceps.* Stand facing a wall with your arms extended so that your palms are against the wall. Lean into the wall, flexing only your arms, like doing a push-up. Keep your body straight. Vary the speed of the push and the degree of lean to strengthen the arm muscles effectively. Repeat several times.

Wrists

1. *Strengthen Wrist Flexors and Extensors.* To strengthen your wrists, hold a broom handle out in front of you as if shaking hands with it. Slowly raise the broom upward

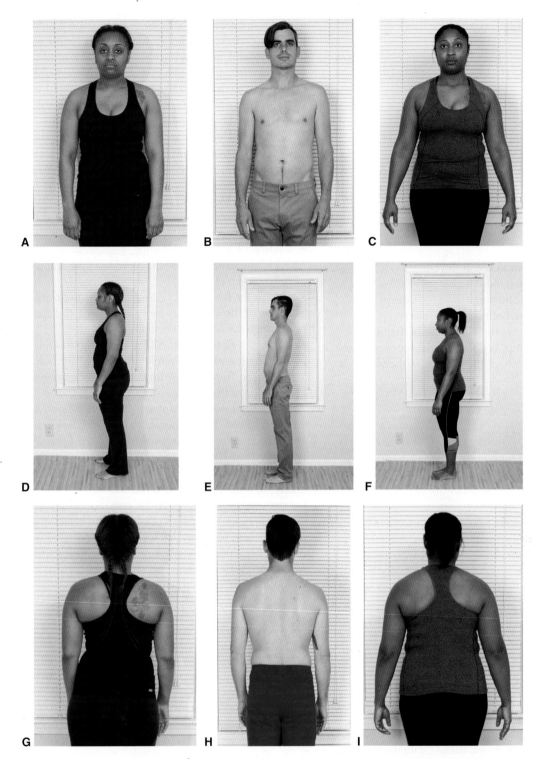

FIGURE 7-3 Postural evaluation: upper extremity.

and downward with the motion of your wrist. To work with less weight, hold the broom closer to the broom head. To use more weight, hold the broom closer to the end of the handle.

2. *Stretch for Wrist Flexors.* Sitting cross-legged on the floor, lean forward slightly from the hip joints. With your arms fully extended in front of you, place the palms on the floor with the fingers turned toward your ankles. Gently press the heel of the palm toward the floor. Hold for at least 10 seconds.

3. *Stretch for Wrist Extensors.* In the same position as above, place the back of the hands on the floor, and press down very gently until you feel a mild stretch in the back of the wrist. Hold for 5 to 10 seconds.

TABLE 7-1 | **Body Reading for the Shoulder Girdle**

Postural Patterns	Muscles That May Be Shortened
Raised shoulder(s)—one or both shoulders are elevated	Scalenes
	Upper trapezius
	Lower trapezius
Rounded shoulders—shoulders are rotated medially	Pectoralis major
	Pectoralis minor
	Anterior deltoid
	Teres major
	Serratus anterior
Retracted shoulders—shoulder blades are pulled back, scapulae winged	Rhomboids
	Trapezius
	Teres minor
	Infraspinatus
	Latissimus dorsi

TABLE 7-2 **Range of Motion (ROM) for the Shoulder and Arm**

Action	Muscles
Shoulder	
Flexion (ROM 170°)	Anterior deltoid
	Biceps brachii
	Pectoralis major
	Coracobrachialis
Extension (ROM 60°)	Posterior deltoid
	Teres major
	Latissimus dorsi
	Triceps brachii
Abduction (ROM 170°)	Supraspinatus
	Deltoids
	Biceps brachii
Adduction (ROM 50°)	Biceps brachii
	Pectoralis major
	Teres major
	Coracobrachialis
	Latissimus dorsi
	Triceps brachii
Medial rotation (ROM 70°)	Anterior deltoid
	Pectoralis major
	Subscapularis
	Teres major
	Latissimus dorsi

Action	Muscles
Lateral rotation (ROM 90°)	Infraspinatus
	Teres minor
	Posterior deltoid
Elbow	
Flexion (ROM 150°)	Biceps brachii
	Brachialis
	Brachioradialis
	Extensor carpi radialis
	Pronator teres
	Flexor carpi ulnaris
	Flexor carpi radialis
Extension (ROM 0°)	Triceps brachii
	Anconeus
Forearm	
Supination (ROM 90°)	Biceps brachii
	Brachioradialis
	Supinator
Pronation (ROM 90°)	Brachioradialis
	Pronator teres
	Pronator quadratus
Wrist	
Flexion (ROM 80°)	Flexor carpi radialis
	Flexor carpi ulnaris
Extension (ROM 70°)	Extensor carpi radialis
	Extensor carpi ulnaris

Hands

1. *Alternately Strengthen and Stretch the Muscles of the Hand.* Exhaling, squeeze the fingers and thumbs of both hands into fists. Inhaling, slowly open them all the way against resistance as if a rubber band were wrapped around the fingers.

▶ SCAPULA ROUTINE

Objectives

- To balance the scapula in relation to the clavicle and humerus
- To reduce tension in muscles affecting the scapula
- To help alleviate painful conditions in the scapular region arising from dysfunction and imbalance
- To explore movement patterns and habits that might be generating stress in the scapular muscles

Energy

POSITION

- The client is lying prone on the table. A bolster may be placed under the ankles.
- The therapist is standing at the side of the table next to the client's shoulder.

POLARITY

Contact the superior angle of the scapula with the index finger of one hand (negative pole on the hand) and the inferior angle of the scapula with the middle finger of the other hand (positive pole on the hand). Envision the scapula floating freely over the underlying ribs. Allow any subtle movements of the scapula to occur. Hold the position for 30 seconds or longer.

SHIATSU

1. Press points along the vertebral border of the scapula with the thumbs or elbow. The outer branch of the bladder channel runs slightly medial to the border of the scapula.
2. With your outside hand holding the shoulder, place the fingers of your inside hand along the lower portion of the vertebral border of the scapula near the inferior angle. The palm of your hand is facing upward. As you circle the shoulder with your outside hand, slide the fingers of your inside hand under the border of the scapula, and point them toward the shoulder joint (Fig. 7-4). Attempt this move only if the musculature feels fairly relaxed.

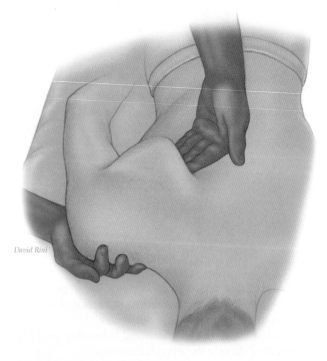

David Ritti

FIGURE 7-4 Shiatsu scapula maneuver.

Swedish/Cross Fiber

1. Use a three-stroke effleurage pattern over the scapula. Beginning at the upper thoracic region of the spine, stroke outward over the upper, middle, and lower scapular region. Alternate hands with each stroke.
2. Apply cross-fiber strokes over the upper back and shoulder area using fingertips and the broad side of the thumb.

Connective Tissue

1. In the myofascial mobilization technique, slide the muscles of the upper back, using the fingers or palms, over the scapula and ribs. Note areas that are not moving freely.
2. Apply the myofascial spreading technique to tight, unyielding musculature.

Deep Tissue/Neuromuscular Therapy

SEQUENCE

1. Trapezius (upper, middle, and lower)
2. Levator scapula (attachment)
3. Rhomboids
4. Subscapularis ▶
5. Pectoralis minor
6. Serratus anterior

Trapezius

Upper Trapezius
Origin: Medial third of the superior nuchal line and external occipital protuberance, ligamentum nuchae, and the spinal processes of C1–C5 vertebrae.
Insertion: Lateral third of the clavicle.
Action: Elevation and upward rotation of the scapula, capital extension.

Strokes
- Using the fingers, perform an elongation stroke down the posterior portion of the neck from the occiput to C7. At the base of the neck, switch to the knuckles or heel of the

Trigger points are best located using the sifting technique. Flexing the client's head in the direction of the side being examined may make palpation of the muscle fibers easier. Trigger points may be found along the border of the muscle, slightly above the lateral portion of the clavicle. Pain is referred up the posterior neck to the mastoid process. Trigger point activity in this muscle is a major source of tension headaches. Complementary trigger points may be located in the supraspinatus and levator scapulae muscles.

hand, and continue stroking outward to the acromiocla-vicular joint (Fig. 7-5).

- Sift the upper trapezius by grasping the belly of the muscle between the thumb and fingers, and roll the fibers, feeling for taut bands. Treat any trigger points that are found (Fig. 7-6).

Middle Trapezius

Origin: Interspinous ligaments and spinous processes of C6–T3 vertebrae.

Insertion: Acromion and superior lip of the spine of the scapula.

Action: Adduction (retraction) of the scapulae.

> A commonly occurring trigger point in the middle trapezius may be located on the superior edge of the spine of the scapula near the acromion process. It shoots pain to the top of the shoulder.

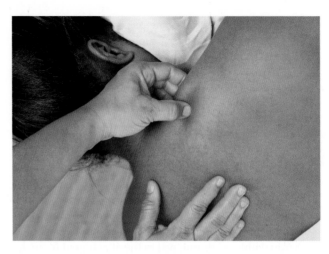

FIGURE 7-6 Sifting the upper trapezius to locate trigger points.

Strokes

- Stand at the side of the table, facing the client's shoulder that is to be treated. Perform an elongation stroke using the knuckles.
- Covering the space between T1 and T3, stroke laterally across the middle trapezius, and end on the lateral edge of the superior lip of the spine of the scapula.

Lower Trapezius

Origin: Interspinous ligaments and spinous processes of T4–T12 vertebrae.

Insertion: Tubercle on the medial end of the spine of the scapula.

Action: Depression and upward rotation of the scapula.

> The lateral border of the middle and lower trapezius should be examined carefully for trigger points. Trigger points in these muscles are best located by rubbing the fibers over the underlying ribs.

Strokes

- Stand at the side of the table, and face toward the client's head. Perform a series of elongation strokes using the forearm. Beginning at T4, stroke diagonally upward to the medial end of the spine of the scapula.
- Repeat the stroke, covering the muscles in strips. The final stroke begins at T12. Cover the muscle completely (Fig. 7-7).

Levator Scapula (Insertion)

Origin: Posterior tubercles of the transverse processes of C1–C4 vertebrae.

Insertion: Vertebral border of the scapula between the superior angle and the root of the spine.

Action: Elevation and adduction of the scapula, rotation causing the lateral angle to move downward.

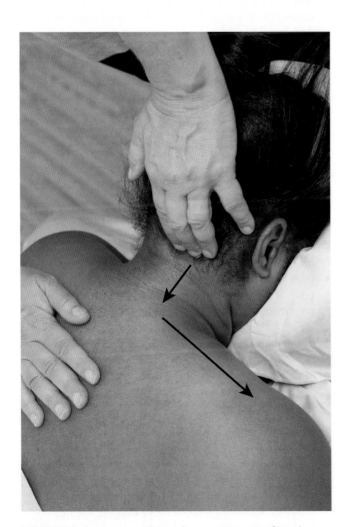

FIGURE 7-5 Elongation stroke on the upper trapezius from the occiput to the acromion process.

To find a trigger point, palpate the fibers slightly lateral to the superior angle (0.5 inch). This trigger point is one of the most common, and it is usually very tender. It refers pain to the surrounding area of the neck.

Strokes

- Sit or stand at the head of the table. The client's arm is flexed at the elbow, with the palm resting against the table next to the shoulder. Using your outside hand, hold the client's elbow. Place the thumb of your other hand against the inferior end of the edge of the superior angle of the scapula.
- Draw the client's arm toward the head of the table. This lifts the superior angle of the scapula. Apply cross-fiber strokes with your thumb pad to the attachment of the levator scapula, just inferior to the superior angle, palpating the tendon for tenderness (Fig. 7-8).

Rhomboids

Rhomboid Minor

Origin: Ligamentum nuchae and spinous processes of C7–T1 vertebrae.
Insertion: Medial border of the scapula at the root of the spine.
Action: Adduction of the scapula; elevation of the scapula; rotates the scapula so that the lateral angle faces downward.

Rhomboid Major

Origin: Supraspinous ligament and spinous processes of T2–T5 vertebrae.
Insertion: Medial border of the scapula below the root of the spine.

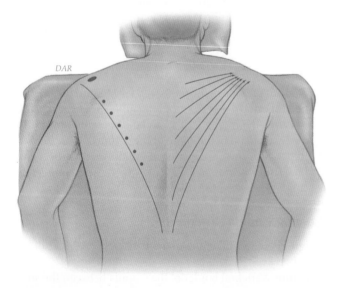

FIGURE 7-7 Elongation strokes on the middle and lower trapezius from origins (T1–T12) to insertion (spine of the scapula).

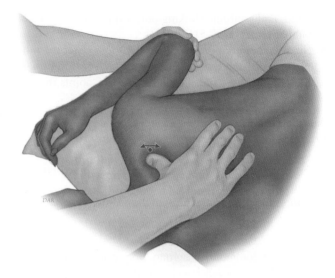

FIGURE 7-8 Cross-fiber stroke on the insertion of the levator scapula (superior angle of the scapula).

Action: Adduction of the scapula; elevation of the scapula; rotates the scapula so that the lateral angle faces downward.

To locate trigger points, check just medial to the vertebral border of the scapula. The pain pattern for these trigger points is local, along the edge of the scapula.

Strokes

- Using thumbs or elbow, do short, up-and-down strokes along the origin of the rhomboids at the sides of the spinous processes of C7–T5 (Fig. 7-9A).
- Perform an elongation stroke with the knuckles along the belly of the muscle, from the upper thoracic spine to the vertebral border of the scapula (Fig. 7-9B). Cover the area from C7–T5.
- Face the client's scapula from the opposite side of the table. The scapula may be raised by placing the client's forearm across the back or by sliding a folded towel under the shoulder of the arm being massaged. Using the thumbs or an elbow, do short, up-and-down strokes on the insertion of the rhomboids (Fig. 7-9C) along the vertebral border of the scapula. Address any trigger points that are found.

Subscapularis

Origin: Subscapular fossa along axillary margin of the anterior surface of the scapula.
Insertion: Lesser tuberosity of the humerus and anterior capsule of the shoulder joint.
Action: Medial rotation of the shoulder; stabilizes the shoulder (glenohumeral) joint by keeping the head of the humerus in the glenoid fossa.

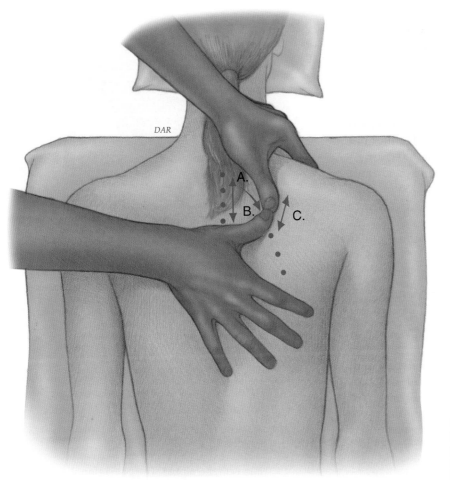

FIGURE 7-9 Strokes on the rhomboids. **A.** Medial attachment (C7–T5). **B.** Belly (spinous processes to the vertebral border of the scapula). **C.** Lateral attachment (vertebral border of the scapula).

Position
- The client is resting in side posture, with the bottom leg extended and the top leg flexed 90° at the hip and knee. A bolster is placed under the knee. A small pillow or folded towel may be placed under the side of the head.
- The therapist is standing behind the client at shoulder level.

> The lateral fibers are the most likely to contain trigger points. These trigger points send pain into the posterior part of the shoulder and, sometimes, down the arm.

Strokes
- To reach the muscle on the client's right side, place the fingers of your right hand on the ribs just in front of the medial side of the scapula, with your left hand grasping the client's upper forearm near the elbow. Pull the client's arm upward to protract the scapula, exposing more of the medial surface (Fig. 7-10). Reverse hand positions for the left side.
- Move the fingers posteriorly along the ribs until the anterior surface of the scapula is felt. Apply short, side-to-side strokes with the fingers along the bone, seeking out tender areas.

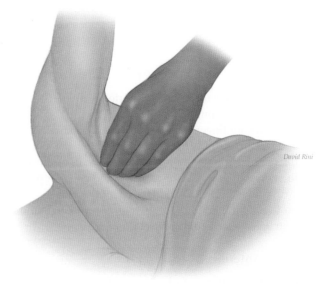

FIGURE 7-10 Contacting the subscapularis along the lateral anterior surface of the scapula.

These fibers often have painful spots, so move slowly, and elicit client feedback often.

⚠ Move slowly, and stay close to the edge of the scapula. The axilla contains several arteries and nerves that are not well protected by muscle, including the axillary, brachial, and cephalic arteries and nerves of the brachial plexus.

- This muscle can also be treated with the client supine. The humerus is abducted 90°, with the forearm flexed 90°. Slide your fingers posteriorly along the ribs until the medial surface of the scapula is felt. Slowly press the fingers into the front side of the scapula, and apply short, side-to-side and up-and-down strokes to treat the subscapularis muscle.

Pectoralis Minor

Origin: Upper and outer surfaces of ribs 3–5.
Insertion: Coracoid process of the scapula.
Action: Protraction of the scapula (moves the scapula forward, with a downward tilt); elevation of the ribs in forced inhalation, with the scapulae fixed.

Position
- The client's top arm rests over a bolster placed in front of the chest.
- The therapist stands behind the client at chest level.

◎ Trigger points will most likely be found in the section of the pectoralis minor that attaches to rib 5. This is the easiest portion of the muscle to palpate. The referral zone is the anterior deltoid. When trigger points are found in this muscle, complementary trigger points almost always are located in the pectoralis major.

Strokes
- To relax the pectoralis major, perform circular friction with the fingers on the muscle.
- Position your fingers under the pectoralis major muscle, and palpate the ribs (Fig. 7-11). Slide along the length of the muscle, from its origins on ribs 3–5 to its insertion on the coracoid process. Move slowly, and pause at painful areas with static pressure. Lift the client's arm that is resting on the bolster, and hold it in your nonworking hand to gain better access to the muscle.

Serratus Anterior

Origin: Outer surfaces of ribs 1 to 8 or 9.
Insertion: Anterior (costal) surface of the vertebral border of the scapula.
Action: Abduction (protraction) of the scapula; upward rotation of the scapula; fixes the medial border of the scapula to the thoracic wall.

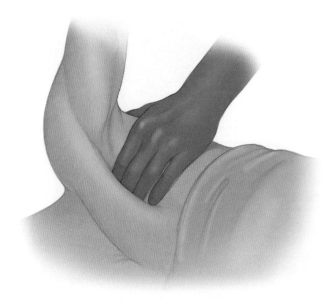

FIGURE 7-11 Reaching the pectoralis minor from underneath the pectoralis major.

Position
- The client's top arm rests on a bolster placed in front of the chest or is extended overhead.
- The therapist stands behind the client.

◎ Examine the section of the muscle that lies over the fifth and sixth ribs, in an approximate line with the nipple. The pain referral zone is surrounding the trigger point. Expect much tenderness in this muscle, even when trigger points are not present.

Strokes
- Use the heel of the hand over the side of the chest when applying pressure during massage strokes.
- Perform an elongation stroke with the heel of the hand from the axillary border of the scapula to the muscle's insertion on the ribs (ribs 1–8). Repeat the stroke several times to cover the entire muscle.
- Perform short, up-and-down and side-to-side strokes on the fibers of the muscle over the ribs (Fig. 7-12).
- Pause to treat trigger points.

STRETCH

Position

- The client is supine.
- The therapist stands at the side of the table facing the client's shoulder.
  1. Hold the client's arm on the upper forearm, just below the elbow. Place the client's arm perpendicular to the table, with the forearm at a right angle to the humerus and facing across the client's chest (Fig. 7-13).

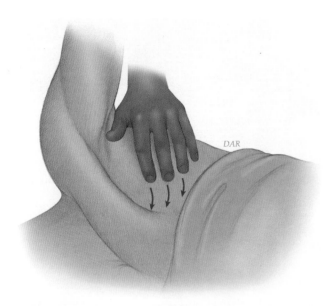

FIGURE 7-12 Contacting the serratus anterior over ribs 1–8.

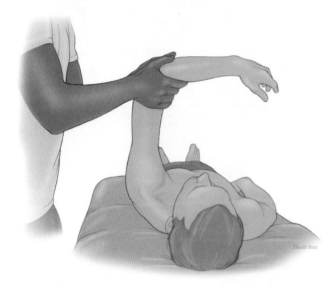

FIGURE 7-13 Stretch for the scapular muscles.

2. Pull up on the arm, protracting the scapula. The humerus may be adducted to stretch the scapular muscles.

ACCESSORY WORK

1. Shiatsu in the chest region (fingertip compression in the intercostal spaces).
2. Trigger point work on the pectoralis major muscle.
3. Circumduction of the arm in both directions.

CLOSING

Sitting at the foot of the table, lightly hold the heels of the client's feet in your hands for 30 to 60 seconds. Remove your hands slowly to complete the session.

▶ SHOULDER AND UPPER ARM ROUTINE

Objectives

- To relieve muscular pulls that may be causing misalignment of the shoulder
- To achieve full range of motion of the humerus in the shoulder joint
- To reduce stress caused by poor posture and movement
- To reduce or eliminate pain resulting from soft tissue damage/dysfunction

Energy

POSITION

- The client is lying supine on the table, with his or her arms at the sides of the body.
- The therapist is standing at the side of the table next to the client's shoulder.

POLARITY

Place the right palm (positive pole) on the posterior side (negative pole) of the shoulder joint; place the left palm (negative pole) on the anterior side (positive pole) of the shoulder joint. Align the two hands along the vertical axis that passes through the center of the shoulder joint. Sense any subtle movements or adjustments that occur in the shoulder, and allow your hands to follow them. Hold for 1 minute or longer.

SHIATSU

Wrap the hands around the upper arm at the shoulder. Compress the arm, and roll it slightly medially, from the shoulder to the wrist (Fig. 7-14). This procedure stimulates the yin channels (lung, pericardium, and heart) and the yang channels (large intestine, triple heater, and small intestine) of the arm.

Swedish/Cross Fiber

1. Perform effleurage strokes on the arm, from the wrist to the shoulder.
2. Perform petrissage strokes from the elbow to the shoulder.
3. Perform circular friction with the heel of hand on the shoulder area.

Connective Tissue

MYOFASCIAL SPREAD

Place the client's upper arm slightly away from the body. Wrap your hands around the upper arm, just above the elbow, with

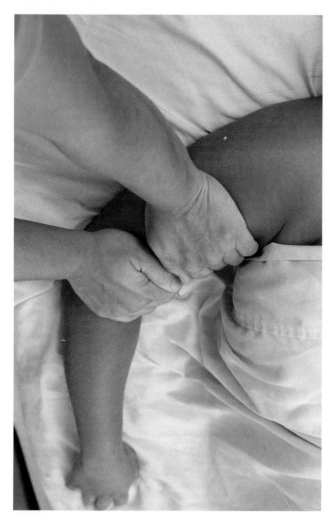

FIGURE 7-14 Shiatsu compression of the upper arm.

the base of the palms at the midline of the arm. Slowly slide the palms apart as the fascia softens, spreading the tissues of the arm with the heels of the hand. Continue, in horizontal strips, to the top of the shoulder.

Deep Tissue/Neuromuscular Therapy

POSITION

- The shoulder sequence is performed with the client in side posture. Place a pillow between the client's knees and a small support under the side of the client's head. The top arm rests along the client's side.
- The therapist stands at the head of the table and cups both hands around the client's shoulder (Fig. 7-15).

SEQUENCE

1. Deltoid
2. Supraspinatus
3. Infraspinatus

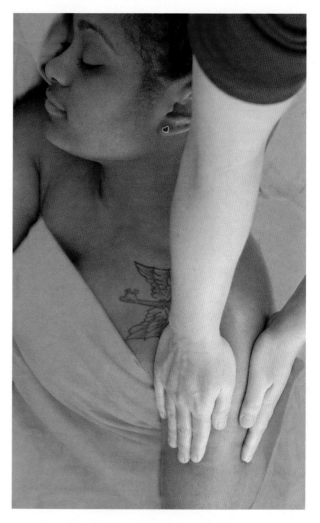

FIGURE 7-15 Beginning hand position for deep tissue massage of the deltoids (posterior, medial, and anterior).

4. Teres minor
5. Teres major and latissimus dorsi
6. Triceps brachii
7. Biceps brachii
8. Brachialis

Deltoids

Posterior Deltoid

Origin: Lower lip of the posterior border of the spine of the scapula.

Insertion: Deltoid tuberosity on the lateral midshaft of the humerus.

Action: Extension and lateral rotation of the humerus.

> To locate trigger points, check along the posterior portion near the border of the muscle. The referral zone is throughout the posterior deltoid and, sometimes, down the arm.

Strokes

- Apply elongation strokes with the knuckles or the heel of the hand from the inferior border of the spine of the scapula to the deltoid tuberosity on the humerus. The hand on the front of the shoulder provides stability and support.
- To palpate trigger points, stand behind the client's shoulder. Grasp the shoulder using both hands, with the fingers in front and the thumb tips touching each other at the level of the posterior deltoid (Fig. 7-16). Perform short, back-and-forth and side-to-side strokes along the entire length of the muscle to seek taut bands.

Medial Deltoid

Origin: Lateral border of the acromion process.
Insertion: Deltoid tuberosity on the lateral midshaft of the humerus.
Action: Abduction of the humerus.

> This section of the deltoid does not develop trigger points as commonly as the other two deltoid sections do. Trigger points may be found in the upper portion, just below the acromion.

Strokes

- Stand at the head of the table, and cup both hands around the shoulder. Using the knuckles or the heel of the hand, stroke down the middle of the upper humerus, from the acromion process to the deltoid tuberosity.
- To palpate trigger points, the hands should remain cupped around the shoulder, with the sides of the thumbs touching. Perform short, back-and-forth and side-to-side strokes along the entire length of the muscle, from the acromion to the deltoid tuberosity (Fig. 7-17).

Anterior Deltoid

Origin: Anterior surface of the lateral third of the clavicle.
Insertion: Deltoid tuberosity on the lateral midshaft of the humerus.
Action: Flexion and medial rotation of the humerus.

> Check for trigger points in the front portion of the muscle, high up, where the muscle covers the head of the humerus. Pain can refer over the anterior and medial deltoid and down the arm.

Strokes

- Apply elongation strokes with the heel of the hand, from the lateral third of the clavicle to the deltoid tuberosity.
- To palpate trigger points, stand in front of the client's shoulder. Grasp the shoulder using both hands, with the fingers wrapped around the back and the thumb tips touching in front, over the anterior deltoid (Fig. 7-18). Perform the techniques to search for trigger points over the entire length of the muscle.

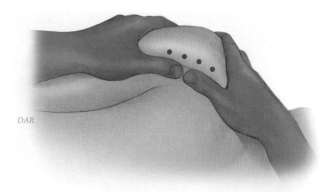

FIGURE 7-16 Locating trigger points in the posterior deltoid along the medial border.

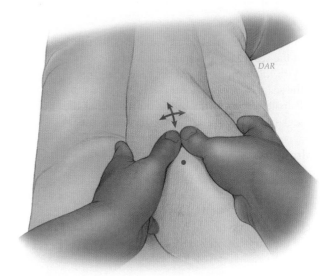

FIGURE 7-17 Locating trigger points in the medial deltoid.

Supraspinatus

Origin: Supraspinous fossa of the scapula.
Insertion: Superior facet of the greater tuberosity of the humerus, capsule of the shoulder joint.
Action: Abduction of the shoulder; stabilizes the head of the humerus in the shoulder joint.

Position

- Stand at the head of the table, and face the client's shoulder. Cup your hands around the shoulder near the base of the neck. The thumbs are placed against the superior border of the spine of the scapula, with one thumb on top of the other to reinforce it.

> Search for trigger points along the superior border of the spine of the scapula. These trigger points refer pain into the medial deltoid and down the side of the arm. A trigger point is often located in the space between the clavicle and scapula, just before they meet at the acromioclavicular joint. The pain referral zone is over the deltoid.

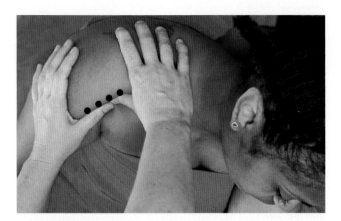

FIGURE 7-18 Locating trigger points in the anterior deltoid beginning along the anterior border.

Strokes

- Perform an elongation stroke along the superior border of the scapula to the acromioclavicular joint (Fig. 7-19). With the thumbs placed slightly superior to the spine of the scapula, repeat the stroke.
- Palpate trigger points in the muscle using the strokes to seek trigger points. Treat any that are found.

Infraspinatus

Origin: Infraspinous fossa of the scapula.
Insertion: Middle facet of the greater tuberosity of the humerus, capsule of the shoulder joint.
Action: Lateral rotation of the shoulder; stabilizes the head of the humerus in the shoulder joint.

> Trigger points tend to accumulate readily in this muscle. Pay close attention to the fibers that run about 0.5 inch below the spine of the scapula. These trigger points refer pain to the deltoid and down the arm. Another trigger point is found about halfway down the vertebral border of the scapula; it refers pain along the medial edge of the scapula.

Strokes

- Using the knuckles or elbow, perform an elongation stroke, from the vertebral border of the scapula to the head of the humerus. The stroke is repeated several times, in strips, over the body of the scapula to cover the entire muscle. Place your nonworking hand on the front of the client's shoulder to provide stability (Fig. 7-20).
- A bolster can be placed in front of the client's chest to prevent the upper body from rolling forward when pressure is applied to the infraspinatus muscle.
- To locate trigger points more effectively, turn the client to the prone position, with the upper arm abducted 90° and the forearm hanging off the table. Use thumb strokes to palpate and treat trigger points.

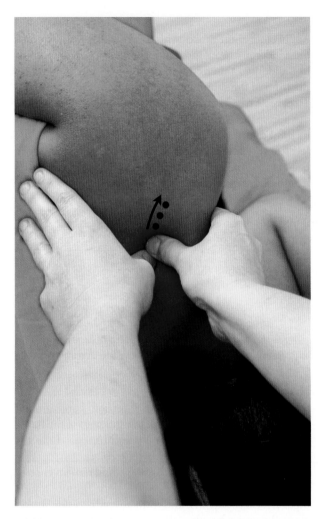

FIGURE 7-19 Elongation stroke on the supraspinatus from origin to insertion.

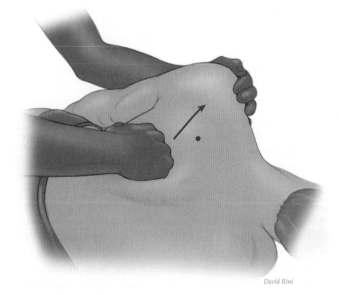

David Rini

FIGURE 7-20 Elongation stroke on the infraspinatus from origin to insertion.

Teres Minor

Origin: Upper two-thirds of the dorsal surface of the axillary border of the scapula.

Insertion: Lowest facet of the greater tuberosity of the humerus, capsule of the shoulder joint.

Action: Lateral rotation of the humerus; weak adduction of the shoulder; stabilizes the humeral head in the shoulder joint.

Position

- The client is lying in side posture, with the side to be treated uppermost.
- The therapist stands at the side of the table, behind the client's shoulder. If treating the right side of the client, the therapist's right thumb is placed along the axillary border of the scapula, and the left thumb is over the top of the client's right shoulder. (When working on the left side, hand positions are reversed.)

 Teres minor is often clear of trigger points. Trigger points are more likely to form in its synergist, the infraspinatus.

Strokes

- Beginning with the thumb one-third of the way up along the axillary border, stroke along the edge of the bone, following the muscle fibers out to the head of the humerus (Fig. 7-21).
- Pause at tender areas, and treat.

Teres Major and Latissimus Dorsi

Teres Major

Origin: Dorsal surface of the scapula near the lateral side of the inferior angle.

Insertion: Medial lip of the bicipital groove of the humerus.

Action: Medial rotation, adduction, and extension of the arm.

Easily confused in palpation with the latissimus dorsi, the teres major is closer to the border of the scapula and more medial. Trigger points are usually close to the scapular border. The pain referral zone is over the posterior deltoid and the long head of the triceps.

Latissimus Dorsi

Origin: Spinous processes of T6–T12 vertebrae, spinous processes of L1–L5 vertebrae and sacral vertebrae, supraspinal ligament, posterior one-third of the iliac crest of the ilium, ribs 9–12, inferior angle of the scapula.

Insertion: Floor of bicipital groove of the humerus.

Action: Extension, adduction, and medial rotation of the arm (most powerful when arm is in the overhead position); active in strong inspiration and expiration.

When using the sifting technique, the latissimus dorsi is the most superficial muscle that is felt. Check the upper portion, particularly near the posterior deltoid. This trigger point, which is found in the axillary fold, refers pain to the midback region.

Strokes

- Standing behind the client's shoulder, grasp the muscles along the posterior border of the axilla, with your thumbs on the surface and your fingers underneath, in the axilla.
- Sift the muscle fibers thoroughly, and feel for taut bands and adhered tissues (Fig. 7-22). Treat any trigger points that are found.

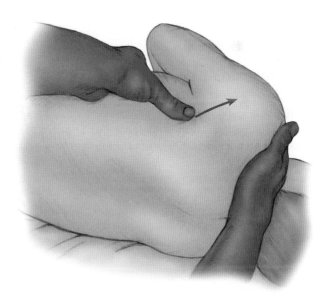

FIGURE 7-21 Elongation stroke on the teres minor from origin to insertion.

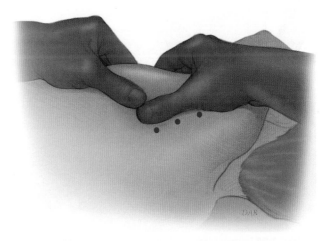

FIGURE 7-22 Sifting the latissimus dorsi and teres major.

STRETCH

The client is in side posture. Lift the client's arm overhead so that the upper arm is resting along the ear, with the forearm flexed. Holding the arm near the elbow, rotate the humerus medially, and allow the forearm and hand to hang off the back of the table (Fig. 7-23). If further stretch is needed, press down on the humerus until an adequate stretch is felt.

Triceps Brachii

Origin:
  Long head—infraglenoid tuberosity of the scapula.
  Lateral head—upper half of the posterior shaft of the humerus.
  Medial head—lower half of the posterior shaft of the humerus.
Insertion: Posterior surface of the olecranon process of the ulna.
Action: Extension of the forearm; when the arm is abducted, the long head aids in adduction.

Position
- The client is placed in prone position. The arm to be worked on is abducted 90°, with the forearm hanging off the side of the table.
- The therapist is standing at the side of the table, next to the client's shoulder.

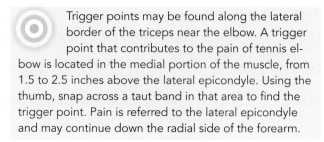

Trigger points may be found along the lateral border of the triceps near the elbow. A trigger point that contributes to the pain of tennis elbow is located in the medial portion of the muscle, from 1.5 to 2.5 inches above the lateral epicondyle. Using the thumb, snap across a taut band in that area to find the trigger point. Pain is referred to the lateral epicondyle and may continue down the radial side of the forearm.

Strokes
- Using the heel of the hand or knuckles, apply elongation strokes from the elbow to the head of the humerus.
- With the thumbs, stroke up the middle of the triceps, between the heads of the muscle (Fig. 7-24).
- Grasp the edges of the triceps between the thumb and fingers. Lift the muscle away from the bone and squeeze. Check for trigger points along its length.

Biceps Brachii

Origin:
  Short head—apex of the coracoid process of the scapula.
  Long head—supraglenoid tubercle of the scapula.
Insertion: Radial tuberosity of the radius, bicipital aponeurosis fusing with the deep fascia over the forearm flexors.
Action: Flexion and supination of the forearm; weak flexion of the arm at the shoulder joint when the forearm is fixed.

Position
- The client is placed in the supine position. The arm to be treated is resting, with the palm supinated, on the table next to the client's side.
- The therapist is standing at the head of the table, superior to the client's shoulder.

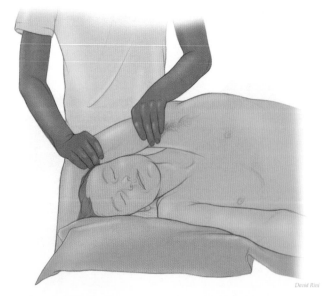

FIGURE 7-23 Stretch for the teres major and minor, latissimus dorsi, and subscapularis.

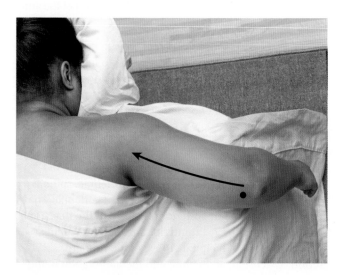

FIGURE 7-24 Direction of strokes on the triceps from the insertion (olecranon process) to origin (upper portion of the humerus).

The lower third of the biceps brachii may contain a trigger point in each head. They may refer pain throughout the biceps and upward into the anterior deltoid. These trigger points are most easily palpated by stretching the biceps fibers. Hold the client's arm at the wrist, and extend it slightly off the table, keeping the forearm fully extended. With your other hand, feel for taut bands in the biceps muscle.

Strokes

- Using the heel of the hand or the knuckles, apply elongation strokes from the elbow to the shoulder joint.
- With the thumbs, stroke up the center of the biceps, between the two heads (Fig. 7-25).
- Grasp the edges of the biceps, between the fingers and thumb. Lift the muscle away from the bone, and squeeze. Check for trigger points along its length.

Brachialis

Origin: Lower two-thirds of the anterior shaft of the humerus.
Insertion: Tuberosity and coronoid process of the ulna.
Action: Flexion of the forearm.

Position

- The client is supine, with the arm to be worked on flexed at the elbow about 45°.
- The therapist stands at the side of the table and holds the wrist of the flexed arm.

 Trigger points are usually located in the distal portion of the brachialis, near the elbow. They refer pain chiefly to the base of the thumb.

Strokes

- The brachialis muscle is deep to the biceps. To reach it, slide your fingers under the biceps brachii muscle, on the medial side of the humerus, about halfway down the upper arm (Fig. 7-26).
- Do the side-to-side stroke, with your fingers along the muscle fibers to the elbow, allowing the muscle to lengthen and relax.

STRETCH

Position

- The client is lying supine.
- The therapist is standing at the head of the table.
1. *Triceps.* Lift the client's arm overhead, with the humerus next to the ear and the forearm hanging over the end of the table. Holding the humerus near the elbow, press the arm toward the table while the client flexes the forearm further by reaching the palm toward the underside of the table (Fig. 7-27).

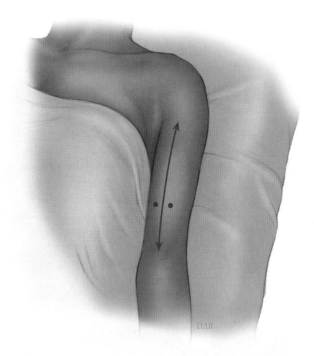

FIGURE 7-25 Direction of strokes on the biceps from insertion (tuberosity of the radius) to origin (coracoid process of the scapula).

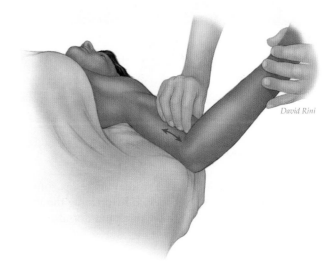

FIGURE 7-26 Contacting the brachialis deep to the biceps brachii.

2. *Biceps and Brachialis.* The client slides to the edge of the table. Bring the client's straight arm off the side of the table, and holding at the wrist, extend it downward, toward the floor, as the client reaches down and back with the hand (Fig. 7-28).

ACCESSORY WORK

1. Circumduct the shoulder, hip, and ankle joints on both sides of the body to help balance the muscles acting on the joints.

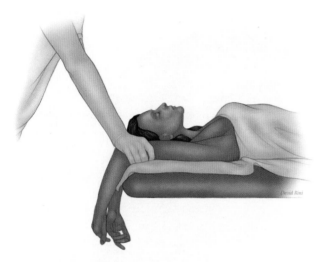

FIGURE 7-27 Stretch for the triceps brachii.

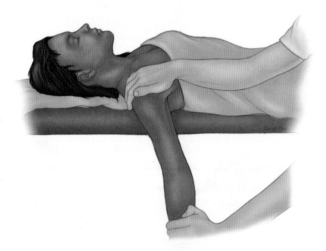

FIGURE 7-28 Stretch for the biceps brachii.

2. Reflexology tradition suggests that the reflex zone for the shoulders may be accessed by pressing the metacarpal heads between the plantar and dorsal surfaces (Fig. 7-29).

CLOSING

Sitting at the foot of the table, lightly hold the heels of the client's feet in your hands for 30 to 60 seconds. Remove your hands slowly to complete the session.

▶ FOREARM AND HAND ROUTINE

Objectives

- To reduce stress and pain in the muscles of the forearm and hand brought about by extended use of the hand in work-related and other activities

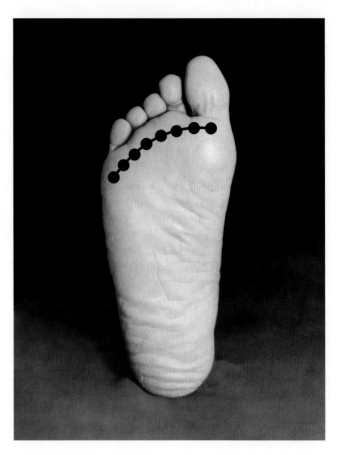

FIGURE 7-29 Reflex zone for the shoulder.

- To improve dexterity and coordination skills of the hand
- To promote general relaxation through hand massage

Energy

POSITION

- The client is lying supine, with the arms to his or her sides.
- The therapist stands at the side of the table and faces the client's forearm.

POLARITY

Lightly contact the wrist and elbow with the palms of the hands. Envision the forearm lengthening and relaxing. Hold for at least 30 seconds.

SHIATSU

1. With both hands, grasping the client's forearm just below the elbow joint, and compress the forearm from the elbow to the wrist. This move stimulates the same meridians as the upper arm shiatsu procedure.
2. Flex the client's forearm 90°. Interlace your fingers with your client's fingers. Holding the client's forearm slightly

inferior to the wrist with your other hand, flex, extend, and circumduct the hand in both directions (Fig. 7-30). Opening up the wrist area stimulates the flow of energy (qi) through the arm channels.

Swedish/Cross Fiber

1. Perform effleurage strokes from the wrist to the elbow.
2. Perform thumb gliding on the palm and the back of the hand.
3. Perform petrissage strokes on the muscles of the forearm.
4. Perform cross-fiber strokes with the broad side of the thumb on the hand and forearm muscles.

Connective Tissue

MYOFASCIAL SPREAD

1. Grasping both sides of the client's hand, curve your fingers, and press them into the center of the palm. Slowly slide the fingers of each hand away from each other, stretching the tissues of the palm.
2. Flex the client's forearm 90° at the elbow. Place your hands around the forearm at the wrist, with the fingers sinking into the midline of the palmar side of the forearm. Slowly spread the fingers away from the midline, stretching the fascia. Continue, in horizontal strips, to the elbow. Repeat on the other side of the forearm.

Deep Tissue/Neuromuscular Therapy

SEQUENCE

1. Palm—superficial muscles, lumbricals, interossei

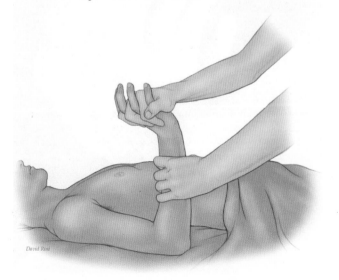

FIGURE 7-30 Hand position for performing shiatsu wrist movements.

2. Thenar eminence—adductor pollicis brevis, flexor pollicis brevis, opponens pollicis
3. Fingers—digital flexors and extensors, ligaments, retinacula
4. Dorsal surface of the hand—extensor digitorum tendon, interossei
5. Wrist—flexor tendons and retinaculum, extensor tendons and retinaculum, pronator quadratus
6. Forearm
   a. Anterior surface—pronator teres, flexor carpi radialis, palmaris longus, flexor carpi ulnaris, flexor digitorum superficialis, flexor pollicis longus, flexor digitorum profundus, and brachioradialis.
   b. Dorsal surface—extensor carpi radialis longus, extensor carpi radialis brevis, extensor carpi ulnaris, extensor digitorum, extensor digiti minimi, supinator, abductor pollicis longus, extensor pollicis brevis, extensor pollicis longus, and extensor indicis.
7. Elbow
   a. Lateral epicondyle—attachments of extensor carpi radialis longus and brevis, extensor digitorum, and supinator.
   b. Medial epicondyle—attachments of the common flexor tendon, brachialis, and pronator teres.

THE PALM

Position

- The client is lying supine, with the arm to his or her side and the palm supinated.
- The therapist is standing at the side of the table, next to the client's hand.

Interossei Muscles

Palmar
Origin:
　　First—entire ulnar side of second metacarpal
　　Second—entire radial side of fourth metacarpal
　　Third—entire radial side of fifth metacarpal
Insertion:
　　First—index finger at base of proximal phalanx on ulnar side
　　Second—ring finger at base of proximal phalanx on radial side
　　Third—entire radial side of fifth metacarpal
Action: Adduction of index, ring, and pinkie fingers toward middle finger

Dorsal
Origin:
　　First—lateral head: first metacarpal of thumb on proximal half of ulnar border, medial head: second metacarpal of index finger on entire radial border

Second—adjacent sides of metacarpals of index and middle fingers

Third—adjacent sides of middle and ring fingers

Fourth—adjacent sides of metacarpals of ring and pinkie fingers

Insertion:

First—radial side of index finger at base of proximal phalanx

Second—radial side of proximal phalanx of middle finger

Third—ulnar side of proximal phalanx of middle finger

Fourth—ulnar side of proximal phalanx of ring finger

Action: Abduction of fingers away from middle finger

> To locate trigger points, have the client spread the fingers wide apart to separate the metacarpal bones. Using your thumb and index finger, squeeze the spaces between the bones. Nodules are often found around active trigger points in these muscles. Pain usually refers into the finger of the adjacent tendon.

Strokes

- Perform an elongating stroke with the fist, lengthwise, from the base of the palm to the fingers, and then horizontally across the palm, from the pinkie side to the thumb side (Fig. 7-31).
- For the lumbricals, perform an elongating stroke along the sides of the finger tendons using the thumbs or tip of the index finger (Fig. 7-32).

Muscles of the Thenar Eminence

Adductor Pollicis Brevis, Flexor Pollicis Brevis, and Opponens Pollicis

Strokes

- Using your thumbs, apply up-and-down and side-to-side strokes over the mound, checking for tenderness and taut bands (Fig. 7-33).

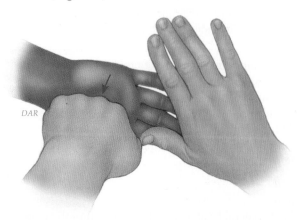

FIGURE 7-31 Elongation stroke from the fifth metatarsal to the first metatarsal.

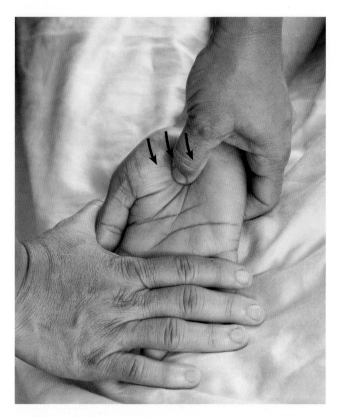

FIGURE 7-32 Contacting the lumbrical muscles between the finger tendons.

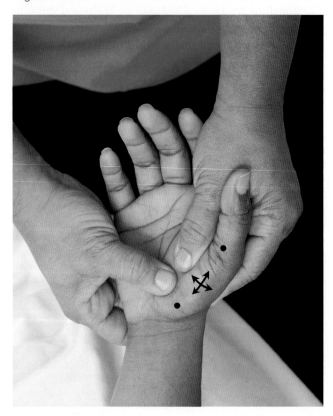

FIGURE 7-33 Deep tissue strokes on the thenar eminence.

Adductor Pollicis

Origin:
    Oblique head—bases of second and third meta carpals, capitate, trapezoid.
    Transverse—distal two-thirds of the palmar side of the third metacarpal.
Insertion: Base of the thumb at the ulnar side of the proximal phalanx.
Action: Adduction of the thumb.

> Trigger points may be located in this muscle by squeezing the webbing between the thumb and index finger. The referral zone is on the thumb, particularly on the lower outside edge near the wrist.

Flexor Pollicis Brevis

Origin: Flexor retinaculum and trapezium, first metacarpal bone.
Insertion: Base of the proximal phalanx of the thumb.
Action: Flexion of the metacarpophalangeal joint of the thumb.

> Place the tip of your thumb against the head of the metacarpal bone. As the client flexes the thumb several times, feel for the tendon, and press. The referral zone is local, around the trigger point.

Opponens Pollicis

Origin: Flexor retinaculum, tubercle of the trapezium.
Insertion: Entire radial side of the first metacarpal bone.
Action: Draws the first metacarpal bone forward and medial, bringing the thumb into opposition to the other fingers.

> Using the thumb tip, roll across the muscle fibers on the thenar eminence, feeling for taut bands and tenderness. Pain is referred to the inside portion of the thumb and to a spot on the radial side of the wrist.

Fingers

Preparation
Begin the following sequence at the base of the proximal phalanx of the thumb. Continue to the tip of the thumb, and then repeat, sequentially, on each of the four fingers.

Strokes
- Grasp the digit with the tip of the thumb on one side and the tip of the index finger on the other side. Alternately move the thumb and index finger up and down along the sides of the bone between the joints.
- Repeat the stroke, grasping the front and back of the bone.

Dorsal Surface of the Hand

Strokes
- Apply the fanning stroke with the thumbs over the entire dorsal surface of the hand.
- Perform short, up-and-down strokes with the tip of the index finger on the interosseus muscles between the tendons of the extensor digitorum muscle (Fig. 7-34).

Wrist (Tendons of Flexor and Extensor Muscles of Fingers)

Strokes
- Apply the fanning stroke, with the thumbs on the palmar and dorsal surfaces of the wrist (Fig. 7-35A).
- With the sides of your thumbs touching, do short, up-and-down and side-to-side strokes on the palmar and dorsal surfaces of the wrist (Fig. 7-35B).

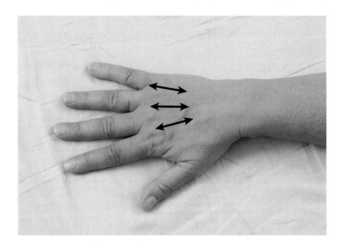

FIGURE 7-34 Direction of strokes on the dorsal interossei.

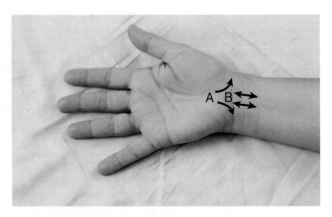

FIGURE 7-35 A. Fanning and **B.** Up-and-down strokes on the tendons of the finger flexor muscles at the wrist.

Forearm

Hand and Finger Extensor Muscles

Trigger points will lodge in the distal portion of the muscles, near the elbow. Pain is referred to the lateral epicondyle and down the forearm to the wrist and hand area.

Hand and Finger Flexor Muscles

Trigger points tend to be located in a line across the muscles, about one-third of the way down the forearm from the elbow. They are best palpated with cross-fiber strokes, feeling for taut bands in the fibers. They refer pain to the wrist and into the fingers.

Strokes

- Using the knuckles, perform elongation strokes from the wrist to the elbow (Fig. 7-34A). Work in strips, with the palm supinated and then pronated, to cover the forearm thoroughly.
- Separate the muscles of the forearm by stroking between them with a thumb, knuckle, or elbow (Fig. 7-36B).
- Using the thumbs or the elbows, perform short, up-and-down and side-to-side strokes on the bellies of the muscles (Fig. 7-36C). Treat areas of tenderness and trigger points.
- Turn the client's forearm so that the thumb side of the hand is up. Grasp the brachioradialis muscle between the thumb and fingers, on the forearm, below the lateral epicondyle of the elbow. Roll the muscle fibers, checking for tenderness and trigger point activity (Fig. 7-37).

Elbow

Supinator

Origin: Lateral epicondyle of the humerus, radial collateral ligament of the elbow joint, annular ligament of the radioulnar joint, supinator crest of the ulna on the dorsal surface of the shaft.

Insertion: Dorsal and medial surfaces of the upper one-third of the radial shaft.

Action: Supination of the forearm and hand.

 A trigger point may be located near its attachment on the lateral epicondyle. The referral zone is the lateral epicondyle. Pain may also shoot to the webbing of the thumb.

Pronator Teres

Origin:

> **Humeral head**—distal supracondylar ridge, medial epicondyle of the humerus.
> **Ulnar head**—coronoid process of the medial ulna.

Insertion: Pronator tuberosity on the lateral surface of the radius.

Action: Pronation and flexion of the forearm.

The median nerve travels between the heads of the pronator teres. Entrapment here can cause symptoms that mimic carpal tunnel syndrome.

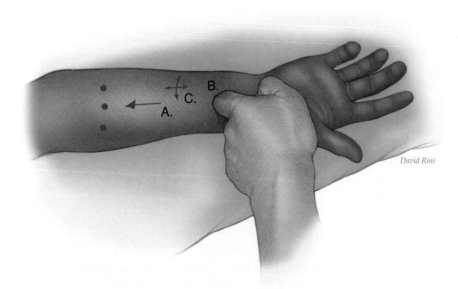

David Rini

FIGURE 7-36 Location and direction of strokes on the hand and finger flexor muscles along the forearm.

A trigger point may be located near its attachment on the medial epicondyle. Pain is felt deep in the radial side of the wrist and may spill over into the forearm.

Strokes

- With the thumb, apply up-and-down, side-to-side, and static-compression strokes around the lateral epicondyle. Treat the attachments of the extensor carpi radialis longus and brevis, extensor digitorum, and supinator muscles (Fig. 7-38). Having the client extend the hand makes these tendons easier to palpate.

Because of the close proximity of the radial nerve, be careful when treating these attachments. If the client experiences a sharp, radiating sensation that is characteristic of nerve stimulation, release the pressure immediately, and shift the location of your thumb.

- With the thumb, apply up-and-down, side-to-side, and static-compression strokes around the medial epicondyle. Treat the attachments of the common flexor tendon, brachialis, and pronator teres muscles. Having the client flex his or her hand makes these tendons easier to palpate. Because of the position of the median nerve at the medial epicondyle, use the same caution as above.

STRETCH

1. With both hands facing each other in front of him or her, the client cups the palms and spreads all the fingers. Touching the tips of the fingers of both hands together, the client begins to push the hands toward each other, keeping the fingers apart and resisting somewhat with the cupped palms. The client continues to press the hands toward each other until a stretch is felt in the fingers and palms. The stretch is held for a minimum of 10 seconds.
2. Place your palm across the palmar surface of the client's fingers, and extend the client's hand until a stretch is felt in the flexor muscles of the fingers and hand (Fig. 7-39).

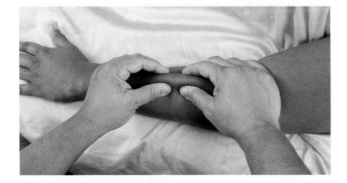

FIGURE 7-37 Rolling the fibers of the brachioradialis muscle.

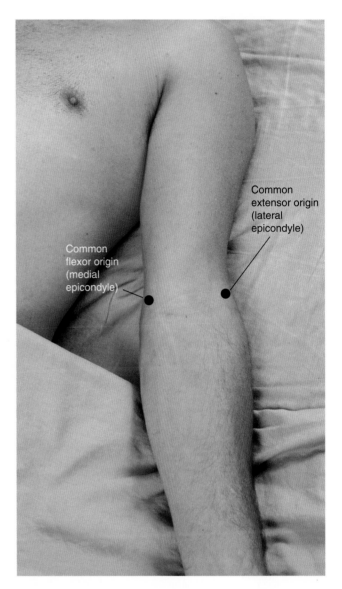

FIGURE 7-38 Location of the forearm muscle attachments.

Common flexor origin (medial epicondyle)

Common extensor origin (lateral epicondyle)

(This and the following stretch are more effective if the client's arm is kept fully straight.)
3. Place your palm across the dorsal surface of the client's fingers, and flex the client's hand until a stretch is felt in the extensor muscles of the fingers and hand (Fig. 7-40).

ACCESSORY WORK

1. "Snapping off" the fingers (a shiatsu technique) will help to draw off accumulated energy that has built up from release of the hand and forearm muscles. An indication of this build-up is sweaty hands. To perform the move, hold the anterior and posterior sides of the client's finger at the base between your index and middle fingers. Gently slide down the finger, gliding straight off at the

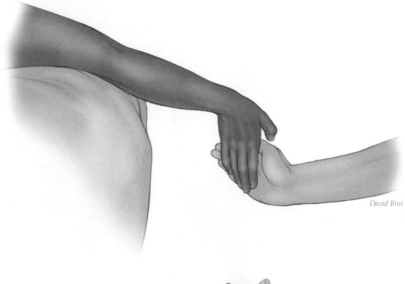

David Rini

FIGURE 7-39 Stretch for the flexor muscles of the fingers and hand.

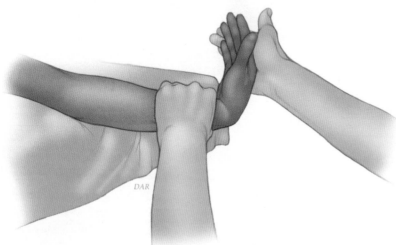

DAR

FIGURE 7-40 Stretch for the extensor muscles of the fingers and hand.

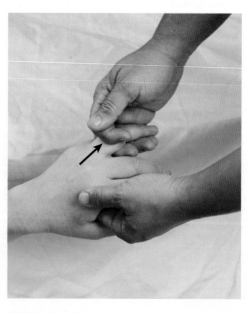

FIGURE 7-41 The shiatsu technique, "snapping off."

tip (Fig. 7-41). Begin with the thumb, and continue with each finger in succession to the pinkie.

2. A thorough foot massage is a good accompaniment to hand and forearm work. It gives the client a sense of integration between the upper and lower extremities.

CLOSING

Sitting at the foot of the table, lightly hold the heels of the client's feet in your hands for 30 to 60 seconds. Remove your hands slowly to complete the session.

SESSION IMPRESSION

THE SHOULDERS AND ARMS

The client is a 43-year-old massage therapist named Doris. She has been practicing massage therapy professionally for 10 years. For the past several months, she has been experiencing tightness and pain in her neck, shoulders, and upper back. The tightness is exacerbated by giving a massage. During the previous 2 weeks, she has begun to experience sharp pains in her right forearm muscles. It is becoming increasingly difficult for her to administer pressure with her right arm; the pain in her forearm becomes intense when she pushes with her right hand.

Doris is a frail-looking woman. She is small-boned and does not have well-developed musculature. She is somewhat stooped over, with a slight kyphosis in her upper back. Her scapulae are protracted, with her arms medially rotated and her upper chest collapsed. She also exhibits a forward position of the head. Based on observing her posture and listening to her describe her situation, it is likely that she may lack the body mechanics skills that she needs for her job. She probably tries to push too much with her arm and back muscles, rather than leaning forward and distributing force throughout her entire body, when applying pressure during massage strokes.

This and future deep tissue sessions will focus on releasing the muscles of the scapulae and relieving tension in the neck, around the clavicles, in the serratus anterior and pectoralis minor muscles, and throughout the muscles of the forearms and hands. She will require a series of integrated deep tissue therapy sessions to address all the problems arising from her posture and lack of proper body mechanics.

Because of the protraction of the scapulae, collapse of the chest, and medial rotation of the arms, her serratus anterior, pectoralis major and minor, and anterior deltoid muscles were emphasized during the first session. Numerous trigger points were encountered, particularly in the lateral section of the pectoralis minor. Working on the right forearm, the common extensor tendon was found to be very tender and perhaps inflamed. It was recommended that the client apply ice to it regularly. The borders of the forearm muscles were carefully traced and separated. The client found that the degree of mobility in both hands was greatly increased following the session. The muscles of the thenar eminence were tender on both hands, but on the right side in particular.

After the session, the likelihood that she is favoring her right arm and hand while performing massage was discussed. Doris is also overusing her arm and hand muscles to apply pressure instead of allowing the weight of her body to flow through her. It was suggested that she diminish her workload of massage clients until the strain in her muscles from incorrect body mechanics is reduced. In addition to receiving deep tissue therapy treatments twice a week for the next month, she is going to engage in daily stretching of the chest, shoulder, arm, and hand muscles. She will also receive coaching in proper body mechanics. Once the initial trauma to the upper body muscles is reduced and better alignment of the shoulder girdle achieved, she will begin a very mild weight-training program to build strength and acquire more kinesthetic awareness of her entire body. ∎

Topics for Discussion

1. Based on the client in the case above, describe some specific exercises that would help to counteract muscular weaknesses and postural distortions.

2. What suggestions regarding body mechanics would you offer to a muscular, male massage therapist who relies exclusively on his strong shoulder and arm muscles to perform massage strokes?

3. Describe the position and movement capacities of well-aligned shoulders and arms in relation to the rest of the body.

4. How would you treat a client who describes difficulty gripping the steering wheel while driving?

REVIEW QUESTIONS

Level 1

Receive and Respond

1. The pectoral girdle includes the. . .
   a. sternum, clavicles, and scapulae.
   b. scapula and humerus.
   c. clavicle, humerus, and scapula.
   d. clavicle and scapula.

2. Where does the shoulder articulate with the axial skeleton?
   a. At the spinoscapular joints
   b. At the glenohumeral joints
   c. At the sternoclavicular joints
   d. At the claviculohumeral joints

3. What is the best description of the glenohumeral joint capsule?
   a. Loose, allowing wide range of motion at the shoulder
   b. Supported by internal cruciate ligaments to stabilize the humerus
   c. Tight, giving important support to the humerus
   d. Supported by external collateral ligaments to stabilize the humerus

4. Which is the strongest flexor of the forearm?
   a. Flexor carpi radialis
   b. Brachialis
   c. Biceps brachii
   d. Flexor palmaris

5. The "funny bone" refers to what endangerment site?
   a. The median nerve at the cubital fossa
   b. The brachial plexus at the lateral neck
   c. The radial nerve at the posterior aspect of the triceps
   d. The ulnar nerve at the medial epicondyle of the humerus

Level 2

Apply Concepts

1. If a client has rounded shoulders, what muscles are likely to be shortened?
   a. Pectoralis major, pectoralis minor, anterior deltoid
   b. Rhomboids, trapezius, latissimus dorsi
   c. Subscapularis, teres minor, infraspinatus
   d. Posterior deltoid, rhomboids, pectoralis major

2. What is the best table position from which to stretch the teres major and minor, latissimus dorsi, and subscapularis?
   a. Supine, arm abducted
   b. Prone, arm abducted
   c. Side-lying, arm abducted
   d. Side-lying, arm adducted across the body

3. What stroke is most effective for finding and treating trigger points in the superior trapezius?
   a. Shiatsu scapula release
   b. Sifting the upper trapezius
   c. Elongation strokes from the occiput to the acromion process
   d. Cross-fiber stroke at the superior angle of the scapula

4. How would you recommend that a client strengthen her triceps?
   a. Teach her how to do modified push-ups, using the wall and varying her angle and speed to increase resistance
   b. Teach her how to do modified pull-ups, using surgical tubing or an elastic exercise band looped around a doorknob for resistance
   c. Encourage her to walk briskly while carrying light weights to help tone her arms
   d. Encourage her to visit a gym where a qualified trainer can assist with her strength-training goals

5. What is the recommended sequence for working with the shoulder?
   a. From a prone position, work with the latissimus dorsi, then deltoid, then trapezius, then supraspinatus
   b. From a side-lying position, work with the deltoid, then supraspinatus, infraspinatus, then teres minor and latissimus dorsi
   c. From a side-lying position, work with the latissimus dorsi, then the teres major, then teres minor, then trapezius
   d. From a prone position, work with the trapezius, then supraspinatus, then deltoid, then brachialis

Level 3

Problem Solving: Discussion Points

1. Amelia is a 22-year-old childcare provider. She works long days with lots of bending and lifting, and she frequently carries heavy bags in each hand. She complains of wrist and shoulder pain. Bruce is a 55-year-old man who works at a desk, using a computer and mouse for many hours each day. He also complains of shoulder and wrist pain. Use the routines described in this chapter to design a treatment plan for each client. While each session will have elements in common, what differences in approach do you predict each client will need?

2. Read the *Session Impressions* piece for the client named Doris. Choose one of the "Topics for Discussion" and work through the question with a classmate. How can you avoid some of Doris's problems in your career as a massage therapist?

Establishing a Firm Foundation

LEARNING OBJECTIVES

Having completed the reading, classroom instruction, and assigned homework related to Chapter 8 of *The Balanced Body*, the learner is expected to be able to. . .

- Apply key terms and concepts related to integrated deep tissue therapy as related to the foot, leg, and knee
- Identify anatomical features of the foot, leg, and knee, including
  - Bony landmarks
  - Muscular and fascial structures
  - Endangerments or cautionary sites
- Identify common postural or movement patterns associated with pain or impaired function of the foot, leg, and knee
- Use positioning and bolstering strategies that provide safety and comfort for clients to receive integrated deep tissue therapy to the foot, leg, and knee

- Generate within-scope recommendations for client self-care relevant to the foot, leg, and knee
- Safely and effectively perform the integrated deep tissue therapy routines as described
- Organize a single session to address the foot, leg, and knee, using the integrated deep tissue therapy approach, customized to individual clients
- Plan a series of sessions to address whole-body incorporation using the integrated deep tissue therapy approach, customized to individual clients

The Foot, Leg, and Knee

❱ GENERAL CONCEPTS

The legs and feet are responsible for efficiently transferring weight from the upper body to the ground with minimal stress. They are also the locomotive structures of the body, providing the means for its movement through space. To perform the multiple tasks of weight transfer and movement, the knees and feet are necessarily complex in design. A balance of muscle, tendon, bone, and ligament in the lower extremity is essential to enable its effective operation without breakdown. Integrated deep tissue therapy in this region seeks to re-establish the precise integration of muscle action with correct bony alignment. Lack of harmony among these body parts results in tension and instability throughout the rest of the body.

The feet form a horizontal platform on which the entire weight of the vertical body rests. The feet are small in proportion to the load they carry, which can create problems for effective weight distribution and support. This dilemma is solved by a series of arches that are located throughout the feet. Architecturally, the arch is used to distribute weight evenly from a smaller, concentrated area over a broad surface. In the case

of the feet, the body forms a vertical column whose weight is focused at the ankle joints and then spread out through the feet and transferred to the ground.

When the body's weight is optimally balanced on the foot, it radiates out from the talus through the bones of the foot. This distribution of weight can be observed in the symmetrical shape of a footprint in the sand. If the arches break down or don't function correctly, the body's weight is more concentrated on the outside or the inside of the foot. This causes a distortion in the footprint and uneven wearing down of the soles of the shoes, which compounds the problem by reinforcing poor weight distribution through the foot. Whether the initial breakdown occurs in the foot itself or further up in the body, it results in a redistribution of weight throughout the body segments in an effort to compensate for the lack of balance. This creates stress and pain around joints, particularly the knee, and loss of full function in the muscles.

The arches of the foot are supported and stabilized by muscles of the lower leg, which attach in various places along the bottom of the foot. These muscles pull up on the plantar surface of the foot, acting as guy wires that suspend the arches from above. Ineffective support of the foot through muscular weakness is evident in legs that lack shape and proportion. Abnormal thickening in the legs denotes lack of fluid flow. This can be a sign of a systemic problem with fluid management like heart or kidney disorders, but it could also be the result of the inefficient pumping action of muscles with poor tone. As effective patterns of action are taught to the leg muscles through integrated deep tissue therapy, diminished arches may be strengthened and raised. This re-education of the foot and leg muscles results in better-coordinated action throughout the body.

The joints of the legs are meant to operate in a relay fashion. In other words, the hip, knee, and ankle should all flex together and extend together during most leg movements. Although these three joints are not all technically hinges, they can be thought of in that way when working as a unit. They work best when they are aligned directly over each other in flexion movements, with the hinge at each joint forming a horizontal platform in relation to the vertical standing body. This alignment allows the muscles of the leg to store power when the joints flex, as in a preparation to jump, and to release that power effectively when the joints extend. Deep tissue work can help to restore this balanced alignment.

▶ MUSCULOSKELETAL ANATOMY AND FUNCTION

See Essential Anatomy Box 8-1 for a summary of musculoskeletal anatomy and function.

The Foot

The ankle and foot should be thought of as a unit, because their functions are interdependent. Structurally, they are similar to the wrist and hand, and they are potentially capable of many of the same movements. The foot is organized as a series of arches that are meant to distribute weight. The foot also acts as a springboard to push the body away from the ground and propel it through space. To accomplish these functions, the foot must be both strong and mobile. It is composed of 26 bones, 31 joints, and 20 intrinsic muscles (Fig. 8-1). The bones of the foot are connected by a series of more than 100 ligaments. These ligaments reinforce the arches and limit movement at the joints so that the foot can maintain its integrity.

The foot has three major arches. The medial longitudinal arch is largely responsible for pushing the foot forward in walking and running. It is made up of the inner portion of the calcaneus, the talus, the navicular, the three cuneiforms, and the first three metatarsals and phalanges. The lateral longitudinal arch is more weight-bearing and weight-distributing. It supports the inner arch by supplying lift and balance, and it is formed by the calcaneus, the cuboid, and the fourth and fifth metatarsals and phalanges. When the outer longitudinal arch is collapsed, the weight of the body is thrown too much onto the outer portion of the foot, the balance of the lower limb is lost, and the risk of lateral ankle injuries increases. The third arch comprises a series of transverse arches across the foot. They are formed by the relationship of the tarsal and metatarsal bones with the surrounding muscles and ligaments.

All the arches of the foot depend on ligamentous support and strong muscular stability. The majority of these muscles have long attachments on the tibia or fibula, providing powerful points of leverage. The long and short plantar ligaments are crucial in maintaining the shape of the arches. They connect the bones that form the ends of the longitudinal arches, like the string of a bow, and prevent them from sliding too far apart when weight is placed on the foot.

The superficial intrinsic muscles on the plantar surface of the foot are the *extensor hallucis brevis*, *abductor hallucis*, *flexor digitorum brevis*, and *abductor digiti minimi*

BOX 8-1 ESSENTIAL ANATOMY | **The Foot, Leg, and Knee Routines**

MUSCLES
Toe tendons
Insertion points of flexor hallucis longus, flexor hallucis brevis, and abductor hallucis
Muscles of the plantar surface of the foot
Muscles of the dorsal surface of the foot
Ankle retinaculum
Flexor digitorum longus
Lateral leg muscles—tibialis anterior, extensor hallucis longus, extensor digitorum longus, and peroneals
Gastrocnemius
Soleus
Knee—ligaments and tendons

BONES AND LANDMARKS
Bones of the foot—phalanges, metatarsals, cuneiforms, cuboid, navicular, talus
Tibia
Lateral malleolus
Medial malleolus
Tibial tuberosity
Fibula
Head of fibula
Patella

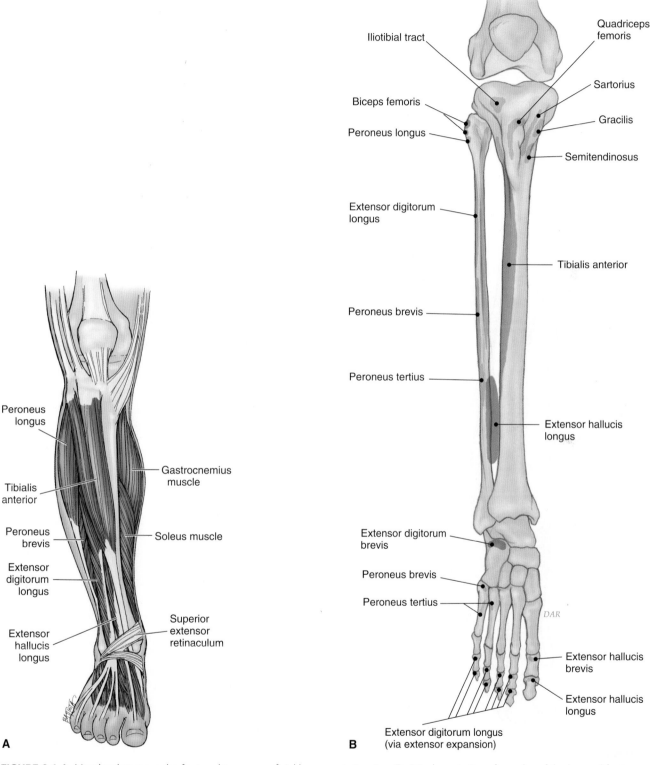

FIGURE 8-1 A. Muscles that move the foot and toes, superficial layer—anterior view. **B.** Attachment sites of muscles of the leg and foot—anterior view. **C.** Muscles that move the foot and toes, superficial layer—posterior view. **D.** Attachment sites of muscles of the leg and foot—posterior view. **E.** Third layer of muscles on the plantar surface of the foot. **F.** Attachment sites of muscles on the plantar surface of the foot.

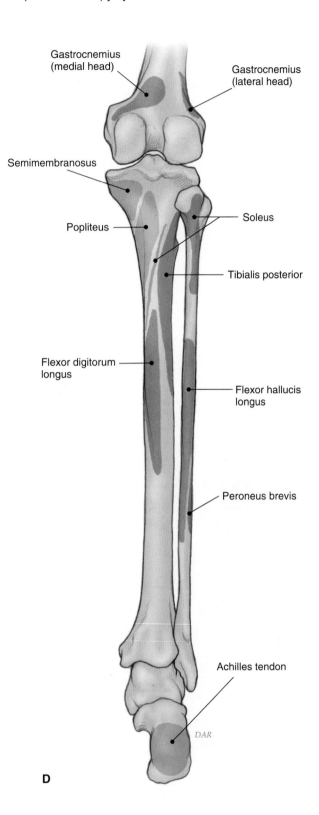

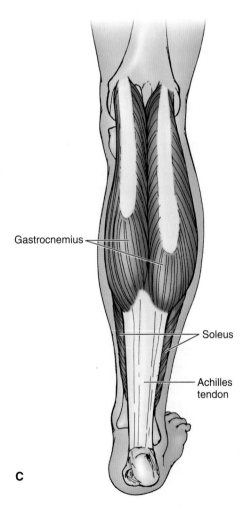

C

D

FIGURE 8-1 (*continued*)

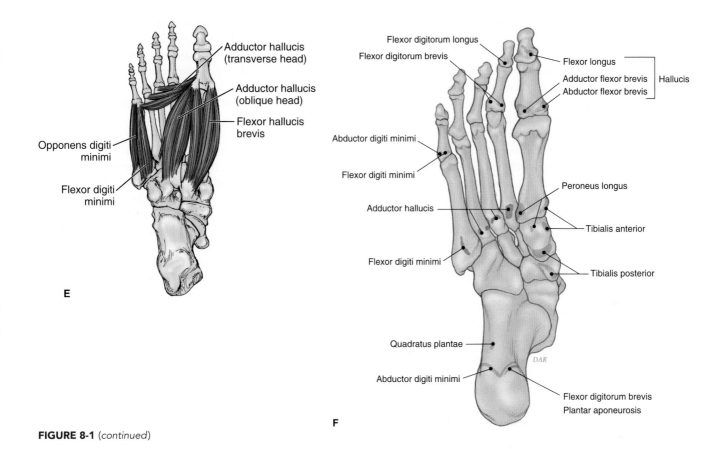

E

F

Adductor hallucis (transverse head)

Adductor hallucis (oblique head)

Flexor hallucis brevis

Opponens digiti minimi

Flexor digiti minimi

Flexor digitorum longus

Flexor digitorum brevis

Flexor longus

Adductor flexor brevis — Hallucis

Abductor flexor brevis

Abductor digiti minimi

Flexor digiti minimi

Adductor hallucis

Peroneus longus

Tibialis anterior

Flexor digiti minimi

Tibialis posterior

Quadratus plantae

DAR

Abductor digiti minimi

Flexor digitorum brevis
Plantar aponeurosis

FIGURE 8-1 (continued)

(Fig. 8-1B). The only intrinsic muscle on the dorsal surface of the foot is the extensor digitorum brevis. Overall, these muscles serve to stabilize the foot when a person is balancing on one leg, and they are used in walking and running. Flexor digitorum brevis is responsible for clutching actions of the foot, where the toe joints are flexed and the person appears to be grasping the ground with the feet. This stance is indicative of tension and instability higher up in the body. Sore feet and pain when walking may indicate the presence of trigger points in the intrinsic foot muscles.

The deep intrinsic muscles consist of the **quadratus plantae** and **lumbricals**, **flexor hallucis brevis**, **adductor hallucis**, **flexor digiti minimi brevis**, and the **interossei** (Fig. 8-1E). Their primary function is to align and stabilize the bones of the foot during propulsion. They guide and move the toes, providing a balanced pulling action on the bones so that the foot tracks forward properly, with the toes not spread too far apart or overlapping each other. Restricted movement or hypermobility of the toes, as well as calluses on them, may indicate tension in the deep intrinsic muscles.

The Ankle

The ankle joint consists of the articulation of the tibia over the talus bone. The medial malleolus, which is a projection

of the tibia, and the lateral malleolus at the lower end of the fibula form the sides of a cavity that fits over the talus, creating a pure hinge joint.

The talus articulates with the calcaneus bone below it, transferring weight to the calcaneus from the tibia and forming another joint capable of inversion and eversion (the lifting and lowering of the medial side of the foot). This joint is extremely important in maintaining the integrity of the foot, because the strength of the arches is largely dependent on the position of the calcaneus. When the calcaneus slides out to the side from underneath the talus, it causes the inner arch to fall and the tibia to rotate medially. In the case of an abnormally high medial arch, the calcaneus has pulled inward under the talus, decreasing the length of the foot and throwing weight to the outside of the foot. An overly high arch inhibits flexibility in the foot, causing the ankle to become looser, because it has to accommodate adjustments that normally would be made by a more flexible foot.

The Leg

The bones of the leg are the tibia and fibula. The tibia supports more weight than the femur, yet the tibia is smaller. The fibula, which is not a weight-bearing bone, attaches to the tibia via an interosseus membrane. It reinforces the tibia, giving increased elasticity and flexibility to the leg, and it provides attachment points for important muscles of the lower extremity.

Several muscles control movements of the foot but have their origins on various places on the leg (Fig. 8-1B). The **extensor hallucis longus** extends and dorsiflexes the big toe and foot, while the **extensor digitorum longus** extends the other four toes. Both muscles help to prevent the entire foot from dropping hard against the ground during walking.

The **flexor hallucis longus** flexes the big toe and dorsiflexes the ankle. It also inverts the foot, and assists support of the medial arch. The **flexor digitorum longus** flexes the four toes and dorsiflexes the ankle, and also provides support for the arches. Both muscles provide stability when a person is standing on tiptoe.

The **tibialis anterior** is the strongest dorsiflexor of the foot, and it also inverts the foot (Fig. 8-1A). It is highly active during running and jumping movements. Attaching on the base of the first metatarsal bone and the medial cuneiform, the tibialis anterior supports the medial arch. Overuse of this muscle is one of the primary causes of shin splints. Regular stretching of the gastrocnemius and soleus, the antagonist muscles on the back of the leg, helps to keep tibialis anterior in proper balance.

The **peroneus longus** and **peroneus brevis** are responsible for plantar flexion, eversion of the foot, and support of the lateral arch (Fig. 8-1A). They oppose the tibialis anterior in their actions. The coordinated action between these muscles is crucial in preventing sideways rolling of the foot.

The **gastrocnemius** crosses both the ankle and knee joints (Fig. 8-1C). When the knee is extended or slightly flexed, it is a strong plantarflexor of the ankle. This muscle also flexes the knee, and when the knee is flexed the gastrocnemius can medially rotate the knee. When the knee is flexed, the gastrocnemius is too slack to be effective in plantarflexion.

The **soleus** is deep to the gastrocnemius. The two muscles act as a unit in their action at the ankle, merging at the Achilles tendon. The soleus attaches broadly on the posterior tibia and fibula.

The Knee

The articulation of the tibia and femur forms the knee joint. The two convex condyles of the femur fit into the two concave condyles of the tibia, allowing flexion, extension, and slight rotation movements at the beginning of flexion because of the uneven size of the condyles. The femur moves on the tibia with a combination of rolling and gliding movements. It is prevented from sliding off the tibia through the reinforcement of cartilage, muscles, and ligaments.

Four ligaments reinforce each knee joint. The anterior and posterior cruciate ligaments make an "x" shape within the joint capsule, and the lateral and medial collateral ligaments connect the femur to the lower leg outside the joint capsule.

Two other structures, the menisci, are crescent moon-shaped shallow cups made of cartilage that are located at the top of the tibia. They provide cushioning, even distribution of weight, and shock absorption between the femur and tibia.

The patella is a small, triangular-shaped bone in front of the knee joint that is held within the quadriceps tendon. It protects the knee, and it provides greater leverage for the action of the quadriceps muscle by acting as a pulley. The patellar cartilage contacts the femoral cartilage when the knee is bent.

Twelve muscles directly affect movement at each knee. Eight of them affect both the knee and another joint: the hamstring group (biceps femoris, semimembranosus, and semitendinosus), the rectus femoris, sartorius, and gracilis all act on both the knee and hip, while gastrocnemius and plantaris act on both the knee and the ankle. The "vastus" group (v. medialis, intermedius and lateralis), along with popliteus cross only the knee joint and have no action at the hip or ankle. All these muscles need to be balanced and coordinated for proper function of the hip, knee and ankle to occur, and all of these muscles should be examined in conjunction with the muscles controlling the hip and the arches of the foot to assure stress-free movements of the knee.

▶ LOWER EXTREMITY ENDANGERMENT SITES

- *Popliteal fossa:* The posterior aspect of the knee houses the popliteal vein and artery, and the tibial nerve (an extension of the sciatic nerve). The small saphenous vein runs between the heads of the gastrocnemius. These structures are somewhat protected when the knee is extended, but when the knee is flexed, as it is when the ankles are supported by a bolster, they are easier to access, so this area must be treated with some caution (Fig. 8-2).
- *Medial lower leg:* The great saphenous vein and saphenous nerve run along the medial aspect of the tibia. The great saphenous vein is often affected with varicosities, and is a site of possible clot formation (Fig. 8-3).
- *Lateral lower leg:* The fibular nerve is accessible just posterior to the head of the fibula. Deep work here can cause nerve pain that radiates into the foot (Fig. 8-4).

▶ CONDITIONS

Feet and Ankles

1. *Pes planus* describes a fallen arch. This can be a result of congenital ligament problems, but it may also have a muscular component. A person with fallen arches may benefit from work on the fibularis muscles, and exercises that strengthen the medial flexors of the lower leg, e.g., picking up marbles with the toes.

POSTERIOR LEG

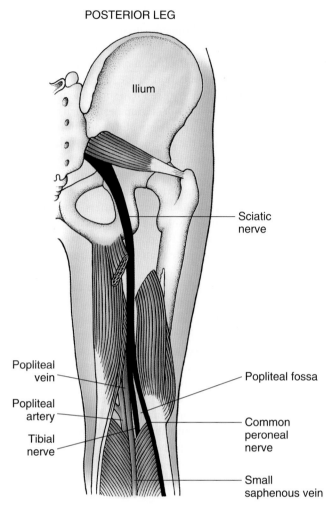

FIGURE 8-2 Endangerment sites at the popliteal fossa.

MEDIAL LEG

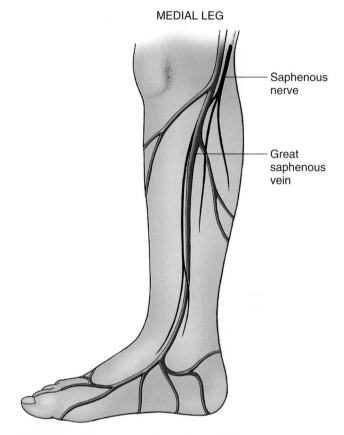

FIGURE 8-3 Endangerment sites at the medial leg.

2. *Callus* is a thickening of the epidermis. It indicates strain or wear on that section of the foot, resulting from misalignment or improperly fitted shoes. Reducing tension in the muscles that pull the toes or metatarsal out of position may help to slow callus growth, or to reduce callus accumulation.

3. *Bunions* occur where the metatarsal-phalangeal joint is distorted. This happens most often at the great toe, where the phalanges are pushed laterally. It can also happen at the little toe, where the phalanges are pushed medially. In either location, the bursae that protect the outside of the joints become inflamed and painful, and thick callus may grow over the area, causing a large bump. Bunions may be a congenital problem, but they are also related to wearing shoes that cause the ball of the foot to be the primary weight-bearing surface, along with a narrow toe box: high heels or cowboy boots. Bunions are easily exacerbated by deep massage and movement, so any touch in this area must avoid these irritations.

4. *Hammertoe* and other toe distortions (claw toe, mallet toe, curly toe) describe situations where the balance between toe extensors and toe flexors is lost. The tendons in the phalanges become permanently shortened and rigid, and their fascial wrappings shrink to fit. This can affect both gait and posture. While massage therapy may be able to prevent or slow this process, it may not be able to reverse it. Massage may help with pain-producing compensations in the rest of the body, however.

5. *Morton neuroma* is a thickening of the fascial wrapping around the common digital nerves of the toes. It is often seen with the other foot problems described here. A person with Morton neuroma has sharp, electrical pain from the ball of the foot into the toes, usually between the 3rd and 4th phalanges, each time he or she steps off. Deep massage therapy in the foot with an emphasis on creating more space between the metatarsals may help with Morton neuroma, but any massage that creates symptoms must be halted.

6. *Plantar warts* are warts that grow on the plantar surface of the foot. They can be painful, and cause people to limp. It is important to differentiate callus from plantar warts, which sometimes look similar. Callus appears only at the site of wear, but plantar warts may develop anywhere on the sole of the foot. Clients should be advised to have a doctor remove plantar warts, because cutting or filing at them may cause them to spread, which contributes to walking pain and movement distortion.

LATERAL LEG

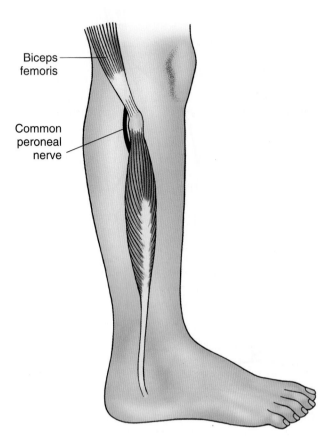

Biceps femoris

Common peroneal nerve

FIGURE 8-4 Endangerment sites at the lateral leg.

may be subject to slight tearing when overused or fatigued, resulting in pain and inflammation. The most common version of this is called medial tibial stress syndrome, and it involves the soleus attachment on the tibia. Treatment consists of rest, application of ice, and massage. Left untreated, shin splints may result in stress fractures to the tibia: this is a frequent result of "running through the pain."

2. *Achilles tendinitis* is an inflammatory condition brought about by overuse of the gastrocnemius and soleus muscles. Rest and ice are the appropriate treatment when the injury is acute, but this situation may not heal well, leading to long-term tendinosis: poor healing, chronic pain, and long-lasting weakness. Shortness of the gastrocnemius muscle is a common cause of strain in the Achilles tendon. Regular massage, exercise, and stretching of this muscle is an excellent treatment and preventive measure.

3. *Muscle cramps* occur frequently in the calf muscles. In this location they may be related to dehydration, over-excitability (especially when they happen with exercise), or nutritional imbalances. To relieve cramping, stretch the muscle by dorsiflexing the foot and holding it for at least 30 seconds. If the cramp does not subside, rest and ice are appropriate treatment.

4. *Compartment syndrome* is a medical emergency that is sometimes seen at the finish line of very challenging athletic events. It involves inflammation within the very tough and unyielding fascial compartments of the lower leg. It can lead to permanent nerve damage, muscle loss, and kidney failure from the cellular debris of dying muscle tissue. One version of this condition, called exertional compartment syndrome, develops with exercise and subsides with rest. This suggests that a person has tight fascia that restricts blood and lymph flow to the deep muscles of the lower leg. Massage therapy to loosen fascia and improve local fluid flow may improve function in this situation.

Knees

1. *Knee pain* may be caused by poor alignment of the leg. Pain on the medial side can be an indication of shearing actions. Pain in the patellar ligament below the knee can be caused by overly deep, forward-lunging actions or hyperextension of the knee, which is often accompanied by pain in the ligaments at the back of the knee.

2. *Patellofemoral syndrome* is the result of roughening of the patellar cartilage. It can be caused by a blow to the knee, unequal pulling by the quadriceps, or by poor muscle tone around the knee. It is accompanied by a grinding or creaking sound when the knee is flexed. Left untreated, patellofemoral syndrome can progress to osteoarthritis at the knee, which can be crippling. Strengthening the quadriceps muscles is recommended.

See Appendix A for more information on these conditions.

7. *Plantar fasciitis* is damage to the plantar fascia leading to poor quality scar tissue and chronic irritation in front of the calcaneus. In many people it is related to age and weight. It can also be caused by overuse of the foot through walking, running, or jumping. It is a stubborn injury that may last for weeks or months before clearing. Massage to the leg muscles that contribute to the maintenance of arches is often recommended.

8. *Ankle sprain* is a common injury: the anterior talofibular ligament is the most frequently injured ligament in the body: this is a classic lateral ankle sprain. Ankle sprains can sometimes mask minor bone fractures, so it is important to have bad sprains checked by a primary care provider. Massage may be helpful after the initial swelling has subsided. Range of motion assessment can indicate more specifically which ligaments have been damaged.

Leg

1. *Shin splints* is a group of conditions that affect the lower leg. Any of the muscles along the lower leg that move the foot

HOLISTIC VIEW

Best Foot Forward, Weak in the Knees

The feet and ankles support and move the entire body. They are also our physical connection to the ground beneath us. Any form of imbalance or distortion in this area may be reflected as a sense of insecurity. How can we take a strong stance in life, or move with grace and fluidity, if we are unsure of our self at our foundation? A person who takes solid steps, who is trusting of firm support underneath his or her feet, exudes a sense of confidence. Such persons know where they belong, and they stand their ground.

A close examination of the feet may predict structural imbalances higher up in the body and may also provide a map of how an individual might compensate for feelings of physical or even emotional insecurity. The way a person's feet relate to the earth mirrors the way that individual relates to the issues of contact and grounding. When we stride forth with confidence we "put our best foot forward." On the other hand, when we make a mistake, this is a "faux pas"—French for a "false step."

The ankle joints are essential for moving the feet. They express, as do all joints, the ability to adapt and change direction. Inflexible ankles prevent the feet from pointing in various directions and stepping on different paths; this may reflect the limited choices a person may feel he or she is able to make in life. Ankles that are weak and buckle under prevent individuals from feeling they can stand up fully and carry their own weight.

The knees are important joints for weight support and transfer. They tie in with a wide variety of emotions. We tend to collapse and shake at our knees in response to a number of emotional stimuli. Fear can cause a person feel "weak in the knees," as can powerful joy and excitement. By contrast, locked knees may denote stress, rigidity, and lack of physical or mental flexibility.

When the knees, ankles, and feet are aligned through the vertical axis, with the feet pointing straight forward, energy and power can flow freely through the lower extremity. The feet relate to the root chakra, dealing with issues of survival and sustenance of the physical body.

Interpretations of body stances are subjective, with many possible nuances of meaning, and these interpretations are offered only as possibilities, not as blanket categorizations of personality or behavior. ■

▶ POSTURAL EVALUATION

1. Check the alignment of the legs (Fig. 8-5).
   - How does the line of gravity flow from the knee to the foot?
   - What is the shape of the legs: straight, bowed, knock-kneed?

2. Observe where the body's weight is concentrated on the feet. Is it forward, back, medial, or lateral? (Fig. 8-6)
3. Compare the directions in which the right and left feet are facing (Fig. 8-7).
4. Describe the shape and configuration of the toes.
   - Are they squeezed together?
   - Are they spread apart?

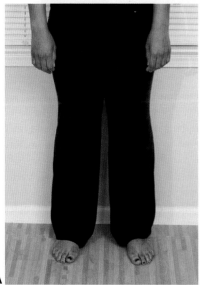 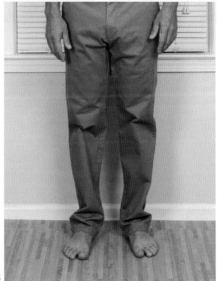 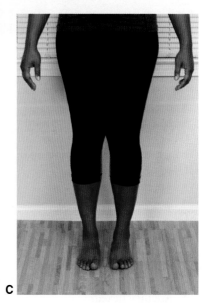

A B C

FIGURE 8-5 Postural evaluation: anterior view.

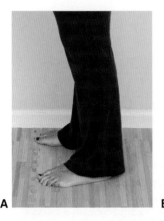
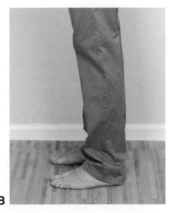
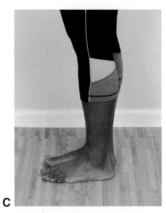

A **B** **C**

FIGURE 8-6 Postural evaluation: lateral view.

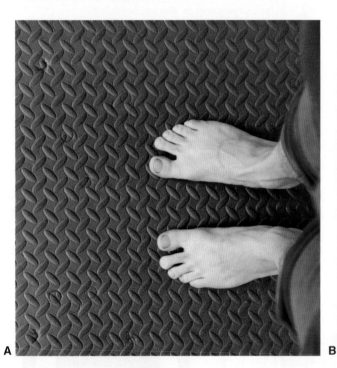
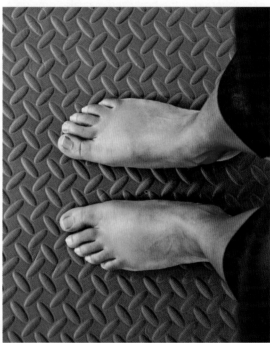

A **B**

FIGURE 8-7 Superior view of feet.

- Are they curled under?
- Does the big toe pull inward?
5. Check for bunions, calluses, and blisters on the feet, which indicate stress points on the feet.
6. Observe the arches (Fig. 8-8).
   - Are they high?
   - Are they collapsed?
7. Observe imbalance and/or weakness in the ankles. Compare the right and left ankles. Are the ankle joints on the same horizontal plane?
8. Describe the positioning of the knees.
   - Are they locked or hyperextended?
   - Are they flexed?

- Are the patellae drawn up?
- Are there bulges on the medial side of the knees, indicating a bracing of the soft tissues against gravity?
9. Examine the shape and muscle tone of the posterior legs (Fig. 8-9).
   - What is the muscular condition of the calves? Are they large, underdeveloped, of equal size and shape on both sides? Are there differences between the right and left legs?
   - Are the Achilles tendons on both legs vertical, or is one (or both) pulling to the side?

Refer to Table 8-1 for a description of common distortions of the feet and possible muscles involved. Refer to Table 8-2 for the range of motion for the knee and ankle.

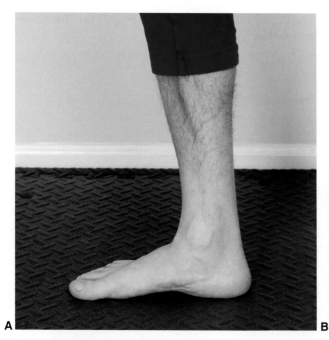 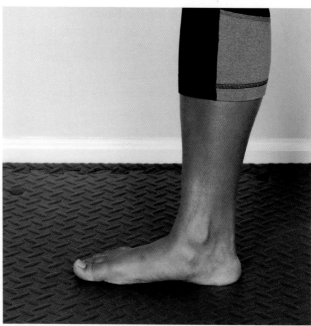

FIGURE 8-8 Medial view of feet.

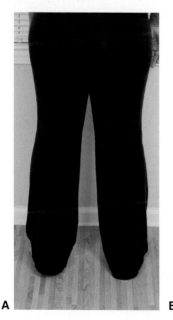 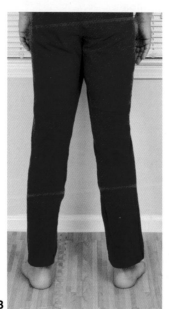 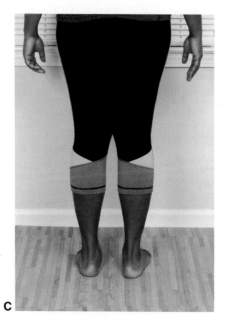

FIGURE 8-9 Postural evaluation: posterior view.

❱ EXERCISES AND SELF-TREATMENT

Feet and Ankles

Lie down on your back, with both knees flexed. Both feet are on the floor and parallel to each other. Bring the right knee to the chest. Place both hands around the knee to stabilize it (Fig. 8-10).

1. *Foot circles* (alternately stretches and strengthens all the muscles that move the ankle joints). Rotate the foot slowly in a full circle, as if tracing the face of a clock. Inhale during the first half of the circle; exhale while completing the circle. Repeat the movement three times in each direction (Fig. 8-11).

2. *Flexing* (alternately stretches and strengthens the intrinsic muscles of the foot and the plantar and dorsiflexor muscles of the ankle). Begin the exercise with the right foot fully flexed. Slowly, and with resistance, point the foot, articulating each joint. Reverse the motion, bringing the

TABLE 8-1 | Body Reading for the Feet

Postural Patterns	Muscles That May Be Shortened
Pigeon-toed—legs rotate medially, feet turn in; a valgus alignment of the knees	Adductors
	Gluteus medius and minimus
	Tensor fascia latae
Duck feet—legs rotate laterally, feet turn out; a varus alignment of the knees	Gluteus maximus
	Iliopsoas
	Piriformis, deep lateral rotators
High insteps	Tibialis anterior
	Tibialis posterior
Fallen arches	Peroneal muscles
Hammer toes	Toe flexor and extensor muscles

foot back to full dorsiflexion. Repeat the movement two more times (Fig. 8-12).

3. *Toe clutching* (alternately stretches and strengthens the flexors and extensors of the toes). Begin with the foot dorsiflexed. Imagine a pencil placed behind the toes. On exhalation, imagine squeezing the pencil with the toes, making a fist with the foot (Fig. 8-13). Inhaling, let go of the flexion of the toes. Repeat the movement three times.

4. Repeat the above three exercises on the left side.

Calf Muscles

Use a 4″ to 6″ stair step, or stack two thick books against the base of a wall. Stand with the balls of your feet on the edge of the step.

1. *Toe raises* (strengthens the gastrocnemius, soleus, tibialis posterior, peroneus longus and brevis, and flexor hallucis longus). Slowly rise up onto the balls of the feet. Hold for three counts. Lower your feet until the heels are parallel to the top of the stair step. Repeat the movement several times.

2. *Calf stretch* (stretches the gastrocnemius, soleus, tibialis posterior, and other plantar flexor muscles). Slowly lower your heels toward the floor, until you feel a stretch in the calf muscles. Hold the stretch for a minimum of 20 seconds.

▶ FOOT, LEG, AND KNEE ROUTINE

Objectives

- To balance the muscles that control the foot so that weight placement and walking patterns can be improved

TABLE 8-2 | Range of Motion (ROM) for the Knee and Ankle

Action	Muscles
Knee	
Flexion (ROM 135°)	Biceps femoris
	Semitendinosus
	Semimembranosus
	Sartorius
	Gracilis
	Gastrocnemius
	Plantaris
	Popliteus
Extension (ROM 0°)	Quadriceps
	Tensor fascia latae
Internal rotation (ROM 10°)	Semitendinosus
	Semimembranosus
	Popliteus
	Gracilis
	Sartorius
External rotation (ROM 10°)	Biceps femoris
Ankle	
Dorsiflexion (ROM 10°)	Tibialis anterior
	External digitorum longus
	Peroneus tertius
	Extensor hallucis longus
Plantar flexion (ROM 65°)	Gastrocnemius
	Soleus
	Plantaris
	Peroneus longus
	Peroneus brevis
	Tibialis posterior
	Flexor hallucis longus
Inversion of the foot (ROM 5°)	Tibialis anterior
	Tibialis posterior
Eversion of the foot (ROM 5°)	Peroneus tertius
	Peroneus longus
	Peroneus brevis

- To relieve stress and uneven pulls on the muscles of the foot so that the formation of bunions, calluses, and other manifestations of foot dysfunction are minimized
- To balance muscular action around the knee, allowing the knee to track properly and thus eliminating strain on the soft tissue components of the joint
- To help relieve painful conditions that manifest in the muscles of the leg, such as spasms, shin splints, and trigger points

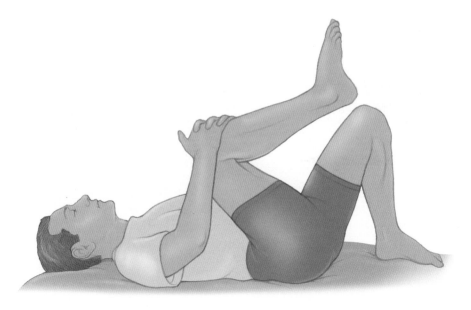

FIGURE 8-10 Body position for performing foot exercises.

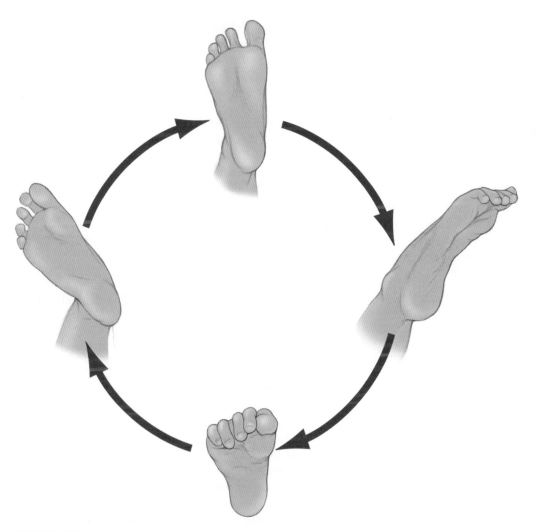

FIGURE 8-11 Foot circle exercise sequence.

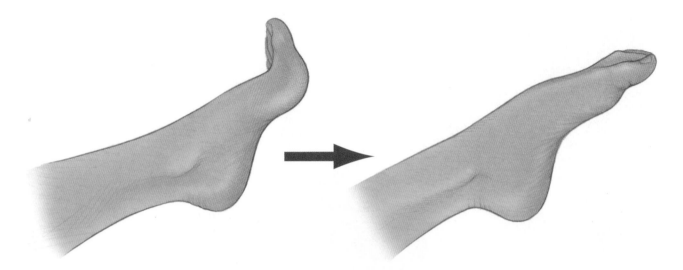

FIGURE 8-12 Sequence of foot positions in flexing exercise.

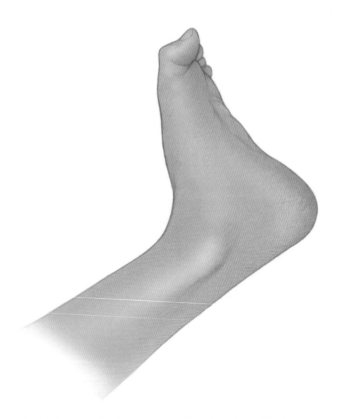

FIGURE 8-13 Toe clutching to strengthen the arches of the foot.

Energy

POSITION

- The client is lying supine on the table. A bolster under the knees is optional.
- The therapist is standing at the foot of the table.

Polarity

Hold the toes of each foot between the thumb and index finger for 10 seconds each, beginning with the fifth toe and ending with the big toe. According to traditional polarity theory, the tip of each toe is the culmination point of a vertical line of force that runs through the body from head to toe. These energy currents stimulate proper physiologic and psychological functioning. Moving from the fifth toe to the big toe, the energy currents are labeled earth, water, fire, air, and ether, respectively, in accordance with ayurvedic terminology. Holding each toe is meant to assist in clearing any blockages along these five energetic pathways.

SHIATSU

1. Compress the leg with both hands from the knee to the ankle. This stimulates the flow of qi through the channels that flow through the leg. The yang channels on the outside of the leg are the gallbladder and stomach. The yin channels on the inside portion of the leg are the spleen, liver, and kidney.
2. Squeeze down the sides of the foot to the toes (Fig. 8-14).

Swedish/Cross Fiber

1. Alternately apply effleurage strokes down the dorsal and plantar surfaces of the foot.
2. Perform knuckle kneading on the plantar surface of the foot.
3. Perform thumb gliding on the dorsal surface of the foot.
4. Perform effleurage and draining strokes from the ankle to the knee.
5. Reach the fingers of both hands underneath the calf, and place the fingertips between the heads of the gastrocnemius

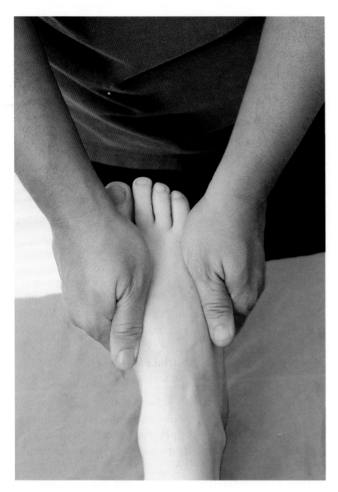

FIGURE 8-14 Shiatsu compression of the foot.

muscles. Rake outward, drawing the hands away from each other. Cover the entire calf, from several inches above the ankle to the knee.
6. Perform thumb gliding around the knee.

Connective Tissue

MYOFASCIAL SPREADING TECHNIQUES

1. Facing the dorsal side of the client's foot from the side of the table, place the hands around the sides of the foot, with the fingertips touching at the midline of the plantar surface. Sink in with the fingers, and spread from the midline to the outside edges of the foot.
2. Standing at the foot of the table, place the fingers on the dorsal surface of the foot at the base of the toes. Sink into the tissues, and slowly glide toward the ankle.
3. Place the heels of the hands at the midline of the leg, above the ankle. Slowly spread the hands apart. Work in horizontal strips to the knee.

Deep Tissue/Neuromuscular Therapy

SEQUENCE

1. Tendons of the toes
2. Insertion points of flexor hallucis longus, flexor hallucis brevis, and abductor hallucis ▶
3. Muscles of the plantar surface of the foot
   a. First layer—abductor digiti minimi, flexor digitorum brevis, abductor hallucis
   b. Second layer—flexor hallucis longus, flexor digitorum longus, four lumbricals, quadratus plantae
   c. Third layer—flexor digiti minimi, adductor hallucis, flexor hallucis brevis
   d. Fourth layer—three plantar and four dorsal interossei; tendons of peroneus longus and tibialis posterior
4. Muscles of the dorsal surface of the foot
   a. Tendons—tibialis anterior, extensor hallucis longus, extensor digitorum longus, peroneus tertius
   b. Muscles—interossei, extensor hallucis brevis, extensor digitorum brevis, abductor digiti minimi
5. Retinaculum of the ankle—anterior portion
6. Medial leg muscles—flexor digitorum longus, soleus, gastrocnemius
7. Lateral leg muscles—tibialis anterior, extensor hallucis longus, extensor digitorum longus, peroneus longus, peroneus brevis, peroneus tertius, soleus
8. Retinaculum of the ankle—posterior portion
9. Gastrocnemius
10. Soleus and deep posterior leg muscles
11. Knee—ligaments and tendons

Tendons of the Toes

- Standing at the foot of the table, grasp the base of the proximal phalanx of the big toe, front and back, with the thumb and index finger (Fig. 8-15). Do short, up-and-down strokes on the flexor and extensor tendons. Repeat on the distal phalanx.
- Repeat the above stroke on each of the other four toes, moving in sequence from the base of the second toe to the fifth toe.

Insertions of Flexor Hallucis Longus, Flexor Hallucis Brevis, Abductor Hallucis, and Adductor Hallucis

Flexor Hallucis Longus
The attachment point is located at the center of the base of the distal phalanx of the big toe, just above the joint, on the plantar surface of the foot.

Strokes
- Do static compression and cross-fiber friction on the attachment with the tip of your thumb or index finger.

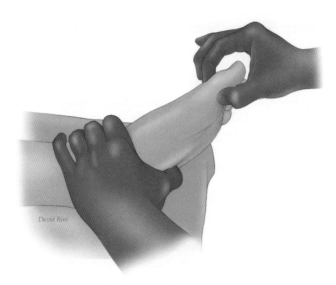

FIGURE 8-15 Contacting the flexor and extensor tendons of the toes.

Flexor Hallucis Brevis
The medial part inserts on the medial side of the base of the proximal phalanx of the hallux. The lateral part inserts on the lateral side of the base of the proximal phalanx of the hallux.

Abductor Hallucis
The abductor hallucis inserts on the medial side of the base of the proximal phalanx of the hallux.

Adductor Hallucis
The adductor hallucis inserts on the lateral side of the base of the proximal phalanx of the hallux.

Strokes
- To contact these attachments, hold the base of the big toe on both sides between your thumb and index finger. Feel for the tender spots on either side of the toe.
- Apply static compression and cross-fiber friction on tender areas.

Muscles of the Plantar Surface of the Foot

Position
- The therapist sits at the foot of the table, with the non-working hand holding the client's foot around the toes and maintaining a dorsiflexed position.

Flexor Hallucis Brevis
Origin: Medial portion of the cuboid bone, lateral cuneiform bone.
Insertion: Base of the proximal phalanx of the hallux on the medial and lateral sides.
Action: Flexes the proximal phalanx of the hallux.

Abductor Hallucis
Origin: Tuberosity of the calcaneus, flexor retinaculum, plantar aponeurosis.

Insertion: Medial side of the base of the proximal phalanx of the hallux.
Action: Abduction of the hallux.

Trigger points tend to develop in the flexor hallucis brevis and abductor hallucis, which are muscles that insert at the medial side of the base of the big toe. The referred pain zone for the flexor hallucis brevis is the region of the head of the first metatarsal and perhaps into the big toe. Trigger point pain from the abductor hallucis can run across the ball of the foot. Check carefully along the toe tendons as well.

Strokes
- Using a soft fist, stroke down the plantar surface of the foot from the base of the toes to the heel (Fig. 8-16).
- To reach the lumbrical muscles, stroke along the sides of each of the toe muscle tendons with the knuckle of the index finger or the thumb, from the base of the toes to the heel (Fig. 8-17). Maintain static compression on tender spots.

Muscles of the Dorsal Surface of the Foot

Extensor Digitorum Brevis
Origin: Anterior and lateral surfaces of the calcaneus, lateral talocalcaneal ligament, and extensor retinaculum.
Insertion: Base of the proximal phalanx of the hallux, joins the lateral sides of the tendons of the extensor digitorum longus on toes 2, 3, and 4.
Action: Extends the hallux (big toe) and toes 2, 3, and 4.

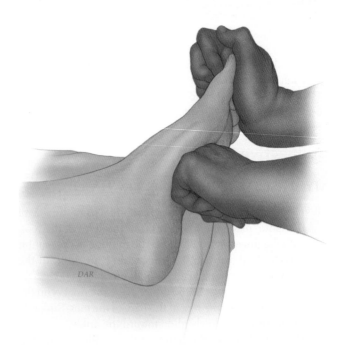

FIGURE 8-16 Deep tissue stroke on the muscles of the plantar surface of the foot.

To check for trigger points, feel for tenderness in the extensor digitorum brevis muscle, near the ankle crease. Pain from trigger points can radiate over the entire dorsal surface but will be most pronounced near the ankle.

Strokes
- With the knuckle of the index finger or the thumb, stroke along the sides of the toe tendons, from the base of the toes to the ankle (Fig. 8-18).

Retinaculum of the Ankle—Anterior Portion

Strokes
- Place both thumbs at the midline of the ankle joint. Simultaneously move both thumbs in short, up-and-down strokes, sliding the retinaculum over the tendon sheaths.
- Separating the thumbs slightly, repeat the stroke (Fig. 8-19). Continue to the medial and lateral malleoli.

Medial Leg Muscles (Flexor Digitorum Longus, Soleus, and Gastrocnemius)

Position
- Stand at the side of the table, and place the fingers of both hands along the medial border of the tibia, behind the medial malleolus.

Strokes
- Perform circular friction strokes with the fingertips on the muscles medial to the edge of the tibia bone. Work from the medial malleolus to the knee.
- Perform short, up-and-down and side-to-side strokes with the fingertips on the borders of the muscles just medial to the edge of the tibia, from the medial malleolus to the knee (Fig. 8-20).

⚠️ Use pressure on the medial leg with great care to avoid trapping or otherwise injuring the lesser saphenous vein. Varicosities here contraindicate intrusive massage.

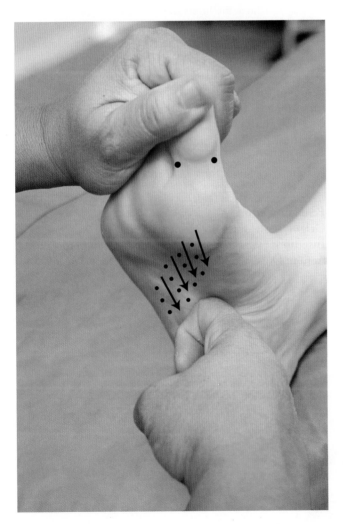

FIGURE 8-17 Stroking the lumbricals muscles between the toe tendons.

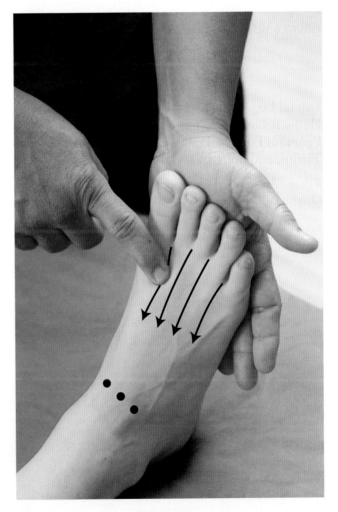

FIGURE 8-18 Direction of deep tissue strokes on extensor digitorum brevis.

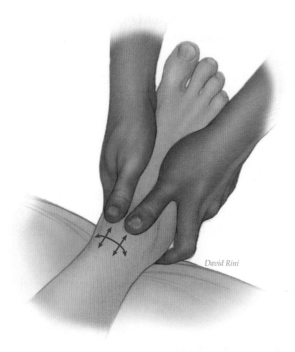

FIGURE 8-19 Directions of strokes on the retinaculum of the ankle.

Lateral Leg Muscles (Tibialis Anterior, Extensor Hallucis Longus, Extensor Digitorum Longus, Peroneus Longus, Peroneus Brevis, Peroneus Tertius, and Soleus)

Tibialis Anterior

Origin: Lateral condyle and proximal two-thirds of the lateral surface of the tibia, interosseus membrane.

Insertion: First medial cuneiform on the medial and plantar surfaces, base of the first metatarsal.

Action: Dorsiflexion of the ankle at the talocrural joint; inversion (supination) of the foot at the subtalar and midtarsal joints.

> Trigger points are most often found in the upper third of the tibialis anterior muscle. The referred pain zone is on the front of the ankle toward the medial side and over the entire big toe (hallux).

Note: It may be easier to work on the tibialis anterior muscle with the client in a supine position.

Peroneus Longus

Origin: Head and upper two-thirds of the lateral shaft of the fibula.

Insertion: Lateral plantar side of the base of the first metatarsal, lateral plantar side of the first cuneiform.

Action: Eversion of the foot; assists plantar flexion of the ankle; support of the transverse arch.

> Check the fibers of peroneus longus approximately 1 inch below the head of the fibula. The trigger point referral zone is around the lateral malleolus, extending along the lateral side of the foot.

Peroneus Brevis

Origin: Distal two-thirds of the lateral surface of the shaft of the fibula.

Insertion: Tuberosity on the lateral surface of the fifth metatarsal.

Action: Eversion of the foot; assists plantar flexion of the ankle.

Peroneus Tertius

Origin: Distal third of the medial surface of the fibula.

Insertion: Dorsal surface of the base of the fifth metatarsal.

Action: Dorsiflexion of the ankle; assists foot eversion.

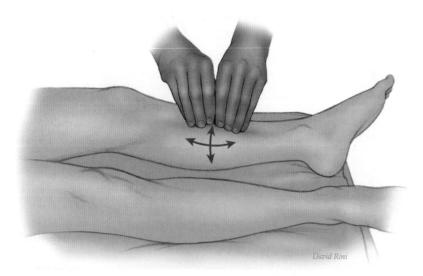

FIGURE 8-20 Directions of deep tissue strokes on the medial leg muscles.

Strokes
- Trace the lateral side of the lateral malleolus with the knuckle or thumb to contact the tendons of the peroneal muscles. Perform the short, up-and-down strokes on the tendons.
- For the tibialis anterior, perform an elongation stroke with the elbow lateral to the shaft of the tibia from the ankle to the lateral condyle of the tibia (Fig. 8-21).

Position
- The client is turned onto his or her side so that the leg to be worked on is uppermost. The top leg is flexed 90° at the hip and knee.
- A bolster is placed under the leg so that the hip does not roll forward.

Strokes
- For the peroneal muscles, perform elongation strokes with the elbow from the lateral malleolus to the head of the fibula (Fig. 8-22).

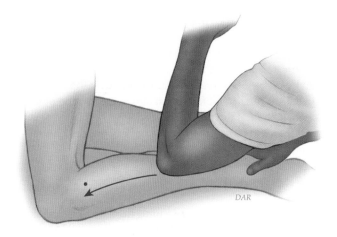

FIGURE 8-22 Elongation stroke on the peroneal muscles.

- Using the elbow, separate the lateral leg muscles by stroking along their borders, from the ankle to the knee.
- A cross-fiber motion with the elbow may be used to locate trigger points.

The Posterior Leg
Position
- The client is placed in the prone position; a bolster is placed under the ankle, if required.
- The therapist is standing at the side of the table next to the client's foot.

Strokes
- The therapist warms up the posterior leg muscles as described above for the anterior leg.

Retinaculum of the Ankle—Posterior Portion

Strokes
- Place the thumbs on either side of the Achilles tendon. Do short, up-and-down strokes on the retinaculum, sliding it over the underlying tendons.
- Separating the thumbs slightly, repeat the stroke. Continue to repeat the stroke, widening the distance between the thumbs, to the lateral and medial malleoli.

Gastrocnemius

Origin:
    Lateral head—lateral epicondyle and posterior surface of the shaft of the femur above the condyle.
    Medial head—popliteal surface of the femur above the medial condyle.
Insertion: Middle posterior surface of the calcaneus via the tendo calcaneus.
Action: Plantar flexion of the foot; assists in knee flexion.

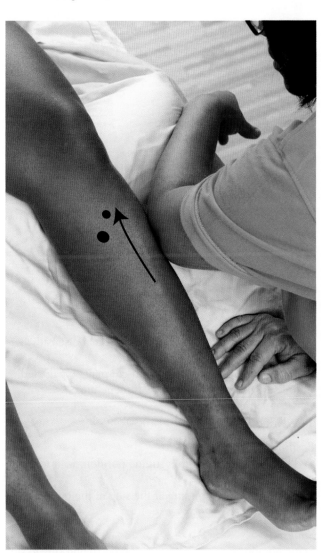

FIGURE 8-21 Elongation stroke on the tibialis anterior.

Clusters of trigger points may form symmetrically in the upper quadrant of the gastrocnemius, in the medial and lateral heads. The referred pain zone is for the most part local, radiating in the upper portion of the muscle and over the knee joint. A trigger point found just above the midline of the medial head of the muscle refers pain primarily to the instep of the foot and along the back of the calf on the medial side.

Strokes

- Perform an elongation stroke using the forearm or knuckles, from the calcaneus to midcalf region (Fig. 8-23A).
- Reposition the forearm or knuckles directly over the lateral head of the gastrocnemius. Continue the elongation stroke to the knee. Repeat on the medial head (Fig. 8-23B).

⚠ Never stroke over the center of the back of the knee (popliteal fossa). Stay on the muscle by stroking on the side of the knee, maintaining your pressure on the muscle fibers of the gastrocnemius.

- Perform an elongation stroke with the thumbs up the midline of the posterior leg to separate the heads of the gastrocnemius (Fig. 8-23C).
- Palpate trigger points in the bellies of the muscle using short, up-and-down and side-to-side strokes with the thumbs. Treat any trigger points that are found.

Soleus and Deep Posterior Muscles

Soleus

Origin: Middle third of the medial side of the shaft of the tibia, proximal third of the shaft on the posterior surface and head of the fibula, fibrous arch between the tibia and fibula.

Insertion: Posterior surface of the calcaneus via the tendo calcaneus (along with the gastrocnemius).

Action: Plantar flexion of the foot; strong stabilizer of the body in standing position, prevents falling forward.

The best way to examine the soleus is to disengage the gastrocnemius by flexing the client's leg 90°. The most frequent trigger point that forms in the soleus is found on the medial side, just above the Achilles tendon. It refers pain primarily into the Achilles tendon and heel, but pain may also radiate up into the medial side of the soleus.

Strokes

- Place thumbs or fingertips on both sides of the Achilles tendon. Working in small sections, apply up-and-down strokes lateral to the gastrocnemius muscle, from the ankle

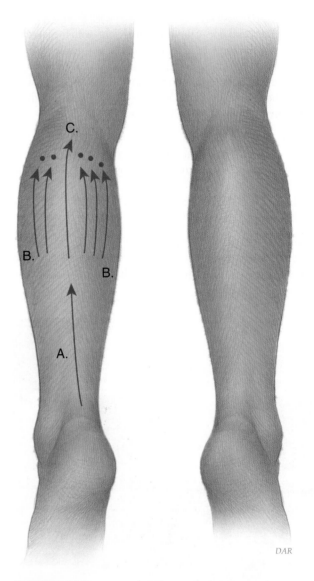

FIGURE 8-23 Sequence of strokes on the gastrocnemius.

to the knee. Seek out areas of tightness and sensitivity to treat in the deeper layers of muscles.
- Trigger points in the soleus muscle may be palpated by pressing deeply through the gastrocnemius.

The Knee

Position

- The client is placed in a supine position, with a bolster under the knee.
- The therapist is standing at the side of the table next to the client's knee.

Strokes

Static compression as well as up-and-down and side-to-side strokes are used on the following attachment points (Fig. 8-24):

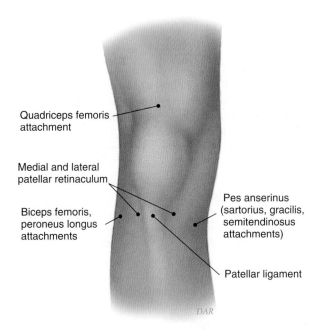

FIGURE 8-24 Muscle attachment sites at the knee.

- **Pes anserinus** (insertion point of semitendinosus, sartorius, and gracilis)—on the head of the tibia, medial to the patella.
- **Biceps femoris and peroneus longus**—on the head of the fibula on the lateral side of the leg.
- **Quadriceps femoris**—on the center of the head of the tibia, slightly superior to the tuberosity.
- **Patellar ligament**—place the thumbs just above the tuberosity of the tibia. Do short, up-and-down and side-to-side strokes on the ligament to the inferior border of the patella.

- **Medial and lateral patellar retinaculum**—place the thumbs on either side of the patellar ligament. Move up and down and side to side, sliding the retinaculum. Pause at tender points.

STRETCH

1. Standing at the foot of the table, grasp the toes of the client's foot with one hand while holding the foot at the heel with the other. Flex and extend the toes several times.
2. Dorsiflex the foot, and hold for several seconds.
3. Plantar flex the foot, and hold for several seconds. (Stretches 2 and 3 above may be performed with the client lying in the supine or the prone position, with the leg flexed 90° at the knee.)
4. Sandwich the foot between the palms. Invert the foot, and hold for a few seconds. Evert the foot, and hold for a few seconds.

ACCESSORY WORK

1. Hand and forearm massage complement this session well, because these areas correspond reflexively to the foot and leg.
2. Neck and cranial massage will help to balance the upper pole of the body after this work.

CLOSING

Sitting at the head of the table, lightly cup the client's head in both your hands, and hold for at least 30 seconds, allowing the client to relax and assimilate the effects of the session.

SESSION IMPRESSION

THE FOOT AND LEG

The client is a 50-year-old man named Eugene, who is the head manager of a fast-food franchise. The duties of his job require that he stand all day. He is constantly moving around the store to ensure the smooth operation of the business. He sought out deep tissue therapy because his feet and legs are becoming extremely sore and swollen, especially by the end of the workweek. Because he is so uncomfortable, it has become increasingly difficult for him to carry out the functions of his job.

Postural evaluation revealed that Eugene has flat feet. This causes the medial side of the knees to fall inward, creating stress on the medial collateral ligaments. He exhibits a high degree of lordosis, and his scapulae are depressed.

His clavicles angle downward, and his arms hang forward of his sides. Eugene also exhibits a forward head position, with his chin held abnormally high.

To deal fully with the problems in his lower body, a series of deep tissue sessions was commenced to align the entire body. Isolated massage to his feet and legs alone would not resolve the problems in his feet, because his problem reflected postural imbalances throughout his entire body. Massage to the feet was performed in every deep session. The current case, however, details the fourth session performed, during which the muscles of the lower limb were emphasized.

Eugene's feet are very stiff and immobile. There is limited movement in the ankles and throughout the

(continued)

SESSION IMPRESSION (continued)

joints of the foot. After the first session, he was shown foot exercises to practice at home to begin to alleviate some of the inflexibility of the foot muscles.

The session focusing on the feet began with work on the intrinsic muscles of the foot. The deep tissue strokes revealed tiny, granular-feeling lumps accumulated along the toe tendons and extreme sensitivity to pressure in many areas on the plantar surface of the foot. Sustained, therapist-assisted flexion and extension of the toes was administered to stretch the muscles and fascia of the foot, along with plantar flexion, dorsiflexion, inversion, and eversion movements.

Low medial arches force both feet into eversion while the client is standing. Therefore, the peroneal muscles, which evert the foot, are extremely contracted. Eugene's felt like concrete. Slow, deep strokes with the elbow were performed on these muscles. A high degree of softening of the peroneal longus and brevis was achieved. To balance the reduced tension in the peroneals, the client was taught an exercise to strengthen the tibialis anterior muscle, which lifts the medial arch. Its action counterbalances that of the peroneal muscles. The lesson took place after the session. Eugene was taught to sit in a chair with his leg flexed at the hip, knee, and ankle. He was to hang a petite-size gift bag containing two soup cans from his flexed foot. He would then slowly invert his foot (turn the plantar surface inward) and hold for 3 seconds. This movement was to be repeated 10 times on the right and left sides.

The gastrocnemius and soleus muscles were also massaged. The heads of the gastrocnemii were sensitive to touch. Extensive Swedish pétrissage and friction strokes were used to relax the muscles. Cross-fiber strokes were incorporated rather than deep tissue elongation strokes, because the muscles were too sensitive to withstand sustained direct pressure. All the muscle attachments around the knee were treated. The muscle attachments of the pes anserinus were particularly sensitive.

Deep tissue therapy to the legs and feet was followed by shoulder, neck, and cranial massage to complete the session. To supplement the foot exercises, additional home care suggestions (including elevation of the legs following a long day at work and regular foot soaks in warm water with epsom salts) were made. ■

Topics for Discussion

1. Describe the likely configuration of the legs and pelvis in a client with fallen medial arches.
2. A client stands with the majority of weight on the backs of the heels. Which muscles of the legs and feet are probably shortened?
3. How would you explain to a client the importance of taking care of the feet?
4. What are some important features of a well-designed shoe to provide support and comfort to the foot?
5. What are some possible indications that a client has plantar fasciitis?

REVIEW QUESTIONS

Level 1

Receive and Respond

1. When the body's weight is optimally balanced on the foot. . .
   a. it passes through the navicular and cuneiform bones to the transverse arch.
   b. it focuses into the calcaneus, the densest weight-bearing bone.
   c. it passes through the talus into the medial longitudinal arch.
   d. it passes through talus to the rest of the foot bones.

2. What bones comprise the ankle joint?
   a. Medial malleolus and lateral malleolus
   b. Tibia and fibula
   c. Talus and tibia
   d. Talus and calcaneus

3. The strongest dorsiflexor and inverter of the foot is the. . .
   a. tibialis anterior.
   b. tibialis posterior.
   c. peroneus longus.
   d. peroneus brevis.

4. Structures in the popliteal fossa are most vulnerable when. . .
   a. the knee is extended.
   b. the knee is flexed.
   c. the knee is medially rotated.
   d. the knee is neutral.

Level 2

Apply Concepts

1. Which joint is most likely to be damaged first if the feet arches are dysfunctional?
   a. The sacroiliac joint
   b. The ankle

c. The hip

d. The knee

2. If a person has feet that point out laterally, what muscles are likely to be shortened?

a. Tibialis anterior, tibialis posterior, peroneus longus

b. Psoas, gluteus maximus, piriformis

c. Adductors, gluteus medius, tensor fascia latae

d. Deep toe flexors, intrinsic foot muscles

3. If a person wants to strengthen her calf muscles, what exercise might be best?

a. Toe raises

b. Calf stretches

c. Toe clutching

d. Foot circles

4. What is the best strategy to access the soleus muscle?

a. With the client supine, have him bend his knee and work on the calf from the anterior side

b. With the client prone, extend the leg fully so the gastrocnemius is as narrow as possible

c. With the client prone, bend the knee to 90° to disengage the gastrocnemius

d. With the client side-lying, access the soleus at the medial aspect of the leg closest to the table

5. What is the recommended sequence of deep tissue/neuromuscular therapy for the foot and leg?

a. Toe flexors, followed by toe extensors, followed by retinaculum ligament

b. Toe tendons, followed by lateral leg muscles, followed by medial leg muscles

c. Plantar foot muscles, followed by dorsal foot muscles, followed by medial leg muscles

d. Toe tendons, followed by insertions of toe flexors and hallucis brevis, followed by plantar surface muscles

Level 3

Problem Solving: Discussion Points

1. Cecilia is a 42-year-old woman who wears narrow-toed, high-heeled shoes. She likes them, and prefers them to other professional footwear. She also has knee pain, low back pain, and bunions on both feet. Plan a session for her using the routines from Chapter 8. Where do you anticipate spending most of your time? What adaptations will she need? What goals can you hope to accomplish in a single session?

2. Given that Cecilia is unlikely to give up on her favorite footwear, what goals can you hope to help her with over a series of integrated deep tissue therapy sessions?

Stabilizing the Core

Having completed the reading, classroom instruction, and assigned homework related to Chapter 9 of *The Balanced Body*, the learner is expected to be able to. . .

- Apply key terms and concepts related to integrated deep tissue therapy as related to the thigh, hip, pelvis, and abdomen
- Identify anatomical features of the thigh, hip, pelvis, and abdomen, including
  - Bony landmarks
  - Muscular and fascial structures
  - Endangerments or cautionary sites
- Identify common postural or movement patterns associated with pain or impaired function of the thigh, hip, pelvis, and abdomen
- Use positioning and bolstering strategies that provide safety and comfort for clients to receive integrated deep tissue therapy to the thigh, hip, pelvis, and abdomen

- Generate within-scope recommendations for client self-care relevant to the thigh, hip, pelvis, and abdomen
- Safely and effectively perform the integrated deep tissue therapy routines as described
- Organize a single session to address the thigh, hip, pelvis, and abdomen, using the integrated deep tissue therapy approach, customized to individual clients
- Plan a series of sessions to address whole-body incorporation using the integrated deep tissue therapy approach, customized to individual clients

This chapter focuses primarily on re-establishing balanced action of the muscles that act on the pelvis. These include many of the thigh muscles as well as the abdominal and pelvic muscles. The thigh/hip and abdominal/pelvic regions are discussed separately to clarify anatomic and functional distinctions. Within the routines, however, these areas are integrated to promote coordination of all the muscles affecting pelvic placement and movement.

The four routines presented in this chapter should be viewed as a progressive unit. To achieve the best results and to prevent imbalance in the pelvic region, they should be performed in the recommended order. The deep-lying psoas and iliacus muscles should never be massaged until the surface abdominal muscles and thigh muscles have been relaxed. Premature work on the iliopsoas is uncomfortable, and can interfere with the effectiveness of integrated deep tissue therapy.

The four sessions described in this chapter work best when they are scheduled at close intervals, with no more than 2 weeks between each one, so that the results from the previous session can be carried over effectively to the next. This work is more effective when the exercises and stretches presented here are incorporated. The integrated deep tissue therapist provides an invaluable service by teaching clients these exercises so they may better and more correctly integrate the muscular changes and increased core awareness achieved within the sessions.

The order of the routines is as follows:

1. The posterior thigh muscles and hip muscles
2. The abdominal muscles, including their attachments on the rib cage and pelvis, and massage to the intestines
3. The lateral and medial thigh muscles
4. The anterior thigh muscles and hip flexors, including the rectus femoris and iliopsoas

The Thigh and Hip

▶ GENERAL CONCEPTS

The thigh consists of the femur, which is the longest and strongest bone in the body, and the muscles that are attached to it. The hip is the articulation of the femur with the pelvis. It is a ball-and-socket joint capable of a broad range of movements, including flexion and extension, abduction and adduction, rotation, and circumduction. The thigh and hip keep the body stable while we stand, and when we initiate movement of the lower limb. The muscles at the front of the thigh, the quadriceps, are among the most powerful in the body, and they are balanced by groups of muscles on the sides and back of the thigh.

A total of 22 muscles are involved in moving the femur at the hip and the knee. Twenty-one of these muscles have an attachment at various places on the pelvis. In a standing position, the legs are fixed in their position over the feet. Therefore, when the anterior or posterior thigh muscles are shortened, the pelvis may be tilted too far in one direction or another. One of the goals of deep tissue work on the thigh muscles is to balance their action so that the pelvis can sit freely over the heads of the femurs without being chronically pulled into a distorted alignment.

The hip joint is reinforced by strong ligaments and muscles. Because of its ball-and-socket design, the hip joint is capable of rotary and circular movements. In walking and running, however, it must direct force to the knee and the ankle beneath it, which are more limited in their ranges of motion. The knee is set up to manage flexion and extension, but it has limited capacity to absorb stress from other directions. It needs the hip to translate that force into a safe range of motion. The knee must also be able to absorb the shock from the impact of weight rising up to it from the ground below in walking and running movements. For these reasons, good mechanics at the hip help to support better health at the knee as well.

When the leg is in optimal alignment, a vertical axis passes from the center of the hip joint at the front of the thigh to the center of the knee joint (Fig. 9-1). This axis is distorted in both knock-kneed (**valgus** alignment of the knee) and bow-legged (**varus** alignment of the knee) conditions, adding additional stress to the joints of the legs (Fig. 9-2). The integrated deep tissue therapist should be aware of this vertical axis when working on the thigh muscles, and pay attention to any asymmetry in the muscles on either side of the axis.

▶ MUSCULOSKELETAL ANATOMY AND FUNCTION

The proximal end of the femur consists of a rounded head, a neck, and two projections, called the greater and lesser trochanters. The head fits into a round cavity in the pelvis, called the acetabulum, which is formed by the junction of the ilium, pubis, and ischium. The entire circumference of the acetabulum is extended by a ring of cartilage called the labrum that wraps around the femoral head. This ring creates a snug fit in the hip joint. Extending from the labrum is a thick sleeve, or joint capsule, that encases the neck of the femur, reinforcing and protecting the joint. (See Essential Anatomy Box 9-1 for a summary of muscles, bones, and landmarks.)

Seven ligaments surround the hip joint, giving it additional strength and support. The strongest of these is the iliofemoral or Y ligament. It attaches in front of the hip joint, at the anterior inferior iliac spine (AIIS), and in the space on the femur between the two trochanters. The ischiofemoral ligament is situated at the posterior aspect of the joint, attaching to the ischium below the acetabulum and to the posterior femoral neck. These ligaments help hold the head of the femur firmly in the hip socket during movements of the thigh.

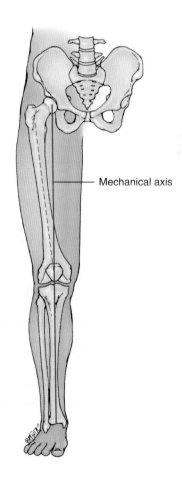

— Mechanical axis

FIGURE 9-1 The mechanical axis of the lower extremity aligns the centers of the hip, knee, and ankle joints.

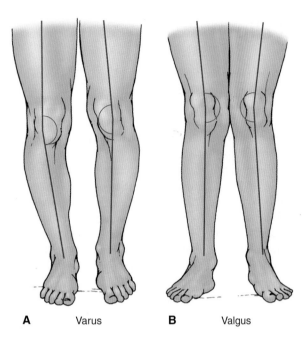

A Varus   **B** Valgus

FIGURE 9-2 Varus and valgus alignment of the knee. **A.** In varus alignment of the knee, the angle formed by lines through the femur and tibia opens medially. **B.** In valgus alignment of the knee, the angle formed by lines through the femur and tibia opens laterally.

The neck of the femur extends diagonally upward from the shaft of the bone. Its design keeps the thigh clear of the pelvis, allowing for greater mobility of the pelvis over the legs. The disadvantage of the shape of the neck is that it is in the form of a bent lever, subjecting it to greater stress than a straight column would receive. It is potentially the weakest point on the thigh. Further, the neck of the femur is composed of trabecular bone, where the bone-thinning effects of osteoporosis are most active. A common injury in older people is a "broken hip," which is usually a break at the femoral neck.

The greater trochanter is the site of attachment for many muscles that initiate movements of the thigh. The six deep lateral rotators as well as the **gluteus medius** and **gluteus minimus** (the medial rotators) have their insertion there. These two sets of muscles oppose each other in rotation of the femur. They must all be in balance to allow the full range of movements of the head of the femur in the acetabulum. Muscular imbalance pulls the head of the femur out of position slightly, and over time, this may result in osteoarthritis of the hip joint. Movement restriction at the hip often has a relay effect, creating stress and imbalance at the knee and sometimes the ankle.

The muscles in front of the thigh, the flexors, move the femur forward in locomotion (Fig. 9-3C and D). The primary hip flexors are the **iliopsoas** and the **rectus femoris**. The rectus femoris is also active in knee extension. Secondary flexors are the **sartorius** and **tensor fascia lata**. Of all these muscles, the iliopsoas is the most important. Because of its location at the body's core, it possesses the greatest power and leverage. It should be the foremost initiator of hip flexion. In a balanced body, walking is not initiated by the legs; rather, it is initiated from the trunk. The movement is then transferred to the legs by means of the psoas. The psoas muscle attaches to the anterior portion of the lumbar spine, and its insertion is on the lesser trochanter on the inner surface of the femur.

The psoas and rectus femoris muscles need to be in balance with each other for a smooth, coordinated walking action to occur. Often, the rectus femoris takes over hip flexion, and the psoas becomes shortened and weak. This tends to increase the lumbar curve and tips the rib cage

BOX 9-1 ESSENTIAL ANATOMY | **The Thigh and Hip Routines**

MUSCLES	BONES AND LANDMARKS
Quadriceps—rectus femoris, vastus lateralis, medialis, and intermedius	Anterior superior iliac spine (ASIS)
	Anterior inferior iliac spine (AIIS)
Adductors—adductor brevis, longus, and magnus, gracilis, pectineus	Sacrum
	Coccyx
Hamstrings—biceps femoris, semimembranosus, semitendinosus	Ischial tuberosity
	Femur
Lateral rotators—piriformis, obturator internus, gemellus superior, gemellus inferior, obturator externus, quadratus femoris	Greater trochanter
	Lesser trochanter
	Patella
Gluteus maximus, medius, minimus	Tibia
Tensor fascia latae and iliotibial band	Tibial tuberosity
Sartorius	Fibula
	Head of fibula

both downward and forward. This causes misalignment in the body segments, with inevitable problems in full-body movement integration.

In hip flexion with a properly functioning psoas, the upper and lower body segments are coordinated around the lumbar spine. When this works well, the lumbar spine allows the pelvis to swing slightly with each step. When this functions poorly, the pelvis is held rigidly: it does not move with the gait, or allow adequate shock absorption through the low back.

Not all of our walking is on smooth, perfect surfaces. We need to be able to walk on irregular surfaces as well. A mobile pelvis helps make this possible. In addition, small, frequent adjustments in the muscles that cross the hip and that cross the ankle help to create a fluid, graceful, effortless gait, whether the surface is hard, soft, or even slightly irregular. Without these adjustments, the gait becomes effortful and jarring, sending unnecessary stress through the foot and leg bones to the low back.

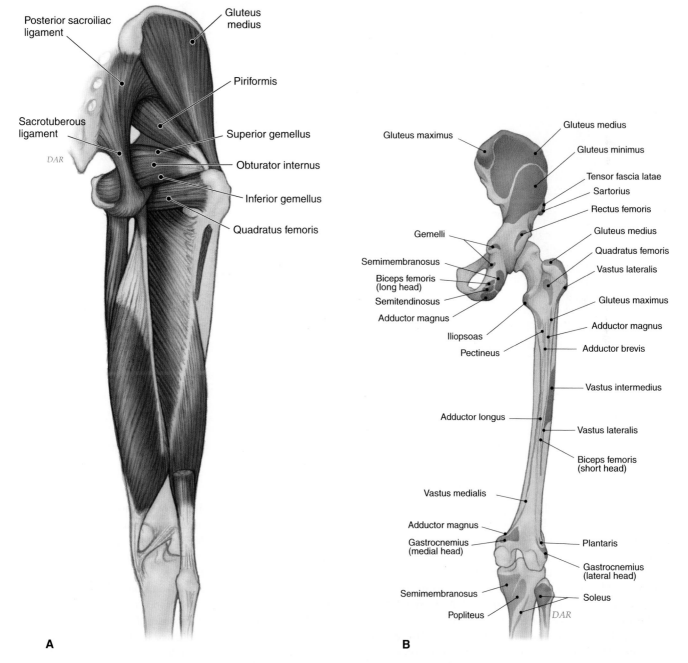

A

B

FIGURE 9-3 A. Muscles of the posterior thigh and hip. **B.** Attachment sites of muscles of the posterior thigh and hip. **C.** Muscles of the thigh, anterior view. **D.** Muscle attachment sites on the thigh and pelvis.

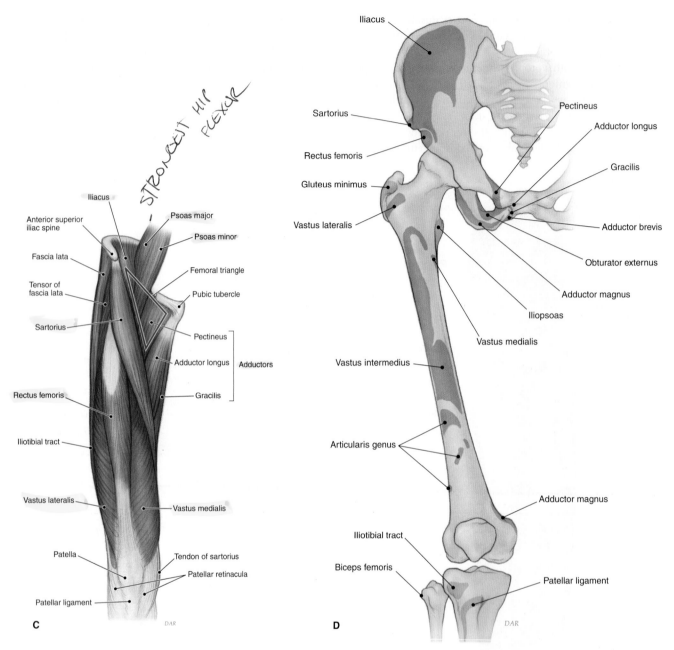

FIGURE 9-3 (*continued*)

In walking on a smooth hard surface, the knees swing forward and back, and the feet roll like the base of a rocking chair, with the weight moving from heels to toes. This connected chain of movement through the body creates a gentle undulation of the spine, which helps to enhance physiologic processes through the increased pumping of fluids through the trunk, including the cerebrospinal fluid that flows through the spinal cord.

The opposing muscles to the hip flexors are the hip extensors, which include the three hamstrings ▶ and the ***gluteus maximus***. The hamstrings are two-joint muscles originating at the ischial tuberosity and inserting on the tibia and fibula. They also serve as knee flexors. Their movement is restricted

by the presence of the iliofemoral ligament in the front of the hip, limiting pure extension to about 45°.

The primary hip abductors are the gluteus medius and minimus, with the tensor fascia latae assisting in abduction when the hip is flexed. The most important function of the tensor fascia latae is to maintain tension in the ***iliotibial band***. ▶ This band of fascia, which is located on the outside of the thigh, assists in absorbing tensile or stretching stresses acting on the femur. Bones are designed to absorb compression, or shortening stresses, better than tension, or lengthening stresses, which are absorbed by the muscles and fascia. Therefore, this additional support is crucial in strengthening the thigh.

The hip adductor muscles are the *pectineus, adductor brevis, adductor longus, adductor magnus,* and the *gracilis.* ▶ The gracilis is the only two-joint muscle of this group, inserting on the medial surface of the shaft of the tibia. For more on the range of motion of the hip joint, see Table 9-1.

TABLE 9-1 | **Range of Motion (ROM) for the Hip**

Action	Muscles
Flexion (knee extended) (ROM 90°)	Psoas major
	Sartorius
	Pectineus
	Adductor longus
	Adductor brevis
	Adductor magnus (anterior)
	Sartorius
	Rectus femoris
Extension (ROM 45°)	Gluteus maximus
	Biceps femoris (long head)
	Semitendinosus
	Semimembranosus
	Adductor magnus
	Gracilis
	Pectineus
Abduction (ROM 45°)	Gluteus medius
	Gluteus minimus
	Iliopsoas
	Tensor fascia latae
	Sartorius
Adduction (ROM 25°)	Adductor brevis
	Adductor longus
	Adductor magnus
	Gracilis
	Pectineus
Internal rotation (sitting) (ROM 35°)	Gluteus medius
	Gluteus minimus
	Tensor fascia latae
	Pectineus
	Adductors—longus, brevis, magnus
External rotation (sitting) (ROM 40°)	Piriformis
	Gemellus superior
	Obturator internus
	Gemellus inferior
	Obturator externus
	Quadratus femoris
	Gluteus maximus

▶ THIGH AND HIP ENDANGERMENT SITES

- *Femoral Triangle.* The femoral triangle is defined by the inguinal ligament, the sartorius muscle, and the medial aspect of the thigh or the gracilis muscle. Within this area the inguinal lymph nodes, femoral nerve, and femoral artery and vein are all vulnerable. The great saphenous vein also travels along the medial side of the sartorius before it joins the femoral vein (Fig. 9-4).
- *Sciatic Notch.* This is a notch in the ilium where the piriformis is located. Deep pressure here can irritate the sciatic nerve, which will cause pain down the leg.
- *Popliteal Fossa.* This area is more of an issue with leg massage (see Chapter 8), but its superior borders are the hamstring muscles. Portions of the sciatic nerve, the popliteal vein and artery, and the lesser saphenous vein are all accessible in the popliteal fossa.

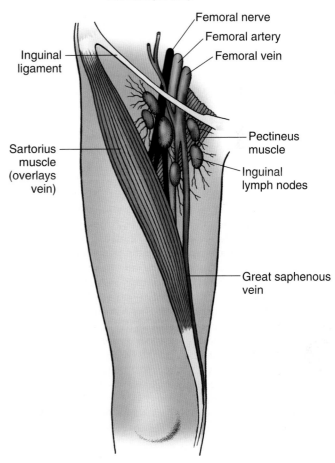

ANTERIOR LEG

Femoral nerve
Femoral artery
Femoral vein
Inguinal ligament
Pectineus muscle
Inguinal lymph nodes
Sartorius muscle (overlays vein)
Great saphenous vein

FIGURE 9-4 Endangerment sites of the femoral triangle.

▶ CONDITIONS

1. *Muscle Strains.* Minor tears are common in thigh muscles. Rest, careful stretching and exercise, and appropriately applied massage techniques are often adequate treatment for good quality long-term healing.

2. *Varicose Veins.* These are usually seen in the superficial veins of the leg and thigh. They are the result of damage to the valves that are meant to direct blood against gravity and toward the heart. While a genetic predisposition is certainly a factor, occupations that require standing without walking, and any physical restraint on the leg or thigh (i.e., a knee brace that is too tight) can contribute to the risk for varicose veins.

   The best home care treatment is elevation of the legs for a period every day, to assist the flow of blood out of the legs. Some people find that alternating hot and cold water on the affected area is helpful. Deep tissue massage is contraindicated in areas with varicosities, but massage with a broad, flat surface, as in light effleurage, is safe if the skin is healthy. See Appendix A for more information on these conditions.

▶ POSTURAL EVALUATION

1. Check the overall alignment of the anterior thigh (Fig. 9-5A–C).
   - Does the line of gravity appear to fall in a straight line between the center of the hip joint in the front of the thigh and the center of the knee?
   - If not, how does the line of gravity deviate?

2. Observe the shape and muscular tone of the thighs.
   - What is the degree of muscular development? Bound, flaccid, well-toned?
   - Do the muscles appear to be pulling in any particular direction?
   - Note any differences between the right and the left thigh.

3. In what direction(s) are the thigh muscles pulling the pelvis? Which muscles are involved? (Fig. 9-6A–C)

4. Check the alignment of the back of the thighs (Fig. 9-7A–C).
   - Where does the line of gravity fall through the back of the thighs?
   - Is the gluteal line at the base of the buttocks horizontal?

5. Observe the muscles of the posterior thigh and hip region (Table 9-1).
   - What is the muscular condition of the back of the thigh? Well-toned, weak, contracted?
   - What is the shape and tone of the gluteal region? Tight, loose, squeezed, overdeveloped, underdeveloped?
   - Are the tendons of the hamstrings prominent at the back of the knees? Do they appear even on the right and left legs?
   - Do the hamstrings appear to be pulling the pelvis downward?
   - Does the degree of muscularity match that of the front of the thighs?

HOLISTIC VIEW

The thighs—a source of momentum

Like the leg and foot, the thigh is involved in moving the body. The muscles of the thigh, being closer to the core of the body, are involved in initiating movement.

The thighs have been called the prime movers of the body. Their shape and tone indicates how a person moves through life. The quadriceps are thick, fiber-dense, and powerful muscles, potentially able to lift more weight than any other muscle group. The hamstring muscles, when chronically contracted, pull the ischial tuberosities of the pelvis downward, restricting pelvic movement and putting strain on the back of the knees.

These two muscle groups must be well-coordinated to orchestrate effectively the movements of flexion and extension at the knee joint and anterior and posterior tipping of the pelvis. The hamstrings are often weak in relation to the quadriceps, allowing the quadriceps to pull too strongly on the front of the pelvis, causing hyperextension of the low back.

Tight adductor muscles often denote a shielding or protective posture. Squeezing the inner thighs blocks access to the pelvic region, and may also reflect a suppressed need to urinate or defecate. Constriction of the outer thigh often accompanies contraction of the gluteal muscles. These muscles sometimes tighten in an effort to contain feelings and sensations.

As the hip and thigh muscles become better balanced through integrated deep tissue therapy sessions, a client may experience a renewed urge to move ahead with life. Reconnecting with the ground gives us a sense of sustenance, momentum, and a feeling of belonging here on the earth. This, coupled with tapping into the vast reserve of personal power that we all contain, as represented by the thighs, is a powerful motivation to create positive changes in one's life. ■

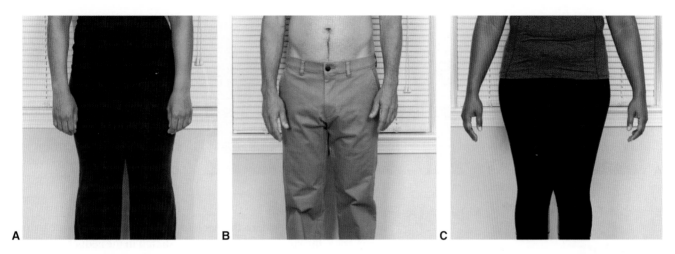

FIGURE 9-5 Postural evaluation: anterior thigh and knee.

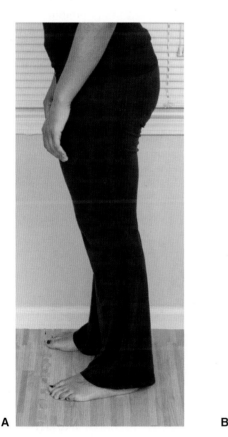 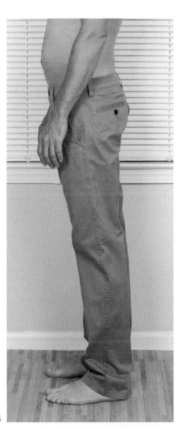 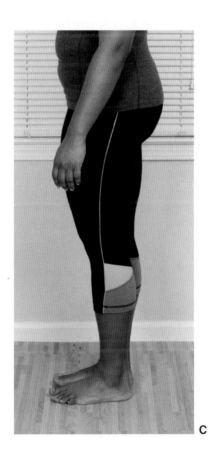

FIGURE 9-6 Postural evaluation: lateral thigh and pelvis.

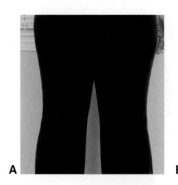
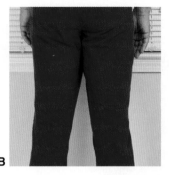
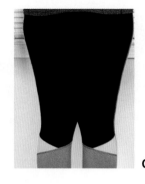

A   B   C

FIGURE 9-7 Postural evaluation: posterior thigh and pelvis.

▶ EXERCISES AND SELF-TREATMENT

Adductors

1. Inner Thigh Lift (Strengthens Adductors)

Preparation
Lie on your right side. The right leg is fully extended along the floor, under you. The left leg is extended straight in front at hip level. Place your left hand on the floor in front of your chest for support. Hold your head in your right hand (Fig. 9-8).

Execution
Exhaling, lift the right leg straight up, keeping the instep parallel to the floor. Think of squeezing the right inner thigh against the left inner thigh. Inhale as you lower the leg. Repeat several times and then reverse the position to do the left side.

2. Inner Thigh Stretch (Stretches Adductors)

Preparation
Lying on your back, bring the soles of your feet together in front of you, close to your pelvis. Wrapping your hands around the outside edges of the feet, turn the knees outward (Fig. 9-9).

Execution
Exhaling, draw the heels toward you as you continue to turn the knees out until you feel a stretch in the adductor muscles. Hold for a minimum of 20 seconds.

Abductors

1. Outer Thigh Lift (Strengthens Gluteus Medius, Gluteus Minimus, and Tensor Fascia Latae)

Preparation
The starting position is the same as for the inner thigh lift above, except that the bottom leg is flexed instead of straight. Medially rotate the leg extended in front of you at hip level so that the toes are pointing downward about 45° (Fig. 9-10).

Execution
Exhaling, lift the leg extended in front of you approximately 2 feet straight up in the air. Hold for a moment and then lower the leg as you inhale until the side of the big toe touches the floor. Repeat several times and then reverse your body position to do the exercise on the other side.

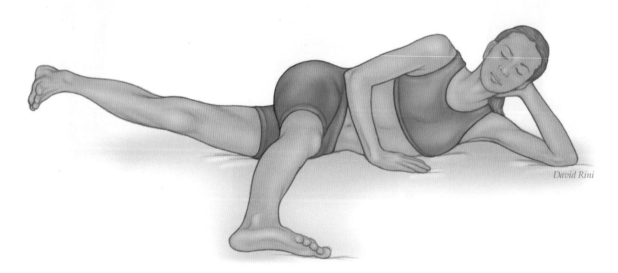

David Rini

FIGURE 9-8 Inner thigh lift.

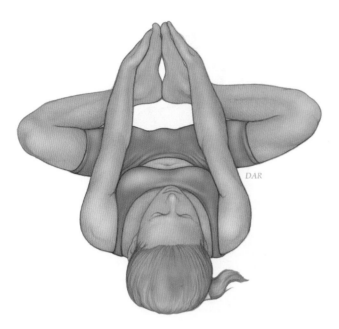

FIGURE 9-9 Inner thigh stretch.

2. Outer Thigh Stretch (Stretches Gluteus Medius, Gluteus Minimus, Tensor Fascia Latae, and Piriformis)

Preparation
Lie on your back, with both legs extended and your arms out to your sides at shoulder level. Circle the right leg along the floor to the left side, bringing it in the direction of your left shoulder.

Execution
Reach down and take hold of the right ankle with your left hand. Slowly bring the leg toward your left shoulder until you feel a stretch in the outer thigh and hip of the right leg. Hold for 30 seconds. Repeat the stretch for the left leg.

Quadriceps

1. Quadricep Strengthener (Strengthens Vastus Lateralis, Vastus Medialis, Vastus Intermedius, and Rectus Femoris)

Preparation
Sit up tall, with the legs extended in front of you. Keeping the right leg extended and the right foot strongly flexed, slide the left thigh toward your chest, keeping the foot on the floor. Hold the left knee with both hands (Fig. 9-11).

Execution
Exhaling, lift the right leg straight up off the ground a few inches while pulling up on the patella. Hold for a few seconds. Inhaling, lower the leg to the floor. Adjust the position of your back, making sure it is straight, and repeat the leg lift a few more times. Reverse your position and then repeat on the left side.

2. Quadricep Stretch (Stretches Vastus Lateralis, Vastus Medialis, Vastus Intermedius, and Rectus Femoris)

Preparation
To stretch your right thigh, lie on your left side. Place your head in your left hand. Flex both legs.

Execution
Lift your right leg, bringing the thigh toward the chest. Reach down and take hold of the top of the right ankle with your right hand. Slowly draw the thigh back until you feel a stretch in the center of your right thigh (Fig. 9-12). Hold for 20 seconds. Reverse the body position and then stretch the left thigh.

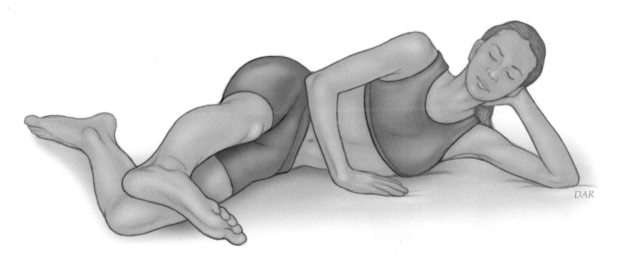

FIGURE 9-10 Outer thigh lift.

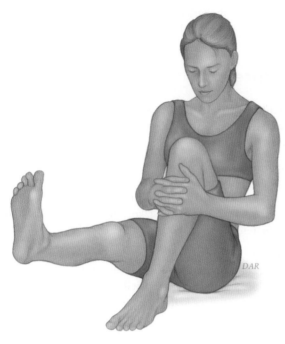

FIGURE 9-11 Quadriceps strengthener.

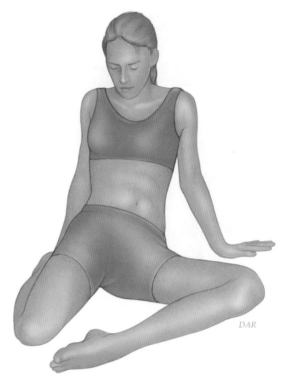

FIGURE 9-12 Quadriceps stretch.

Hamstrings

1. Hamstring Strengthener (Strengthens Biceps Femoris, Semitendinosus, and Semimembranosus)

Preparation
Lie face down on the floor, and turn your head to one side. Flex your right leg at the knee. Place your left foot behind the right ankle (Fig. 9-13).

Execution
Try to draw the right heel toward your hip as you resist the movement by pressing against the right ankle with your left leg. With resistance, flex the right leg toward the hip several times. Then, hold an isometric contraction of the right hamstring muscles for up to 30 seconds.

2. Hamstring Stretch (Stretches Biceps Femoris, Semitendinosus, and Semimembranosus)

Preparation
Have a belt or a tie handy. Lie on the floor on your back, with the left knee flexed and the left foot placed on the floor. Bringing your right thigh to your chest, loop the belt around the ball of the foot.

Execution
Exhaling, slowly extend the right leg toward the ceiling. Push upward with the heel as you flex the foot by pulling down on the sides of the belt (Fig. 9-14). Hold for 30 seconds.

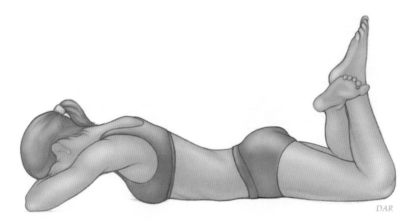

FIGURE 9-13 Hamstring strengthener.

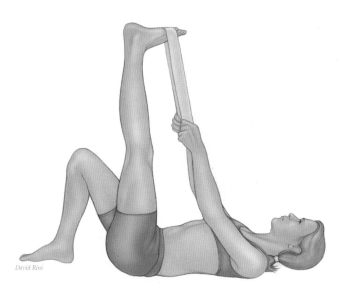

David Rini

FIGURE 9-14 Stretching the hamstrings using a belt.

Hips

1. Gluteal Strengthener (Strengthens Gluteus Maximus)

Preparation
Position yourself on your forearms and knees, with the right leg extended straight back and turned out so that the big toe is touching the floor.

Execution
Exhaling, lift the right leg straight up until you feel the gluteus maximus tighten (Fig. 9-15). Do not arch your back. Lower the right leg, and repeat several more times. Reverse the leg position, and repeat the lifts with the left leg.

2. Gluteal Stretch (Stretches Gluteus Maximus and Piriformis)

Preparation
Sit cross-legged, with the right heel placed in front of the left. Leaning forward slightly from the hip joints, place both hands on the floor in front of the legs.

Execution
Exhaling, slide the hands forward, slowly folding the trunk toward the floor until you feel a stretch in the back of the right hip (Fig. 9-16). Make sure both hips are touching the floor. Hold the stretch for 30 seconds and then repeat with the left foot in front to stretch the left hip.

3. Hip Relaxation

Preparation
Lying on the floor on your back, flex both knees, keeping the soles of the feet on the floor.

Execution
Bring your right thigh to your chest, and place both hands around the knee. Circle the thigh slowly as you imagine breathing into the right hip joint. Keep the thigh muscles totally relaxed. Let your arms guide the movement. Circle a few times in the other direction, then repeat the hip circles with the left leg.

▶ POSTERIOR THIGH AND HIP ROUTINE

Objectives

- To reduce restrictions in the hamstring muscles and their attachments, which can contribute to low back problems and pelvic distortion.

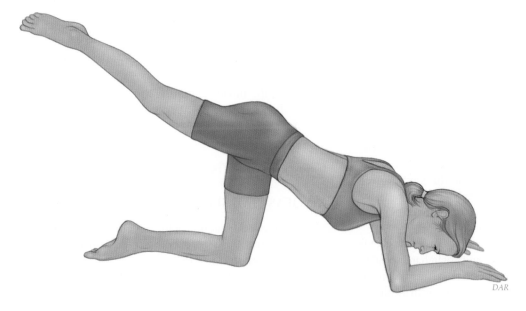

DAR

FIGURE 9-15 Gluteal strengthener.

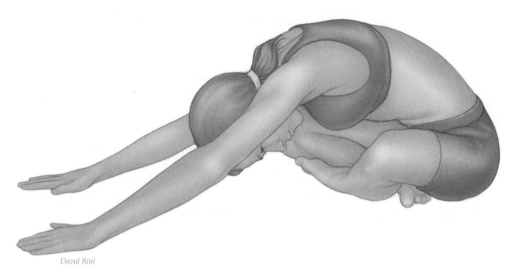

David Rini

FIGURE 9-16 Position to stretch the gluteal and piriformis muscles.

- To reduce unnecessary tension in the gluteal muscles.
- To help the deep lateral rotators to relax, which helps to improve the walking pattern.
- To reduce sciatic pain generated by a tight piriformis muscle.
- To help heal injuries in the sacral ligaments, a frequent contributor to low back pain.
- To bring balance to the soft tissues acting on the sacrum, allowing it to find its natural position. This brings greater ease throughout the body, as the upper and lower halves balance around the sacrum.

Energy

POSITION

- The client is lying prone on the table. A bolster may be placed under the ankles.
- The therapist is standing on the left side of the table and is facing the client's back.

POLARITY

Sacral Rock

1. The left hand contacts the C7–T1 area of the upper back. The palm of the right hand contacts the sacrum. Gently rock the sacrum with the right hand while stabilizing the upper back with the left hand. Continue for at least 30 seconds.

    This procedure helps to mobilize the lumbar vertebrae by freeing constrictions around the joints as well as by relaxing the muscles of the pelvis. It also helps the client to experience a feeling of continuity throughout the length of the spinal column.
2. The therapist's left hand (negative pole) contacts the client's sacrum (positive pole). The therapist's right hand (positive pole) rests on the back of the client's left knee (negative pole). This polarity procedure integrates the pelvis with the thighs.

a. Rock the sacrum with the left hand.
b. Place the right hand (positive pole) on the right knee (negative pole), and continue to rock the sacrum.

SHIATSU

1. Compress the back of the left thigh with both hands, from the hip to the knee. Repeat on the other leg. This shiatsu move stimulates qi flow through the bladder channel, which runs down the back of the leg.
2. Roll both fists across the muscles in the gluteal area. The bladder and gallbladder channels run through the back of the pelvis.

Swedish/Cross Fiber

1. Perform effleurage strokes on the posterior thigh and gluteal area.
2. Perform petrissage strokes on the posterior thigh and gluteal area.
3. Perform friction strokes on the posterior thigh and gluteal area.
4. Using the broad side of the thumb and/or the heel of the hand, apply cross-fiber strokes across the hamstrings and gluteal muscles.

Connective Tissue

MYOFASCIAL SPREADING TECHNIQUES

1. Starting at the midline of the posterior thigh, spread outward, using the heels of both hands. Work in horizontal strips, from the knee to the hip.
2. Using the heels of the hand and/or fingertips, spread the gluteal muscles.

Deep Tissue/Neuromuscular Therapy

SEQUENCE

1. Hamstrings—bellies and attachments
2. Gluteus maximus, medius, and minimus
3. Lateral rotators—piriformis, obturator internus, obturator externus, gemellus superior, gemellus inferior, and quadratus femoris ▶
4. Sacral ligaments—sacrotuberous and posterior sacroiliac

Hamstrings

Biceps Femoris
Origin:
    Long head—ischial tuberosity (inferior and medial aspects, sharing same tendon as semitendinosus), sacrotuberous ligament.
    Short head—entire length of the lateral lip of the linea aspera on the femur, proximal two-thirds of the lateral supracondylar ridge, lateral intermuscular septum.
Insertion: Lateral aspect of the head of the fibula, lateral condyle of the tibia.
Action: Knee flexion, knee external rotation.
    Long head—hip extension.

Semitendinosus
Origin: Ischial tuberosity (inferior medial aspect).
Insertion: Shaft of the tibia on the proximal medial side.
Action: Knee flexion, knee internal rotation, hip extension; assists hip internal rotation.

Semimembranosus
Origin: Ischial tuberosity (superior and lateral aspects).
Insertion: Medial condyle of the tibia on the posterior medial aspect, lateral condyle of the femur (posterior aspect via fibrous expansion, forming part of the oblique popliteal ligament).
Action: Knee flexion, knee internal rotation, hip extension; assists hip internal rotation.

◎ Trigger points tend to cluster in the distal portion of all three hamstring muscles above the knee. Checking along the borders of the muscles will often reveal trigger points. Referral patterns can be up to the gluteal area, around the ischial tuberosity, and around the back of the knee.

Position
- The client is lying prone on the table. A bolster may be placed under the ankles.
- The therapist is standing at the side of the table next to the client's knees.

Strokes
- Flexing the client's knee, follow the tendons of the hamstrings across the knee joint to their insertions on the leg, and apply static compression and cross-fiber techniques with your thumbs or fingers (Fig. 9-17).
- Perform an elongation stroke with your forearm from the knee to the ischial tuberosity. Repeat, covering each of the three hamstring muscles.
- Using the elbow, separate the three hamstring muscles. Follow the tendon of each muscle from the knee to find its border on the posterior thigh. Stroke from the knee to the ischial tuberosity along the edge of each muscle.
- Apply short, cross-fiber strokes with your thumb or knuckle to the origins of the hamstrings at the ischial tuberosity.

Gluteus Maximus, Medius, and Minimus

Gluteus Maximus
Origin: Posterior gluteal line and crest of the ilium, posterior surface of the sacrum and coccyx, aponeurosis of the erector spinae, sacrotuberous ligament.
Insertion: Iliotibial band of the fascia lata, gluteal tuberosity of the femur.
Action: Hip extension, lateral hip rotation, extension of trunk when insertion is fixed.
    Upper fibers—hip abduction.
    Lower fibers—hip adduction.

◎ The most common trigger point in gluteus maximus is found in the fibers slightly above the ischial tuberosity. The referred pain zone can be over the entire gluteal region. Another trigger point can be located in the fibers next to the lower portion of the sacrum. Activity here can refer pain along the gluteal line at the base of the muscle. A third trigger point has been found in the most medial and inferior fibers of the muscle, near the coccyx. This third trigger point refers pain to the coccyx so that when active, people often mistakenly think they have a problem with the coccyx.

Strokes
- Standing at the side of the table next to the client's pelvis, perform elongation strokes with the forearm, fist, or heel of the hand. Work in strips, from the ilium and sacrum to the greater trochanter (Fig. 9-18).
- Taut bands may be palpated by rolling across the fibers of the muscle with the fingertips or elbow. Treat trigger points as they are found.

Gluteus Medius
Origin: Outer surface of the ilium inferior to the iliac crest.
Insertion: Oblique ridge on the lateral surface of the greater trochanter of the femur.

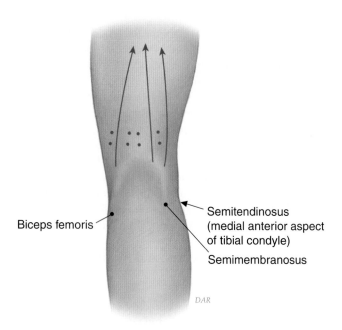

Biceps femoris

Semitendinosus
(medial anterior aspect
of tibial condyle)

Semimembranosus

DAR

FIGURE 9-17. Insertions of hamstrings and direction of deep tissue strokes.

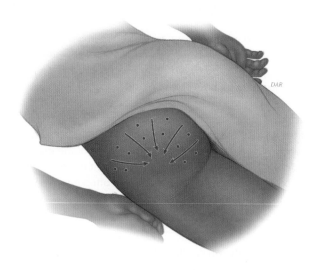

DAR

FIGURE 9-18 Direction of deep tissue strokes on gluteal muscles.

Action: Hip abduction.
> **Anterior fibers**—medial rotation of the hip.
> **Posterior fibers**—lateral rotation of the hip. The action of the gluteus medius prevents the pelvis from sliding laterally and tilting during the walking motion.

The three most common trigger points in the gluteus medius are located along the iliac crest, each in one of the three portions of the muscle. The first trigger point is found along the underside of the crest, near the sacroiliac joint. The pain pattern is along the iliac crest and over the sacroiliac joint and sacrum. The second trigger point is at the center point of the iliac crest (dividing it in two equal portions, front and back) and just below the lip. It refers pain to the middle of the gluteal region and sometimes down the outside of the thigh. The third point is much less common than the other two. It is found near the anterior superior iliac spine (ASIS), again just below the lip of the iliac crest. Pain is referred along the iliac crest to the lower lumbar region and the sacrum.

Gluteus Minimus
Origin: Outer surface of the ilium between the middle and inferior gluteal lines.
Insertion: Anterior border of the greater trochanter of the femur.
Action: Hip abduction, medial rotation of the hip.

Trigger point pain from the gluteus minimus is characteristically deep and quite severe. It projects down the leg more intensely than referred pain from the other gluteal muscles. There are two portions of the muscle. Trigger points in the anterior portion lie along the fibers vertically in a line to the greater trochanter. They refer pain to the lower buttock region and along the side of the thigh, sometimes all the way down to the ankle. Trigger points in the posterior portion accumulate in a fan-shaped pattern across the muscle, near its origin on the ilium. The pain pattern will cover the buttock and run down the back of the thigh, over the knee to the posterior calf region.

Strokes
- Perform elongation strokes with the forearm, elbow, or fist. Work in strips, from the lateral portion of the iliac crest to the upper portion of the femur just below the greater trochanter.
- Taut bands may be palpated by rolling across the fibers of the muscle with the fingertips or elbow. Treat trigger points as they are found.

Lateral Rotators (Piriformis, Obturator Internus, Gemellus Superior, Gemellus Inferior, Obturator Externus, and Quadratus Femoris)

Piriformis
Origin: Anterior surface of the sacrum, sacrotuberous ligament.

Insertion: Superior border of the medial aspect of the greater trochanter of the femur.

Action: Lateral rotation of the hip.

Obturator Internus

Origin: Margin of the obturator foramen on the pelvis, ramus of the ischium, inferior ramus of the pubis, pelvic surface of the obturator membrane.

Insertion: Medial surface of the greater trochanter of the femur.

Action: Lateral rotation of the hip.

Gemellus Superior

Origin: Gluteal surface of the ischial spine.

Insertion: Superior border of the greater trochanter.

Action: Lateral rotation of the hip.

Gemellus Inferior

Origin: Superior surface of the ischial tuberosity.

Insertion: Superior border of the greater trochanter.

Action: Lateral rotation of the hip.

Obturator Externus

Origin: Medial margin of the obturator foramen formed by the rami of the pubis and ischium.

Insertion: Trochanteric fossa of the femur.

Action: Lateral rotation of the hip.

Quadratus Femoris

Origin: Lateral border of the ischial tuberosity.

Insertion: Quadrate tubercle on the posterior aspect of the femur.

Action: Lateral rotation of the hip.

Strokes

- Apply short, side-to-side strokes with the elbow or thumbs next to the border of the sacrum to contact the medial portion of the piriformis near its origin on the anterior sacrum (Fig. 9-19A).
- Perform an elongation stroke with the elbow, fist, or heel of the hand, from the border of the sacrum to the greater trochanter, following the length of the piriformis from origin to insertion (Fig. 9-19B).

 Be careful while doing this move, because the piriformis covers the sciatic notch, where the sciatic nerve surfaces from the pelvis. Pressure on the sciatic nerve causes a shooting pain down the posterior thigh and should be avoided.

- Roll across the fibers of the lateral rotator muscles with the fingertips or elbow, from the border of the sacrum to the greater trochanter. Treat trigger points as they are found.
- Using the elbow or thumbs, apply static compression and cross-fiber strokes against the insertion points of the muscles on the greater trochanter (Fig. 9-19C).

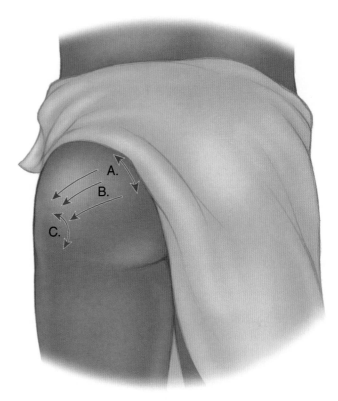

FIGURE 9-19 Directions of strokes on the piriformis and the attachment sites of the lateral rotator muscles on the greater trochanter.

Sacral Ligaments

The sacral ligaments are responsible for supporting the most moveable joints at the pelvis: the sacroiliac joints. In this role they are subject to frequent compressive and/or twisting forces, and may become irritated and inflamed: a contributor to low back and hip pain. Not every client will need work on the sacral ligaments, but for those who do, the following strategies work well.

Sacrotuberous Ligament

Strokes

- Palpate the lateral edge of the sacrum just above the coccyx. Next, palpate the ischial tuberosity on the same side of the pelvis. The ligament runs between these two locations (Fig. 9-20).
- Starting just lateral to the sacral edge, slide both thumbs under the gluteal muscles and then press up in a superior direction until you feel a dense, taut band of tissue.
- Move the thumbs slowly from side to side along the ligament, checking for tenderness. Hold painful areas with static compression for 8 to 12 seconds.

Posterior Sacroiliac Ligament

Injuries to this ligament will project pain across the low back and perhaps into the groin, thigh, and leg on the injured side.

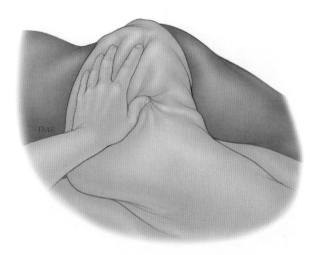

FIGURE 9-20 Contacting the sacrotuberous ligament.

Strokes

- Locate the posterior superior iliac spine with your thumbs. Press in and up on the underside of it with the thumb pads (Fig. 9-21). Perform short, cross-fiber strokes against the edge of the bone.
- With your fingertips, do short, up-and-down and side-to-side strokes on the sacrum, covering the entire surface.

STRETCH

Position

- The client is lying supine, with the leg to be stretched extended along the table and the other leg flexed with the sole of the foot against the table.

- The therapist stands at the side of the table near the client's foot.
  1. *Hamstrings.* Using your inside hand, hold the client's foot behind the heel, and lift the straight leg off the table. You may place the client's leg against your shoulder for additional support. Place your other hand on the client's anterior thigh. Stretch the leg by pressing forward and upward on the heel. Press against the anterior thigh with your other hand or forearm to encourage the knee to straighten (Fig. 9-22).
  2. *Gluteus Maximus.* The client's knee is brought to his or her chest. The client and therapist both place their hands over the knee. As the client draws the knee toward his or her chest, lean forward to apply additional impetus to the stretch (Fig. 9-23).
  3. *Gluteus Medius and Minimus.* Holding the client's ankle, bring the client's straight leg across his or her body to an adducted position. Rotating the leg laterally so that the toes and knee are facing upward, press the leg downward, in the direction of the table, until a stretch is felt in the gluteals (Fig. 9-24).
  4. *Lateral Rotators.* The leg of the side to be stretched is flexed at the knee and hip. The other leg is also flexed at the knee and hip, with the sole of the foot against the table. Holding the client's knee and ankle, turn the knee out, and place the client's foot against the thigh of the client's other leg. As the foot rests there, take hold of the knee and ankle of the supporting leg, and bring it toward the client's chest, sandwiching the foot of the stretched side between the client's chest and shoulder. Continue to bring the thigh toward the chest until a stretch is felt in the lateral rotator muscles (Fig. 9-25).

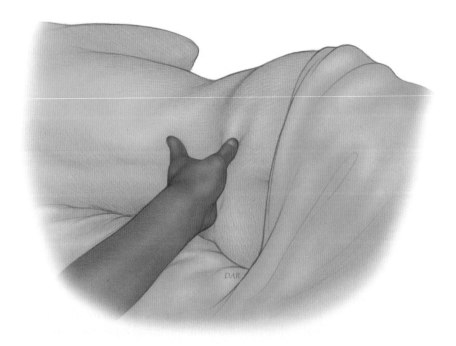

FIGURE 9-21 Contacting the posterior sacroiliac ligament.

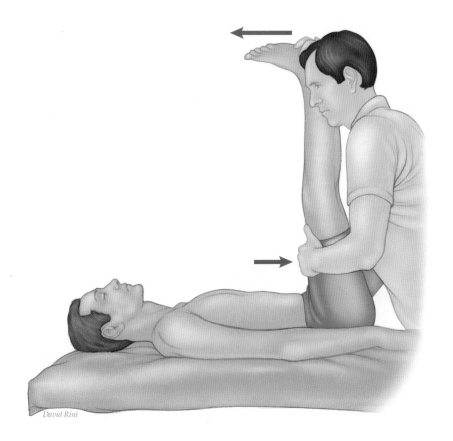

FIGURE 9-22 Hamstring stretch.

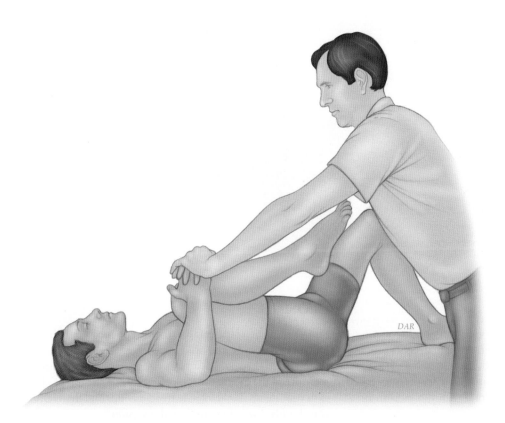

FIGURE 9-23 Gluteus maximus stretch.

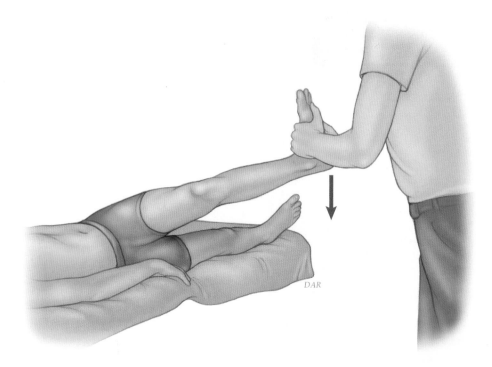

FIGURE 9-24 Stretch for gluteus medius and minimus.

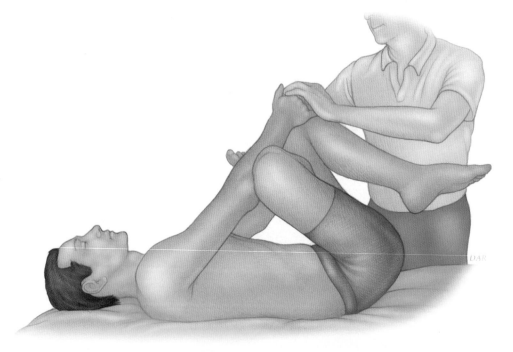

FIGURE 9-25 Stretch for the lateral rotators.

ACCESSORY WORK

1. This session is complemented with work on the rectus abdominus muscle, which, when shortened, contributes to posterior pelvic tilt along with shortened hamstrings.
2. Polarity balancing of the cranium and feet reinforces the alignment work that was done with the sacrum in this session.

CLOSING

Sitting at the head of the table, lightly cup the client's head in both of your hands, and hold for at least 30 seconds, allowing the client to relax and assimilate the effects of the session.

Move to the foot of the table. Lightly cup the client's heels with your hands. Hold for at least 30 seconds and then remove your hands slowly to complete the session.

SESSION IMPRESSION

THE HIP

This case demonstrates the pervasive effects that an injury can have on the soft tissues. The client is a 31-year-old homemaker named Mia, who is a former ballet dancer. She sustained an injury to her left hip while stretching in a dance class when she was 16 years old. At the time, she was sitting in a spread open-leg position on the floor, with her upper body flexed forward and her arms extended along the floor in front of her. After a few seconds in the stretch, she felt a shift of the left femur in the hip socket and a sharp pain running down the inside of her left thigh.

For several months after the injury, Mia experienced sharp pains extending down the inside of her left thigh. Over time, the pain has become less pronounced, but she still experiences a dull throbbing in that area. The most dramatic effect of the injury was a loss of full turn-out of the left leg, as a result of restriction of the femur in the hip socket. Mia found that this lack of turn-out on the left side affected her knee; it was difficult to plié (flex) the left leg while keeping the left knee properly aligned over the foot. She would experience pain and swelling in that knee after dancing.

The bracing of the muscles around the left hip has caused a build-up and hardening of connective tissue on the left side of the body, extending well up into the back. A hardened mass of connective tissue is found along the lateral border of the iliocostalis muscle under the 12th rib; this mass of connective tissue feels like another rib. Viewing the hips from the anterior position, the left hip appears to be narrower and posteriorly rotated. Mia walks with a small but noticeable limp on the left side.

The plan for the session was to attempt to improve the alignment of the muscles on the left side, which have been strained over the years in bracing the hip. These include the adductor muscles, gluteus medius and minimus,

and erector spinae (particularly the iliocostalis). Deep tissue strokes along the borders of these muscles were incorporated extensively to relieve adhering of the muscles. Connective tissue spreading techniques and deep tissue elongation strokes were also applied to the muscles where a build-up of connective tissue was found. Deep tissue techniques were used to reduce tension in the lateral rotator muscles of the posterior hip. Therapist-assisted stretches for the left hip included flexion, adduction, and abduction. The client was encouraged to continue to perform these stretches regularly between sessions.

A visit to a chiropractor or an osteopath was recommended to evaluate the condition of the hip. An adjustment to the left hip joint may alleviate some of the stress around the joint. Although the problem was not resolved by the deep tissue session (i.e., the left hip joint did not become unrestricted), the client felt much more range of motion in the left hip after the session and wishes to continue to receive deep tissue therapy. She feels that it will be of great benefit in halting the further build-up of connective tissue above the left hip. ∎

Topics for Discussion
1. Describe several ways of evaluating restrictions in hip movement.
2. Design an exercise program to achieve greater lateral rotation of the thigh.
3. How would you explain to a client why connective tissue tends to accumulate around a misaligned joint?
4. If a client walks with both legs and feet laterally rotated, which muscles are probably short? Which muscles are weak?
5. Specify two functions of the gluteus medius muscle.

The Pelvis and Abdomen

▶ GENERAL CONCEPTS

The pelvis forms the body's core. Functionally, it is analogous to the hub of a wheel, with the spine and the lower limbs acting as spokes radiating from it. The pelvis serves four main purposes:
1. It houses and protects vital organs.
2. It provides attachment sites for the muscles that control the trunk, legs, and arms.
3. It absorbs and distributes the shock that is transferred up the lower limbs in percussive activities like walking and jumping.
4. It transfers the weight of the upper body to the legs and feet.

The pelvic bones create a series of arches and curves that, when joined together, form a bowl. This shape allows weight to be moved easily around and through the pelvis without jarring the bowl's contents. The pelvis is a highly mobile structure, able to alter its position to accommodate weight shifts brought about by the movement of the body segments above and below. The pelvis moves freely between the spine and the heads of the femora, with its position mostly determined by muscular action.

The muscles of the thigh and trunk that attach to the pelvis must be balanced for correct pelvic alignment. Chronic shortness in any of these muscles creates compensatory tightening in other muscles, ligaments, and fascia, leading to stress and dysfunction in the hips and low back. Identifying and relieving chronic muscular tension patterns in the pelvis are the primary concerns of the integrated deep tissue therapist. The body as a whole cannot become integrated until the process of relaxing the core is initiated.

The primary pelvic muscle group is the iliopsoas: the iliacus, psoas major, and psoas minor. The psoas group connects the spine to the thigh, and by blending with fibers of the diaphragm, it connects the thorax to the legs. Its level of tension helps to determine the position of the pelvis. When the psoas group is functioning properly, the body's movements initiate from the core, giving increased power, grace, and stamina.

The abdomen joins the pelvis to the rib cage. The entire region is wrapped in muscles and fascial sheaths. The muscles of the abdominal wall are responsible for the movements of forward and lateral flexion as well as rotation of the trunk. They also support and protect the abdominal organs. These muscles attach along the ribs and the pelvic rim. The abdominal muscles work in conjunction with the back muscles to maintain pelvic alignment from above.

Correct alignment of the pelvis is crucial for maintaining the health and vitality of the abdominal organs. Poor posture compresses the organs and diminishes their efficiency. Sluggish or irregular function of the intestines is a major problem and affects many people. The factors contributing to intestinal dysfunction include poor diet, lack of exercise, stress, inadequate intake of water, and lack of tone and balance of the abdominal muscles. Abdominal massage is often helpful to promote healthy intestinal activity.

▶ MUSCULOSKELETAL ANATOMY AND FUNCTION

The Pelvis

Each whole pelvic bone is called an os coxa. The left and right os coxae are connected anteriorly at the pubis symphysis, and posteriorly by way of the sacroiliac joints with the sacrum.

The pelvis is made up of three pairs of bones: the ilia, the ischia, and the pubic bones. The ilium bones brace the sacrum, which is situated in the center of the back of the pelvis. The articulation of the ilium and the sacrum is the sacroiliac joint; it is a gliding synovial joint. The ilia flare in the back in a fan shape. They taper as they curve around to the front, fusing with the pubic bones. The pubic bones join in the

front of the pelvis at the pubic symphysis, a slightly moveable joint with a disk between the two bones. The ilia and pubic bones join seamlessly with the ischia. The acetabulum is the hollowed out cavity, the socket of the hip joint, formed where the three pelvic bones fuse. It consists of equal portions of the ilium, pubic bone, and ischium. This arrangement allows equal forces from all three bones in the pelvis to pass to the hip joint (Fig. 9-26). (See Essential Anatomy Box 9-2 for a summary of muscles, bones, and landmarks.)

The sacrum is the keystone for the human skeleton. Weight from the upper body accumulates at the sacrum and then passes from the sacroiliac joints across the ilia to the hip joints and, when a person is standing, from there to the heads of the femora. In a seated position, the weight is transferred to the ischial tuberosities, which are ring-shaped projections at the base of the ischia. This balanced weight transfer depends on soft tissue interaction to keep the joints aligned. Subtle movement at the sacroiliac joints make the sacrum subject to a variety of displacements, including slight rotation and posterior deviation, but the most common aberration by far is anterior displacement.

Weight pressing on the sacrum tends to shift the upper portion forward between the left and right os coxae, causing it to become pushed forward, below the fifth lumbar vertebra. This tendency is counteracted by strong ligaments that wrap the sacrum and prevent it from sliding. The attachment of the *piriformis* muscle to the front side of the sacrum also contributes to its stability. When the sacrum shifts, it causes irritation and pain in the sacroiliac joints and ligaments, and it disrupts the sequence of weight transfer through the lower body. The piriformis muscles become contracted as they attempt to

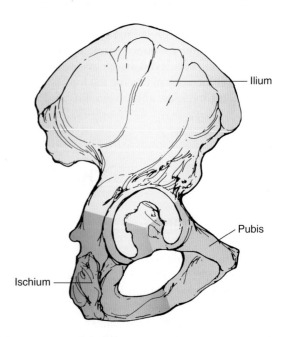

FIGURE 9-26 The acetabulum is formed by the convergence of the ilium, ischium, and pubis.

MUSCLES
Psoas major and minor
Iliacus
Rectus abdominus
Obliques—external and internal
Gluteus maximus, medius, and minimus
Inguinal ligament

BONES AND LANDMARKS
Ilium
Iliac crest
Ischium
Pubic symphysis
Sacrum
Sacroiliac joint
Lesser trochanter of the femur

stabilize the sacrum and pass this tightness to the other lateral rotator muscles. External rotation then alters how weight is passed through the knee, and so on to the foot. During massage work, the therapist should never press down hard toward the floor on a client's sacrum, because this may cause it to slide anteriorly, creating the problems described above.

The musculature at the base of the pelvis composed of muscles and ligaments known as the pelvic floor or pelvic diaphragm. The principal muscle is the levator ani, which operates like a sling that supports the pelvic organs above it. It attaches to the inner surfaces of the pubic bones and ischia in the front and then runs posteriorly, around the genitals and anus, to attach in the back to the coccyx. The fascia that wraps this muscle is a continuation of the fascia of the inner thigh muscles, thus creating an essential bond between the pelvis and the inner thigh. In this way, the degree of restriction in the inner thighs affects the condition of the internal pelvic structures. The strength, proper muscle tone, and elasticity of the pelvic floor are essential to good health. The perineum can form trigger points that refer pain to pelvic organs; this may be a factor in chronic pelvic pain for men and women. Urination and defecation rely on proper tone in this muscle. Impact injuries to the coccyx are common, and they may create problems in the perineum. For women, childbirth is much easier when the pelvic floor is able to relax; this is the final barrier through which the baby passes and if it is too tight it may tear. After childbirth, it is important that muscle tone be restored to the pelvic diaphragm for bladder control.

The iliopsoas is made up of three muscles, the *iliacus*, *psoas major*, ▶ and *psoas minor*, with each having a slightly different purpose (Fig. 9-27E). The psoas major muscle attaches to the bodies of the 12th thoracic vertebra and the five lumbar vertebrae. It passes over the front of the pelvis like a sling, and inserts on the lesser trochanter on the inside of the femur.

When the hip joints are stable, the psoas major flexes the trunk toward the legs, as in the action of a sit-up. In this capacity, the psoas works in conjunction with the rectus abdominis muscle. Flexion of the spine should be initiated by the psoas, because it is positioned closer to the spine for the best mechanical advantage. Flexion is then reinforced by the action of the abdominal muscles. When movement patterns become inefficient, the rectus abdominus muscle does most of the work while the psoas remains inactive.

The range of influence of the psoas major muscle is extensive. The origin of the psoas on the 12th thoracic vertebra blends with the attachments of the crura of the diaphragm. Inadequate functioning of the psoas can influence the action of the diaphragm, thus affecting respiration. The psoas may also affect autonomic function, because nerves of sacral plexus pass through it. Some of these nerves exert autonomic control the abdominal viscera. Therefore, the general health and well-being of the body is tied to the condition of the psoas.

The psoas minor has its origin at the 12th thoracic vertebra and inserts on the ilium bone. It connects the spine with the pelvis, and it assists in flexion of the trunk and lumbar spine.

The iliacus muscle originates on the iliac crest and the anterior surface of the ilium. It joins the psoas major as it glides over the front of the pelvis and inserts on the lesser trochanter of the femur. The iliacus connects the pelvis with the legs, giving increased power to hip flexion movements, like running and kicking. These three muscles, acting as a group, provide force and stability to the body's central core.

The Abdomen

The muscles of the abdomen are the *rectus abdominus*, *external obliques*, ▶ *internal obliques*, and *transverse abdominus*. In addition to providing support for the abdominal contents, they are important accessory breathing muscles. As they collectively contract during forced exhalation, they push the diaphragm back up into position for inhalation. (See Essential Anatomy Box 9-3 for a summary of muscles, bones, and landmarks.)

The left and right rectus abdominus muscles form the most central part of the abdominal wall, connecting the rib cage to the pelvis at the pubic bone (Fig. 9-27A). When they contract, they draw the base of the pelvis upward, causing the top of the pelvis to tip posteriorly. In this action, the rectus abdominus is the antagonist to the psoas major when a person is standing. In the standing position, when the psoas major

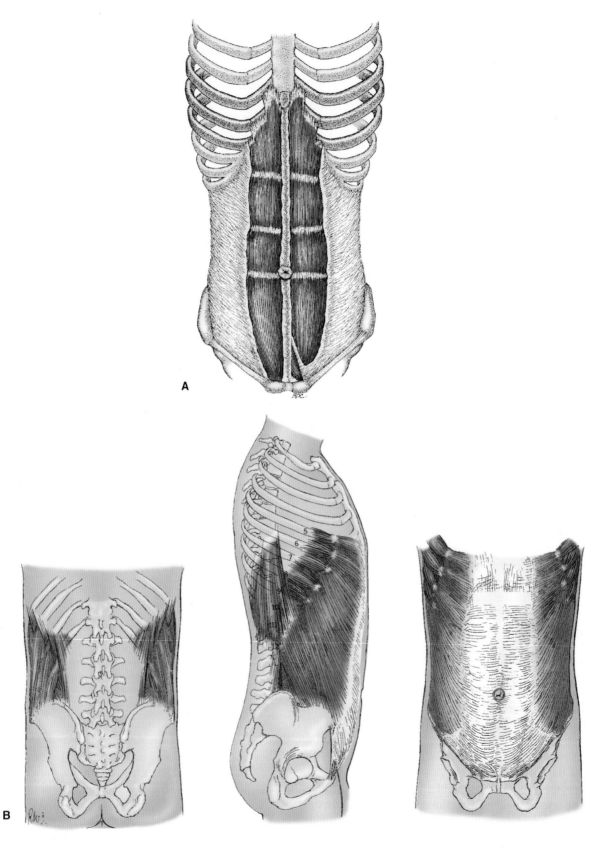

FIGURE 9-27 A. Rectus abdominus. **B.** External obliques. **C.** Internal obliques. **D.** Transverse abdominus. **E.** The iliopsoas group. **F.** Quadratus lumborum.

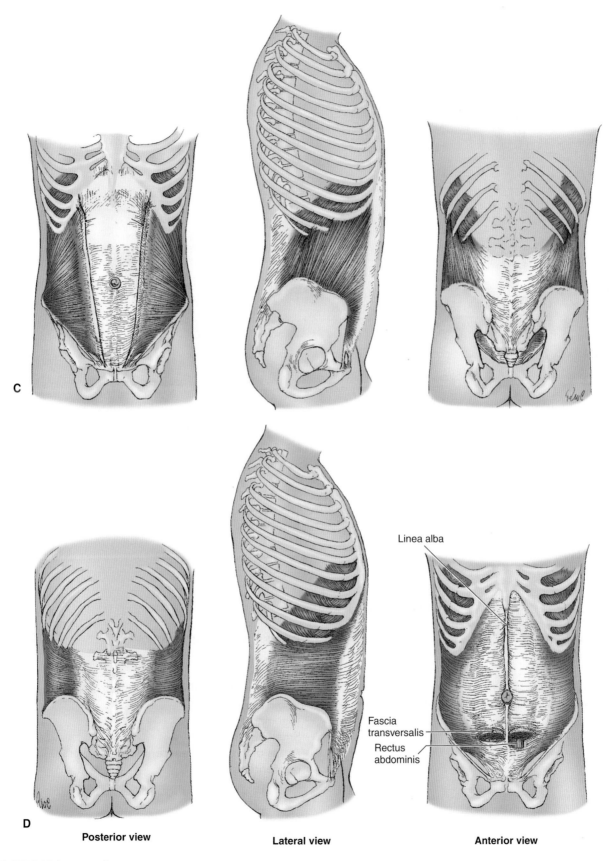

Linea alba

Fascia transversalis

Rectus abdominis

Posterior view   **Lateral view**   **Anterior view**

FIGURE 9-27 (continued)

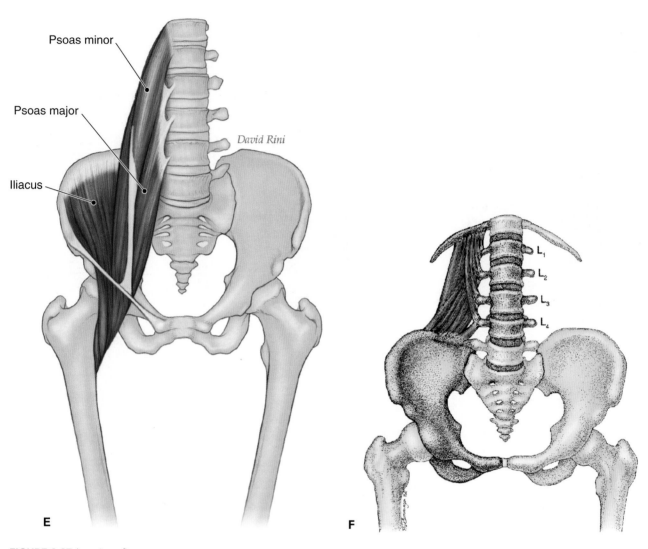

FIGURE 9-27 (continued)

BOX 9-3 ESSENTIAL ANATOMY | **The Abdominal Routines**

MUSCLES	**BONES AND LANDMARKS**
Rectus abdominus	Costal cartilage
External obliques	Ilium
Internal obliques	Anterior superior iliac spine (ASIS)
Transverse abdominus	Pubic bone
	Inguinal ligament
	Small intestine
	Areas of the colon—ascending, transverse, descending
	Ileocecal valve
	Appendix
	Hepatic and splenic flexures
	Sigmoid colon and rectum
	Aorta

contracts, it pulls the lumbar spine forward, causing the top of the pelvis to tilt anteriorly. The balancing action of the rectus abdominus and psoas muscles as an agonist–antagonist pair is essential for proper alignment and coordinated movement of the body as a whole.

The left and right external obliques, acting together, also flex the spine (Fig. 9-27B). Unilaterally, they laterally flex the trunk and cause rotation to the opposite side. The fibers of the external obliques angle toward the midline, matching the direction of the external intercostal muscles.

The internal obliques duplicate the actions of the external obliques, except that when acting unilaterally, they rotate the trunk to the same side (i.e., the right internal oblique rotates the trunk to the right, and the left internal oblique rotates the trunk to the left). The fibers of the internal obliques angle away from the midline, matching the direction of the internal intercostal muscles (Fig. 9-27C).

The transverse abdominus is the deepest of these three muscles. Its fibers run in a horizontal direction (Fig. 9-27D). It acts to compress the abdominal contents. Its strong contraction causes forced exhalation and regurgitation.

The fascial sheaths that separate the external intercostals, internal intercostals, and transversus abdominus merge as they come medially to form the fascial sheath that wraps the left and right sides of the rectus abdominus.

The **quadratus lumborum** forms the posterior wall of the abdomen (Fig. 9-27F) and is situated behind the psoas muscle. The quadratus lumborum consists of three sections, which have their origin on the inner lip of the iliac crest and the iliolumbar ligaments. The insertions are on the lower border of the 12th rib and the transverse processes of the first four lumbar vertebrae. The muscle is wrapped in thoracolumbar fascia.

The quadratus lumborum is a strong stabilizer of the lumbar spine. It prevents excessive lateral bending to the opposite side. Acting bilaterally, the quadratus lumborum extends the spine, and when overly contracted, it contributes to increased lordosis. Unilaterally, the muscle assists in lateral flexion to the same side. The quadratus lumborum is known as "the hip hiker." In a standing position, if the upper border of one of the iliac crests is higher than the upper border of the other, the quadratus lumborum on that side is often shortened.

▶ ABDOMINAL ENDANGERMENT SITES

- *Xyphoid Process.* This bony prominence can be broken with any sharp, downward pressure; a broken xyphoid process can damage the liver.
- *Floating Ribs:* While massage is unlikely to damage the 11th and 12th ribs, deep work in this area can pin soft tissues on them, which is very uncomfortable.
- *Inguinal Canal.* This is the opening where a man's spermatic cord and supporting blood vessels pass into the pelvic cavity. This area is a weak spot in the abdominal wall, and if a man has any history of inguinal hernias, special care must be taken here to not stretch the tissues beyond a comfortable level.
- *Abdominal and Pelvic Organs.* The liver, ovaries, spleen, kidneys, and the large intestine are all potentially vulnerable to damage with deep abdominal work (Fig. 9-28).

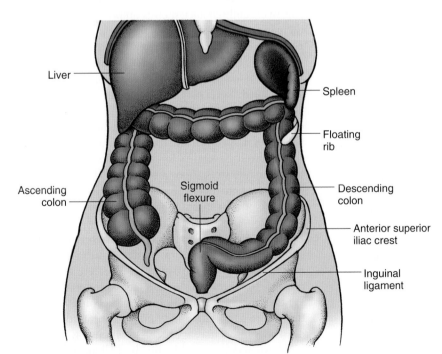

FIGURE 9-28 Endangerment sites of the abdomen and pelvis.

▶ CONDITIONS

1. *Anterior Pelvic Tilt.* This is a forward tipping of the ilium that creates an increased lumbar curve and often a protrusion of the abdomen. If the pelvis is visualized as a bowl that is filled with water, the water would be spilling out in front of the person. The iliopsoas and the rectus femoris on both sides will be shortened, causing compression of the vertebral disks and strain on the soft tissues of the low back. This is the pattern seen with hyperlordosis.

2. *Posterior Pelvic Tilt.* This is a backward tipping of the ilium. It causes the buttocks to appear tucked under and is often accompanied by contraction in the gluteal muscles, a tight rectus abdominus, and shortened hamstrings. The erector spinae muscles will be pulled downward, and the lumbar curve will be diminished, which will affect the transfer of weight through the spine.

3. *Short Leg.* This is a general term, describing a lateral tilt of the pelvis, presumably because one leg is shorter than the other, causing the pelvis to lean toward the short side. In most cases, however, the unevenness of the pelvis is caused by spinal curves or twists. The shortened side is often indicative of a tight psoas and quadratus lumborum muscle.

   Differences in length between the right and left psoas can also lead to pelvic rotation. The pelvis will be pulled forward and down on the side of the shortened psoas.

4. *Sciatica.* This is an irritation or inflammation of the sciatic nerve, which is made of nerves that emerge from L4–S3. The sciatic nerve, the largest nerve in the body, goes through the sciatic notch in the pelvis, and runs down the back of the leg. Spinal problems or disk damage can irritate the nerve. If this is the case, the pathway of pain usually extends down the back of the leg and sometimes even to the ankle.

   In some cases, the source of irritation is at the site of the piriformis muscle at the back of the hip, under which the sciatic nerve passes. (In some people, the sciatic nerve passes *through* the piriformis.) If tightness in the piriformis is the source of the irritation, the pain is usually localized at the hip and back of the thigh.

5. *Psoas Strain.* The psoas muscle is difficult to injure, but it may become strained from extreme stretching motions of the trunk and groin, as in a jump initiated from a crouched position. This kind of injury is common in basketball players reaching for the hoop and in volleyball players. To test for psoas impairment, have the client sit on the edge of the table, with the feet hanging toward the floor. Place your hand on the thigh of the side you are checking, and have the client try to lift the thigh as you resist. If the psoas is injured, the client will experience pain in the groin area.

   Another form of psoas injury can occur as a groin pull: irritation to the psoas insertion on the lesser trochanter. This injury is often seen in hurdlers and other track athletes.

6. *Menstrual Cramps.* Painful menstrual cramps are usually a multifactorial problem involving spasms of the uterus, irritation of pelvic ligaments and fascia, and referred pain to the groin and low back. A woman who is having cramps will probably not welcome intrusive abdominal massage during her period, but she may benefit from it at other times of the month. Gentle work on the fascia of the low back and sacrum however is often helpful for easing the pain of menstrual cramps. This is a rare example of a referred pain arc that seems to work in both directions: organ pain refers to the skin of the low back, and soothing touch appears to refer back to the over-working organ.

7. *Abuse Issues.* It is not uncommon for both male and female clients to have experienced sexual abuse, either as children or adults. As a result, they may be afraid of having their pelvic area touched. In fact, this work can be sensitive for anyone to receive because of the societal taboos imposed on the pelvic region, as result of our attitudes about sex and the eliminative functions. As a therapist, always approach this work sensitively, and respect the client's limitations. Agree ahead of time on what you plan to do together, and be ready to change tactics if your client changes his or her mind during the session. It may take time for the client to come to terms fully with all the emotional responses to being touched in the low abdomen. Be patient and nurturing, and allow healing to unfold at its own pace.

   Abdominal massage should be introduced slowly to a client who has a history of abuse or concerns about having the abdominal area touched. It may take several sessions before the client is comfortable with work being done on that area. Initial contact with the abdomen may consist of gentle contact; such as simply holding the hands there over the drape while the client relaxes. Keeping the abdomen covered with a drape while touching it often adds to the client's sense of safety. This contact may be included in several sessions before full abdominal massage is attempted. Never perform abdominal work without the client's willingness and permission.

8. *Constipation.* Constipation occurs when peristalsis in the colon slows down and fecal material does not move through well. Several factors contribute to constipation; these include stress, poor diet, lack of abdominal tone, and inadequate intake of water. Deep tissue massage is often helpful in stimulating intestinal contractions so that material moves through more easily.

9. *Diverticulitis.* This is an inflammatory condition of the colon. Diverticula are tiny pouches in the colon wall that are filled with fecal matter. They are created by pressure from straining to push feces through the colon. When these sacs of waste material become inflamed, they cause pain. This condition is a contraindication to deep abdominal massage therapy, which may be able to pin down and damage this already challenged structure.

10. *Other Pelvic Pathologies.* Many other conditions can affect the muscular function of the pelvis, or they can impact the safety of pelvic or abdominal massage therapy. These include undiagnosed conditions, ovarian cysts, enlarged prostate, pregnancy, any type of pelvic cancer, and any infections that may cause inflammation in the pelvis. These conditions can range from being annoying to being life-threatening. Massage therapists need to understand how a client may be affected by these possibilities before proceeding with intrusive pelvic or abdominal massage.

See Appendix A for more information on these conditions.

HOLISTIC VIEW

The center of power

The pelvis is the body's structural center and its optimal point of leverage. All parts of the body come into equilibrium when they are correctly balanced around the pelvis. Muscles function with their maximum efficiency in this alignment, and signals from the nervous system that are unimpeded by hypertonic muscles lead to smooth, flowing, elegant action.

When our power emanates from this centered place, we can move with freedom and grace, without unnecessary inhibition, pain, or inefficiency. We can live experience the natural power of the body, and enjoy the vitality that such balance offers.

Few of us, however, function at this level. For the most part, we identify our core and initiate our actions from higher in the spine. The emphasis placed on intellectual processes draws most people's awareness up toward the head. Muscular initiation of movement tends to occur more from the chest and thoracic region of the spine. This recruits the muscles that are responsible for breathing in fruitless effort, and it also disconnects us from the more powerful and effective muscles of motion that originate in the pelvis, hips and thighs.

The pelvis houses the organs of reproduction and elimination. Many cultures are not comfortable with recognizing these functions as a normal part of a healthy life. Many societal constraints are placed on both the act of elimination and sexuality. From early childhood we are taught to squeeze our sphincters and hold our eliminations for a more convenient time. Then in young adulthood we are bombarded with conflicting and often unhealthy messages about sexuality and attractiveness, just as our bodies are rapidly changing and growing. This forms the basis of a potentially lifelong pattern of associating strong emotions and a sense of control with tightening the pelvic floor, inner thighs, gluteal and deep lateral rotator muscles, and the low back. In essence, we cut ourselves off from the most powerful part of our body.

The pelvis is designed to swing freely between the hip joints and the lumbar spine. This capability is limited by chronic muscular contractions in and around the pelvic region. Muscle action is controlled by the nervous system, and it is inevitable that our mental attitudes and beliefs play an important part in determining our body's freedom of movement, and limitations of movement.

Because pelvic positioning is largely determined by muscle tension, we have a tremendous capacity to distort pelvic placement and movement through our responses to emotional and physical issues associated with this body segment. Common patterns include the anterior tilt of the pelvic bowl, tucking under of the hips, and constriction across the lumbar muscles. All of these denote some form of muscular imbalance that inhibits complete mobility of the pelvis.

The abdominal wall is a cylinder of muscle and fascia covering the viscera. Having no bony protection, the belly is commonly perceived as being vulnerable and weak. A feeling of apprehension is often associated with receiving touch in this area, partly because of a sense of defenselessness, and self-consciousness over not having a perfectly toned, magazine-model type of abdomen. In short, exposing the abdomen makes many people feel protective, unsafe, and even ashamed. These emotional responses to abdominal and pelvic massage cannot be completely untangled from our attitudes about ourselves: our self-acceptance or self-judgment.

The image of the tight, washboard abdomen is considered to be desirable by many people. We are enticed by TV commercials and videos extolling the virtues of a trim, tight midsection. But by overly tightening the abdominal muscles, we effectively create a shield of armor around our perceived vulnerabilities in an attempt to protect ourselves from the world—both physical threats and emotional ones.

A truly balanced abdomen has a slightly rounded contour. It is supple and toned, not cinched in tight and rigid. Neither is it flaccid and lifeless, allowing the abdomen to protrude and weakening the alignment of the lumbar spine and rib cage.

A lot of people have tight pelvic muscles, and weak abdominal muscles, and rigid, overworked low back muscles. They are vulnerable to the pain and injuries that occur when these structures are out of balance. But when the muscles of the pelvis, abdomen, and low back coordinate with each other to maintain the integrity of the trunk, we have more strength and the flexibility to adapt to the many demands of life. Balance in the pelvis reflects a quality of poise, self-confidence and integrity that allows one to experience fully the kinesthetic unity of the body. ■

▶ POSTURAL EVALUATION

The Pelvis and Abdomen: Front View

1. Check the level of the iliac crests. Are they on the same horizontal line? (Fig. 9-29A–C)
2. Look for rotation of the pelvis. If one ASIS is more prominent than the other, it indicates that side of the pelvis is rotated forward.
3. Does the rib cage float over the iliac crests, or does the waist area seem compressed, forming bulges at the sides (i.e., love handles)?
4. When the client's knees are flexed, do they align over the feet properly? Incorrect tracking of the knees over the feet affects psoas function.
5. Does the pelvis seem too large or too small for the rest of the body?
6. Check the position of the lower ribs. Are they. . .
   * Squeezed together, pulling downward?
   * Spread apart, lifted, protruding?
7. What is the general shape of the abdomen?
   * Tight, withdrawn, held in?
   * Distended?
8. Describe the distribution of fat content: does most fat seem to be in the abdomen (apple shape), or in the superficial fascia around the lower belly, hips and thighs (pear shape)?
9. Does the belly move with the breath?

The Pelvis: Side View

1. Observe the direction and degree of pelvic tilt, if any (Fig. 9-30A–C).
2. During walking and standing, can the pelvis swing forward and backward freely? If not, in which motion is it restricted?

Please refer to Table 9-2 for a list of variations in pelvic alignment and possible muscles involved.

The Abdominal Region

Please refer to Table 9-3 for a list of common tension patterns found in the abdominal region and possible muscles involved.

▶ EXERCISES AND SELF-TREATMENT

Pelvis

Pelvic Opening (Integrates Muscular Action in the Pelvis and Low Back Regions)

Preparation
Sit on the edge of a chair, with both feet flat on the floor, or sit in a cross-legged position on the floor. Do each movement slowly and consciously. The purpose of the exercise is to increase awareness of the pelvic region.

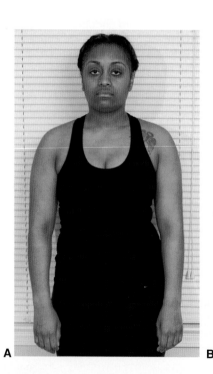
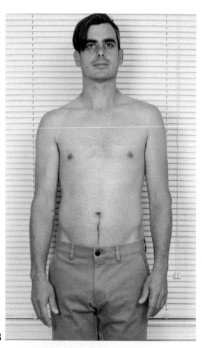
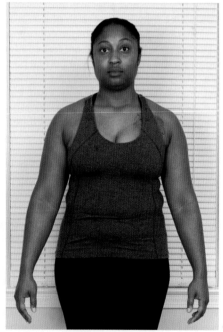

FIGURE 9-29 Postural evaluation: anterior pelvis and abdomen.

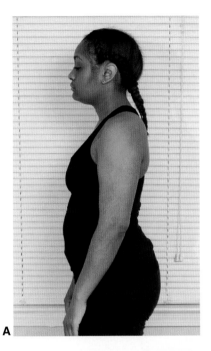 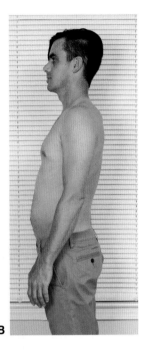 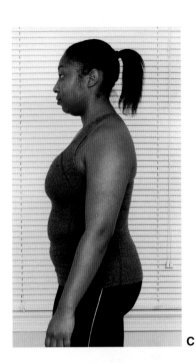

A   **B**   **C**

FIGURE 9-30 Postural evaluation: lateral pelvis and abdomen.

TABLE 9-2 | Body Reading for the Pelvis

Postural Patterns	Muscles That May Be Shortened
Anterior tilt—the iliac crests are tipped forward	Iliopsoas
	Rectus femoris
	Erector spinae
	Quadratus lumborum
Posterior tilt—the iliac crests are tipped backward	Rectus abdominus
	Gluteus maximus
	Lateral rotators
	Hamstrings
Lateral tilt—one iliac crest is higher than the other	Gluteus medius
	Quadratus lumborum
	Abductors on high side
	Adductors on low side

TABLE 9-3 | Body Reading for the Abdomen

Postural Patterns	Muscles That May Be Shortened
Distended belly—accompanied by anterior tilt of the pelvis	Quadratus lumborum
	Iliopsoas group
	Rectus femoris
	Erector spinae
Tight midsection—rectus abdominus is overly defined, lower ribs are pulled in and down; rigid abdominal wall	Rectus abdominus
	Transverse abdominus
	Hamstrings
Bladder belt—upper abdominal area is distended; lower area is pulled in, as if wearing a tight belt	Obliques
	Pelvic floor muscles

Execution

- Roll the pelvis posteriorly, rounding the low back and taking your weight off the ischial tuberosities (Fig. 9-31A). Let your chin drop forward naturally. Return the pelvis to the vertical position, and repeat a few more times.
- Roll the pelvis anteriorly, arching the low back slightly (Fig. 9-31B). Return to the upright position, and repeat several more times.
- Combine the two movements above, creating a fluid, forward and backward, rocking motion of the pelvis. Rest briefly afterward, and note any changes in your level of awareness in the pelvic region.

- Beginning with your weight distributed evenly over the base of the pelvis, shift slightly to the right, increasing the weight on the right ischial tuberosity. Keep the left hip on the chair or floor. Return to the center position, and repeat the shift to the right several more times.
- Beginning with your weight distributed evenly over the base of the pelvis, shift slightly to the left, increasing the weight on the left ischial tuberosity. Keep the right hip on the chair or floor. Return to the center position, and repeat the shift to the left several more times.
- Combine the previous two movements, rocking your weight from side to side several times. Rest briefly afterward, noting any changes in your level of awareness in the pelvic region.

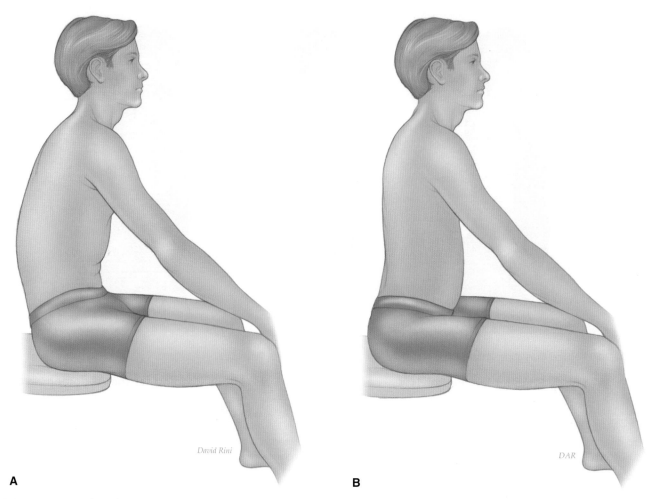

A

B

David Rini

DAR

FIGURE 9-31 A. Tilting the pelvis posteriorly. **B.** Tilting the pelvis anteriorly.

Abdomen

Sit-Downs (Strengthens Rectus Abdominus, External and Internal Obliques, and Transverse Abdominus)

Preparation
Sitting on the floor, bring your knees to your chest, with both feet remaining on the floor. Place your hands under the thighs just above the knees.

Execution
Exhaling, pull in your abdomen, and tuck your pelvis under as you roll down the back slightly (Fig. 9-32). Hold for a few seconds as you breathe normally. Exhale strongly, and roll down the back a little farther. Continue to roll toward the floor in small increments. If your back begins to hurt or the abdominal muscles cannot support the rolling motion any further, lie down on your back and rest.

Abdominal Stretch (Stretches Rectus Abdominus, External and Internal Obliques, and Transverse Abdominus)
Lying on your back on the floor, extend your arms overhead. Exhaling, press the low back to the floor as you reach the

arms behind you, until you feel a stretch in the abdominal muscles (Fig. 9-33). Hold for 20 seconds. Slightly arching the back increases the stretch. Laterally flex the trunk to the right by reaching both arms slightly to the right. Hold for 20 seconds. Laterally flex the trunk to the left by reaching both arms slightly to the left. Hold for 20 seconds.

▶ ABDOMINAL MUSCLES ROUTINE

Objectives

- To elongate the portion of the trunk that connects the thorax and pelvis
- To normalize tension in the attachments of the trunk muscles along the pelvis and the lower ribs
- To normalize tension in the quadratus lumborum muscle, which can contribute to low back pain and misalignment of the pelvis
- To improve the function of the intestines
- To further open the abdominal cavity

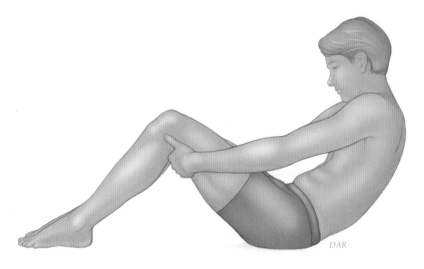

FIGURE 9-32 Sit-down exercise to strengthen rectus abdominus.

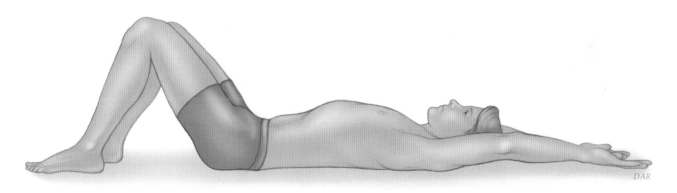

FIGURE 9-33 Stretch for rectus abdominus.

Energy

POSITION

- The client is lying supine on the table, with a bolster under the knees. Female clients are covered with a separate chest drape.
- The therapist is standing at the side of the table next to the client's waist.

POLARITY

Place the left palm (negative pole) on the abdomen (positive pole). Slide the right palm (positive pole) underneath the client's back to contact the lumbar spine (negative pole). Your palms should be aligned to each other vertically through the client's trunk. Keep your hands relaxed, allowing them to mold to the contours of the client's body and to be moved by the motions generated by the client's breathing action. During this polarity hold, focus on feelings of trust and nurturing, allowing the client to become accustomed to being touched in the abdominal region. Hold for at least 1 minute.

SHIATSU

Slide the fingers of both hands under the client's back, palpating the lateral edge of the erector spinae in the lumbar region with your fingertips. Straighten the fingers, allowing the weight of the client's trunk to rest on your fingertips. Repeat on the other side of the back. The outer branch of the bladder channel runs along the lateral border of the erector spinae. This move helps to relax tightness in the muscles of the low back, allowing the lumbar spine to decompress.

Swedish/Cross Fiber

1. Perform circular effleurage on the abdomen.
2. Perform two-handed petrissage on both sides of the torso, between the rib cage and pelvis.
3. Perform circular friction around the abdomen in a clockwise direction.
4. Perform fingertip raking across the abdominal muscles.

Connective Tissue

Place your right palm on the abdomen, over the navel area. Place your left palm on top of your right hand. Make a slow, clockwise spiraling motion, moving the skin over the underlying tissues. Do not glide over the skin. Gradually increase the size of the spiral, stretching the skin and fascia as far as they can comfortably go.

Deep Tissue/Neuromuscular Therapy

SEQUENCE

1. Abdominal muscle attachments on the iliac crest
2. Inferior border of the costal cartilage of the ribs
3. Abdominal muscle attachments on the ribs ▶
4. Rectus abdominus ▶
5. Obliques—external and internal
6. Transverse abdominus
7. Quadratus lumborum ▶
   a. 12th rib attachment—tendon
   b. Iliac crest attachment—tendon
   c. Belly—muscle fibers

> ◎ Trigger point patterns in the abdominal muscles are not as predictable as those in other muscle groups. The referred pain from these trigger points is often mistaken for visceral pain. Trigger points in these muscles often cause pain bilaterally.
>
> Check all muscle attachments thoroughly, feeling for strings and lumps that are frequently found around trigger points. The origin of the rectus abdominus at the pubic symphysis often harbors trigger points, as does its insertion along the inferior border of the rib cage, just lateral to the xiphoid process.

Abdominal Muscle Attachments on the Iliac Crest (External and Internal Obliques and Transverse Abdominus)

Strokes
- Stand at the side of the table, and face the upper border of the client's iliac crest. Placing one or both thumbs on the upper border of the iliac crest, apply short, side-to-side strokes against the inner edge of the bone.
- Continue around the pelvis as far as your hand can reach.

Inferior Border of the Costal Cartilage of Ribs 7 to 10 (Transverse Abdominus)

Strokes
- Placing the thumbs just lateral to the xiphoid process, apply short, side-to-side strokes along the inferior border of the rib cage to the tip of rib 11.

Abdominal Muscle Attachments on the Ribs

See Figure 9-34 for muscle attachments on the ribs.

Rectus Abdominus

Strokes
- Place your fingers on the costal cartilages of ribs 5 to 7, next to the xiphoid process.
- Using short, up-and-down and side-to-side strokes with your fingertips, try to reduce tension in the muscular attachments.

External Obliques

Strokes
- The attachments for this muscle are on the lower eight ribs, interweaving with the serratus anterior. Place your fingers on rib 5, near the sternum. Perform short, up-and-down and side-to-side strokes on the rib.
- Continue to work the attachments on each rib, in succession. On each rib, slide your fingers a little further laterally to make contact with the muscle insertion. Use the border of the serratus anterior for a guideline.

Internal Obliques

Strokes
- The muscle attaches on the costal cartilages of ribs 8 to 10. Place your fingers or thumbs along the lower portion of rib 8, just lateral to the rectus abdominus. Apply short, side-to-side and up-and-down strokes on the attachment.
- Moving slightly lateral, slide down to rib 9. Repeat the same strokes on the attachment and then repeat once more on the rib 10 attachment.

Rectus Abdominus

Origin: Medial tendon from the pubic symphysis, lateral tendon from the crest of the pubis.
Insertion: Costal cartilages of ribs 5 to 7, xiphoid process.
Action: Flexion of the spine, posterior tilt of the pelvis; compresses abdominal contents.

Strokes
- Place your fingers next to the midline of the upper abdomen, just below the rib cage.
- Using a spreading technique, slide your fingers across the fibers of the muscle (Fig. 9-35). Pause and work on abnormalities in the muscle tissue with side-to-side strokes. Address trigger points as they are found. Continue, working in strips, down the rectus abdominus. Be sure to palpate the tendinous sheath between each section of the muscle.

> ⚠ Avoid pressure on the linea alba, which is the fascial line running down the midline of the rectus abdominus that joins its right and left halves. The aorta runs down the center of the trunk just deep to this area. If you feel a strong pulse under your fingers when massaging the rectus abdominus, immediately move off it.

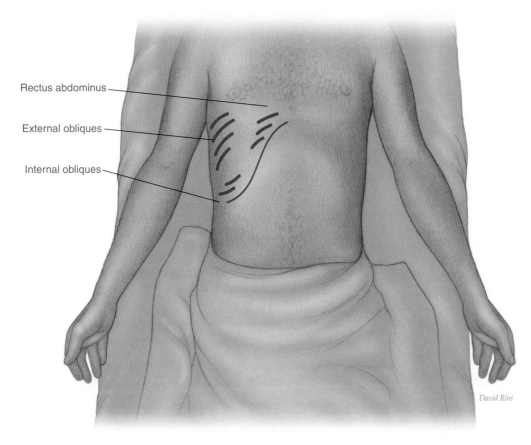

David Rini

FIGURE 9-34 Abdominal muscle attachments on the ribs.

Rectus abdominus

External obliques

Internal obliques

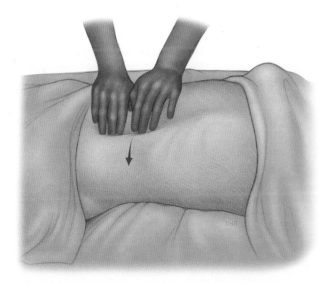

FIGURE 9-35 Cross-fiber technique on the rectus abdominus.

- Place your thumb or fingers along the upper border of the pubic symphysis. Using short, side-to-side strokes, contact the attachment of the rectus abdominus.

⚠ Be sure that the client is comfortable with this procedure before attempting it. Describe the move to the client and establish permission in the presession interview. Then repeat this question during the session before proceeding.

External and Internal Obliques

Obliquus Externus Abdominis
Origin: Ribs 4 to 12, interdigitating with the serratus anterior.
Insertion: Anterior part of the iliac crest, abdominal aponeurosis.
Action: Flexion of the trunk (bilaterally), lateral flexion of the trunk and rotation of the trunk (unilaterally), support and compression of abdominal viscera; assists in forced exhalation.

Obliquus Internus Abdominis
Origin: Thoracolumbar fascia, lateral two-thirds of the inguinal ligament, anterior two-thirds of the iliac crest.
Insertion: Cartilages of ribs 9 to 12, abdominal aponeurosis to the linea alba.

Action: Flexion of the trunk (bilaterally), lateral flexion of the trunk and rotation of the trunk (unilaterally), support and compression of abdominal viscera; assists in exhalation.

Strokes

- Begin lateral to the border of the rectus abdominus. Do a spreading stroke, with your fingers across the direction of the fibers, as described above. Remember that the fibers of the external obliquus angle on a lateral diagonal, so cross-fiber strokes on the muscle are performed on a medial diagonal perpendicular to the fibers (Fig. 9-36A). The fibers of the internal obliquus angle on a medial diagonal, so cross-fiber strokes on the muscle are performed on a lateral diagonal that is perpendicular to the fibers (Fig. 9-36B).
- Continue outward to the lateral border of the latissimus dorsi on the side of the body. Cover the muscles thoroughly, pausing at tender areas and working in detail on tissues that feel aberrant. It is important to visualize the muscle you are working on under your fingers to be able to palpate it effectively, because the abdominal muscles overlap each other.

Transverse Abdominus

Origin: Lateral third of the inguinal ligament, anterior two-thirds of the lip of the iliac crest, thoracolumbar fascia, costal cartilages of ribs 7 to 12.
Insertion: Abdominal aponeurosis to the linea alba.
Action: Compresses the abdomen, assists in forced exhalation.

Strokes

- Place your fingers next to the lateral border of the rectus abdominus, facing in a superior direction. Apply short, up-and-down strokes across the muscle fibers, covering the area between the base of the rib cage and the iliac crest thoroughly (Fig. 9-37).

Quadratus Lumborum

Origin: Inner lip of the iliac crest, iliolumbar ligament.
Insertion: Lower border of the 12th rib, transverse process of L1–L4 vertebrae.
Action: Extension of the lumbar spine (bilaterally), lateral flexion of the spine (unilaterally), fixation and depression of the 12th rib.

Trigger points in the superficial layer of the muscle are located in the lateral section, with one near the attachment on the 12th rib and the other near the attachment on the iliac crest. Pain from the 12th rib attachment point is referred along the iliac crest and gluteus medius region. The referral zone for the iliac crest attachment point is to the greater trochanter and outer thigh area.

Two trigger points in the deeper layer are found near the transverse process of L3 and between the transverse processes of L4 and L5. The trigger point at L3 refers pain to the sacroiliac joints and across the upper sacral region. The second trigger point lower down refers pain to the lower gluteal area.

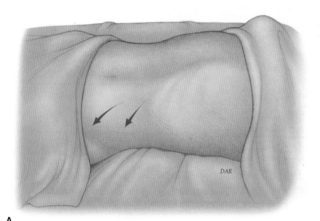

A

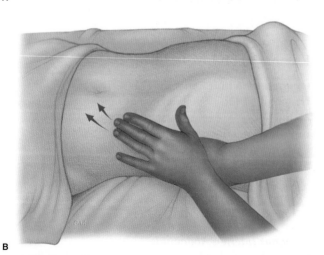

B

FIGURE 9-36 A. Cross-fiber technique on external obliques.
B. Direction of cross-fiber strokes on internal obliques.

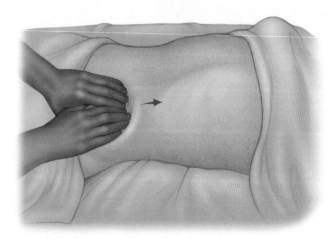

FIGURE 9-37 Cross-fiber technique on the transverse abdominus.

Position

- Place the client in side posture. Place a bolster between the knees and a small support under the side of the head. A bolster may also be placed between the side of the client's waist and the table. Have the client stretch the topmost arm overhead.
- The therapist stands behind the client.

Strokes

- Place your front hand on the client's hip for support. Using the heel of your back hand, do deep, circular friction on the muscles from the 12th rib to the iliac crest.
- Slide your thumbs upward, along the lateral border of the erector spinae, until the 12th rib is felt. Using the thumbs or a knuckle, do short, side-to-side strokes across the underside of the rib to the spine. It is likely that knotted areas and trigger points will be found here.
- Turn to face the iliac crest. Apply short, side-to-side strokes along the superior border of the iliac crest with the knuckle or thumbs, pausing at tender points.
- Standing behind the client's waist, place both palms on the side of the torso with the thumbs pointed downward toward the spine. Finding the edge of the erector spinae, slide the thumbs slightly anterior, and press downward toward the transverse processes of the spine (Fig. 9-38). Be careful not to push into the tips of the bones. Perform short, up-and-down and side-to-side strokes along the quadratus lumborum. Work between the 12th rib and the iliac crest.

STRETCH

1. *Quadratus Lumborum and Obliques.* The client is lying in side posture and slides to the edge of the table near the therapist. The bottom leg is flexed at the knee. The top leg is straight, and the uppermost arm is stretched overhead, grasping the end of the table. Place one hand on the client's uppermost arm and the other hand on the client's top leg.

   The straightened top leg is positioned behind the bottom leg so that it can hang off the side of the table. As you push down on the top arm, press the leg toward the floor until a stretch is felt in the quadratus lumborum (Fig. 9-39).

2. *Rectus Abdominus.* The client is lying supine and slides the heels toward the hips, keeping the feet flat on the table and with both knees flexed. The arms are stretched overhead, reaching toward the head of the table (Fig. 9-40). If further stretch is required, a bolster may be slid under the client's back.

ACCESSORY WORK

1. This work should be done in conjunction with the pelvic session.
2. Reflexologists claim that the solar plexus reflex point is located on the sole of the left foot slightly inferior to the bases of the metatarsal bones of the first through third toes (Fig. 9-41). Pressing this point is intended to bring relaxation to the upper abdominal region.

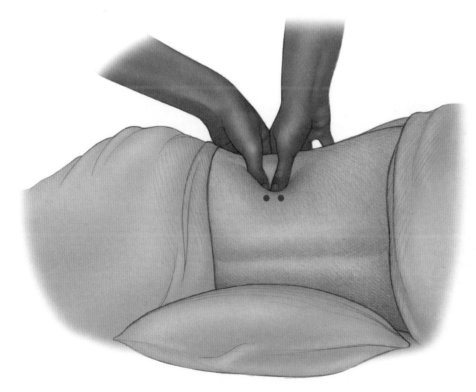

FIGURE 9-38 Contacting the lateral border of the quadratus lumborum.

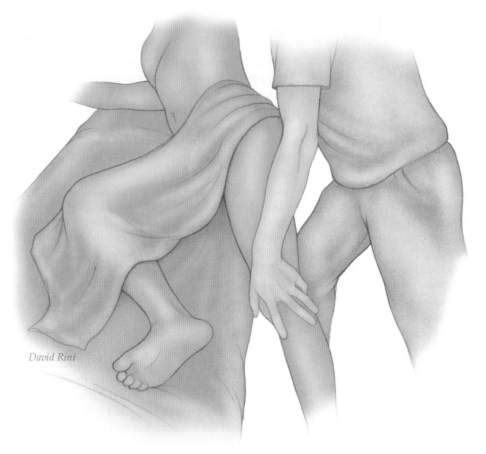

FIGURE 9-39 Stretch for the quadratus lumborum and obliques.

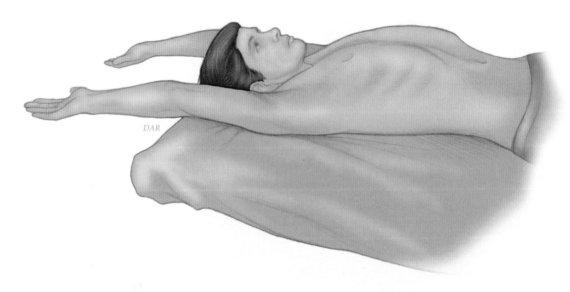

FIGURE 9-40 Stretch for the rectus abdominus.

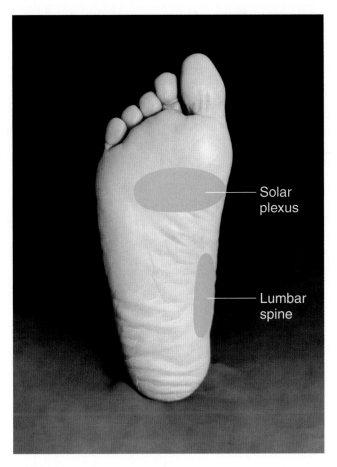

FIGURE 9-41 Reflex zones on the foot to accompany an abdomen session.

3. The traditionally recognized reflex zone for the lumbar spine is along the medial side of the instep on both feet, in the space between the first cuneiform bone and the calcaneus. Press this point to help relieve low back stress and pain.

CLOSING

Sitting at the foot of the table, lightly hold the heels of the client's feet in your hands for 30 to 60 seconds. Remove your hands slowly to complete the session.

▶ INTESTINES ROUTINE

Swedish/Cross Fiber

POSITION

- The client is lying supine on the table with a bolster under the knees. Female clients are covered with a separate chest drape.
- The therapist is standing at the side of the table at the level of the client's waist.

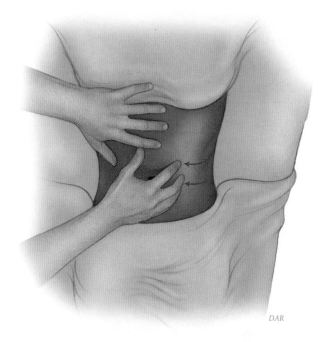

FIGURE 9-42 Cross-fiber fingertip raking on the rectus abdominus.

1. Perform circular effleurage on the abdomen.
2. Perform cross-fiber fingertip raking on the abdominal muscles (Fig. 9-42).

Connective Tissue

Placing the right palm on the abdomen over the navel and the left palm over the right hand, begin an outward spiraling, clockwise motion, stretching the fascia of the abdomen.

Deep Tissue/Neuromuscular Therapy

Large Intestine

Strokes
- Reach across the table, and place your fingers lateral to the ascending colon, on the right side of the client's abdomen (Fig. 9-43). Gently draw the fingers inward, against the edge of the large intestine, without gliding over the skin. Continue tracing the border of the colon with your fingers, pulling it away from the outer edge of the abdomen until you reach the midline of the body. Walk around to the right side of the table, and continue pulling the fingers inward, along the border of the large intestine, until you reach the left ASIS.
- Beginning at the ileocecal valve, do slow, circular fingertip friction over the large intestine, tracing its entire length around the abdominal cavity (Fig. 9-44).

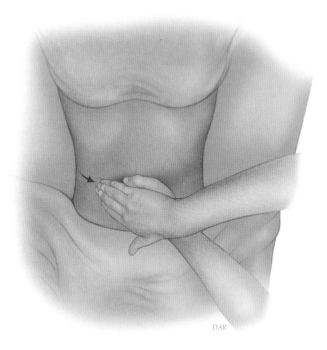

FIGURE 9-43 Contacting the lateral border of the large intestine.

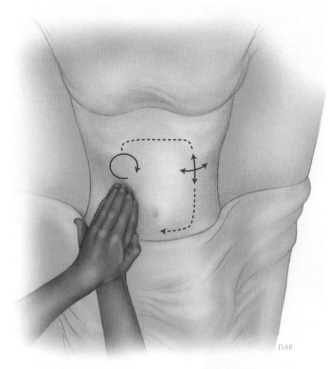

FIGURE 9-44 Sequence of deep tissue strokes on the large intestine.

- Repeat the same path as above, doing short, up-and-down and side-to-side strokes with your fingers over the large intestine. Spend extra time on impacted areas.

⚠️ Discuss your plans for abdominal massage with your client in the presession interview, and ask permission again before beginning work in this area. Pay close attention when applying pressure over the intestines. Never push against resistance. Elicit client feedback often, and move very slowly.

Small Intestine

Strokes
- Cupping your palm, curve and spread the fingers. Place your fingertips on the abdomen, over the small intestine. Press down, and circle the fingers (Fig. 9-45).

ACCESSORY WORK, INTESTINES

Reflex Points on the Feet

Reflexology tradition associates these areas of the foot with parts of the abdominal organs. See Figure 9-46 for an illustration of the reflex zone of the large intestine.

1. *Ileocecal Valve Point.* This point is located on the heel line on the lateral side of the right foot. Support the heel of the client's right foot with your right hand as you press the ileocecal valve point with your left thumb.
2. *Intestinal Reflex Zone.* To locate this zone, divide the sole of the foot into quarters, excluding the toes. The intestinal

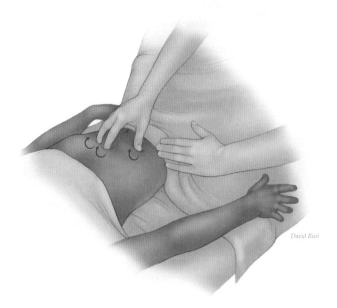

FIGURE 9-45 Massaging the small intestine.

zone is located in the third quadrant, just above the heel line. To cover the area thoroughly, begin at the ileocecal point on the right foot. Press on the point with the pad of your left thumb. Move the thumb slightly forward, and press on the next point (approximately one-sixteenth of an inch in front of the first point). The thumb hinges slightly from the joint of the first phalanx.

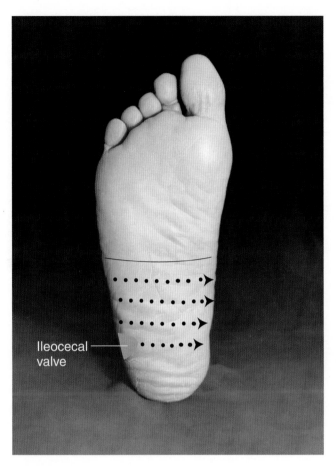

FIGURE 9-46 Reflex zone for the large intestine.

Continue to move with the thumb tip across the foot in a horizontal direction toward the medial side, covering all points. To access the next strip of points, begin again on the lateral edge of the foot, above the first horizontal line. Repeat the sequence until the entire zone is covered. Switch hands, and repeat the entire sequence, with the exception of the ileocecal point, on the left foot.

CLOSING

Sitting at the foot of the table, lightly hold the heels of the client's feet in your hands for 30 to 60 seconds. Remove your hands slowly to complete the session.

▶ LATERAL THIGH/INNER THIGH ROUTINE

Objectives

- To balance the muscular action of the inner and outer thighs
- To address uneven pulls on the pelvis coming from thigh muscles that attach on it

Energy

POSITION

- The client is in side posture, with a small pillow under the head. The leg lying against the table is slightly flexed. The top leg is flexed 90°, with a bolster placed under the knee.
- The therapist is standing behind the client's hip.

POLARITY

Place the palm of your top hand on the client's hip and your bottom hand on the side of the knee. Breathe deeply and rhythmically, envisioning the client's thigh area relaxing between your two hands. Hold for at least 30 seconds.

SHIATSU

1. *Top Leg.* Using your forearm, perform shiatsu compression movements along the side of the hip, from the iliac crest to the greater trochanter (Fig. 9-47). Both you and the client should exhale each time you lean your forearm into the hip. Continue the compression movements down the side of the leg to the knee. The gallbladder channel traverses this area.
2. *Bottom Leg.* Using your palm or the tiger's mouth position of the hand (the webbing between the thumb and index finger), perform shiatsu compression movements on the inner thigh, from the pelvis to the knee (Fig. 9-48).

Deep Tissue/Neuromuscular Therapy

SEQUENCE

Lateral Thigh

1. Vastus lateralis
2. Iliotibial tract
3. Tensor fascia latae

Inner Thigh

1. Pes anserinus
2. Adductor muscles—adductor magnus, brevis and longus; pectineus, and gracilis

▶ LATERAL THIGH

Swedish/Cross Fiber

POSITION

- The therapist moves to the front side of the table and faces the client's top leg.

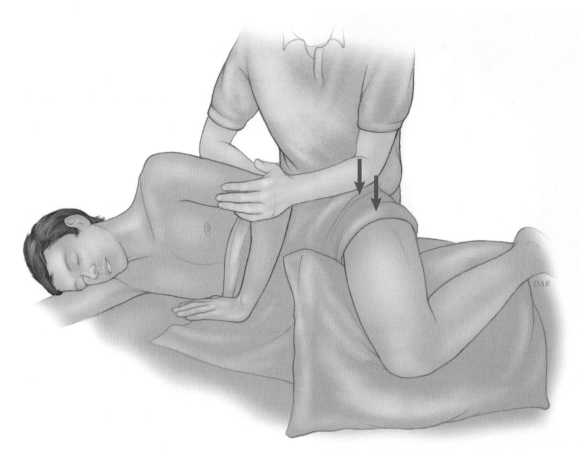

FIGURE 9-47 Forearm compression down the side of the hip.

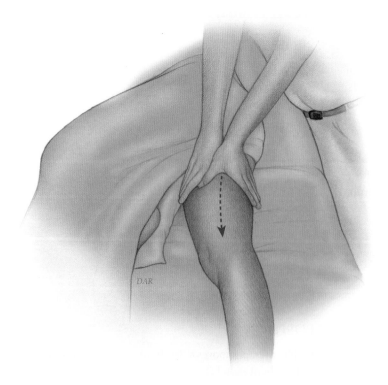

FIGURE 9-48 Tiger's mouth position on the inner thigh.

1. Perform effleurage strokes on the top leg from the knee to the iliac crest.
2. Perform circular friction with the heel of your hand from the knee to the iliac crest.

Connective Tissue

MYOFASCIAL SPREADING

Place the heels of your hands on the midline of the thigh at the knee. Stroke outward with both hands, spreading the tissues in opposite directions. Continue, working in strips, to the iliac crest.

Deep Tissue/Neuromuscular Therapy

POSITION

- The client remains in side posture.
- The therapist stands at the front side of the table and faces the client's flexed thigh.

Vastus Lateralis

Origin: Intertrochanteric line, greater trochanter, gluteal tuberosity, lateral lip of the linea aspera, lateral intermuscular septum.
Insertion: Lateral border of the patella, patellar ligament to the tibial tuberosity.
Action: Extension of leg at the knee joint.

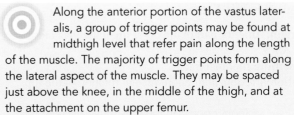

Along the anterior portion of the vastus lateralis, a group of trigger points may be found at midthigh level that refer pain along the length of the muscle. The majority of trigger points form along the lateral aspect of the muscle. They may be spaced just above the knee, in the middle of the thigh, and at the attachment on the upper femur.

Trigger points in the superficial fibers fire more locally. Trigger points in the deeper layers shoot pain throughout the muscle and down to the side of the knee.

Strokes
- Perform elongation strokes with the forearm or knuckles along the lateral thigh in the space between the rectus femoris and iliotibial tract. Pause to treat trigger points (Fig. 9-49A).
- Perform elongation strokes with an elbow or the thumbs along the distal half of the lateral thigh, in the space between the iliotibial tract and biceps femoris (Fig. 9-49C).
- Pause to treat trigger points.

Iliotibial Tract

Strokes
- With your thumbs or elbow, press a line of points along the iliotibial tract, from the knee to the greater trochanter (Fig. 9-49B).

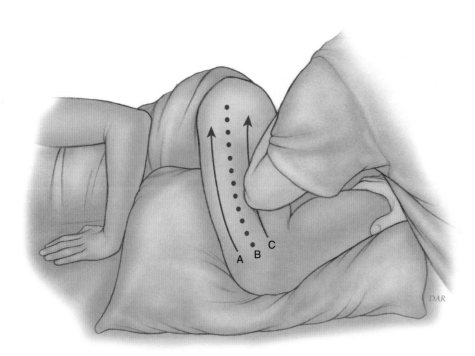

FIGURE 9-49 Deep tissue strokes on the vastus lateralis and iliotibial tract.

Tensor Fascia Latae

Origin: Anterior part of the outer lip of the iliac crest, ASIS.
Insertion: Iliotibial tract.
Action: Flexion, abduction, medial rotation of the hip.

 Trigger points in this muscle usually refer pain along the iliotibial tract.

Strokes

• Standing behind the client at the level of the hip, place your elbow on the anterior surface of the hip. Apply short, up-and-down and side-to-side strokes along the fibers of the muscle, between the iliac crest and greater trochanter (Fig. 9-50).
• Pause to treat trigger points.

▶ INNER THIGH

Swedish/Cross Fiber

POSITION

• The client remains in the same position as above.
• The therapist works on the inner thigh muscles of the leg that is against the table.
  1. Perform effleurage strokes from the knee to the pelvis.

2. Perform circular friction on the muscle attachments at the knee.
3. Perform cross-fiber fingertip raking on the adductor muscles.

Connective Tissue

MYOFASCIAL SPREADING

Standing at the front side of the table and facing the client's bottom leg, place the fingertips of both hands along the fibers of the adductor muscles, slightly above knee level. Using the spreading technique, slowly glide the fingers in a posterior direction, perpendicular to the direction of the fibers. Continue, working in strips, to the pelvis.

Deep Tissue/Neuromuscular Therapy

POSITION

• The client remains in side posture.
• The therapist stands at the front of the table and faces the inner thigh of the client's leg, which lies against the table.

Pes Anserinus (Attachment Points of Sartorius, Gracilis, and Semitendinosus)

Location: on the medial side of the proximal end of the tibia.

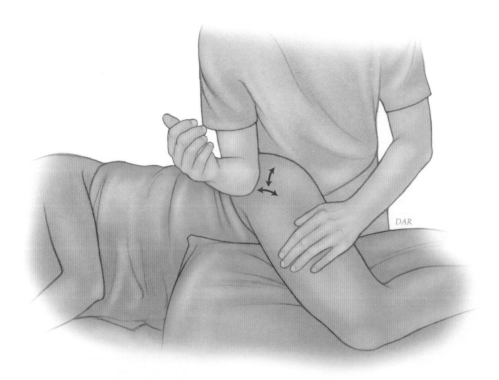

FIGURE 9-50 Position for contacting the tensor fascia latae.

Strokes

- Press down on the insertion points on the bone with your thumbs or fingers. Move slowly up and down and side to side.
- Pause at the tender areas until the pain decreases or subsides.

Adductor Muscles

Adductor Magnus

Origin: Inferior ramus of the pubis, inferior ramus of the ischium, inferior and lateral part of the ischial tuberosity.

Insertion: Linea aspera of the femur.

Action: Hip adduction; assists in hip extension and lateral rotation.

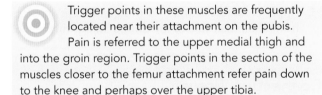
The trigger points in this muscle will probably be found in the middle portion. They project pain deep into the groin and pelvic region.

Adductor Brevis

Origin: Inferior ramus of the pubis.

Insertion: Proximal third of the medial lip of the linea aspera, distal pectineal line.

Action: Hip adduction.

Adductor Longus

Origin: Anterior part of the pubis.

Insertion: Middle third of the medial lip of the linea aspera.

Action: Hip adduction; assists in lateral rotation when the hip is in extension.

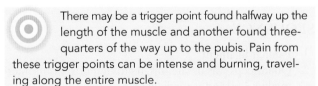
Trigger points in these muscles are frequently located near their attachment on the pubis. Pain is referred to the upper medial thigh and into the groin region. Trigger points in the section of the muscles closer to the femur attachment refer pain down to the knee and perhaps over the upper tibia.

Gracilis

Origin: Inferior ramus of the pubis near the symphysis.

Insertion: Medial surface of the shaft of the tibia below the tibial condyle.

Action: Hip adduction, knee flexion; assists in medial rotation of the knee when the leg is flexed.

There may be a trigger point found halfway up the length of the muscle and another found three-quarters of the way up to the pubis. Pain from these trigger points can be intense and burning, traveling along the entire muscle.

Pectineus

Origin: Pectineal line on the superior ramus of the pubis.

Insertion: Femur from the lesser trochanter to the linea aspera.

Action: Hip adduction; assists in hip flexion.

The common trigger point is palpated on the attachment of the muscle on the pubis. It sends pain deep into the groin.

Strokes

- Place the fingertips of both hands along the fibers of the adductor muscles, as in the connective tissue technique above. Use short, up-and-down and side-to-side strokes on the muscle bellies to reduce tension in adherent fibers and locate trigger points (Fig. 9-51).
- Find the borders of the muscles with your fingers. Slide in between the muscles, and move the fingers up and down along the borders to separate the muscles from each other. Work from the knee to the pelvis.

Avoid any pressure in the femoral triangle, which is located in the upper third of the medial thigh. The femoral nerve, artery, and vein pass through this area.

- Place your fingers or the broad side of the thumb against the pubis, and move slowly side to side across the bone to contact the adductor muscle attachments on the pelvis (Fig. 9-52).

Obtain the client's permission during the presession interview, and again during the session before performing this stroke. Some clinicians find that inviting the client to make contact through the therapist's hand can be a helpful way for the client to feel safe and in control.

STRETCH

Tensor Fascia Latae

Position

- The client is lying in side posture, with the leg to be stretched positioned on top.
- Standing behind the client, take hold of the ankle of his or her top leg. Abduct the leg, medially rotate the thigh by letting the knee drop somewhat toward the bottom leg, and extend the thigh until a stretch is felt on the front of the hip at the location of the tensor fascia latae (Fig. 9-53).

Adductors

Position

- The client is lying supine on the table, with both legs extended.
- The therapist stands at the foot of the table. Holding the client's ankle, laterally rotate the leg slightly, and move the leg into abduction, keeping it straight, until the client feels a stretch in the adductor muscles (Fig. 9-54).

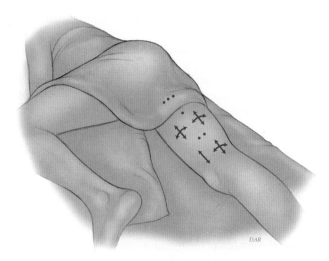

FIGURE 9-51 Direction of strokes on the adductor muscles.

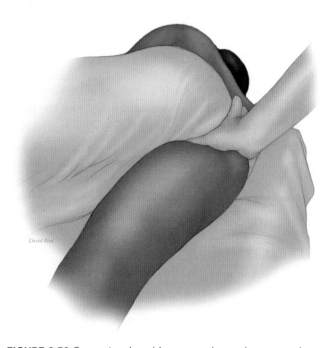

FIGURE 9-52 Contacting the adductor muscle attachments on the pubis.

▶ ANTERIOR THIGH/ILIOPSOAS ROUTINE

Objectives

- To relax and lengthen the quadriceps muscles
- To help correct anterior tilt of the pelvis
- To complete the opening and balancing of the pelvic region
- To achieve more efficient movement patterns, originating from the core muscles

Energy

POSITION

The client is lying supine, with the leg to be worked on fully extended. A bolster may be placed under the knee of the other leg, if desired.

The therapist is standing at the side of the table and is facing the client's pelvis.

POLARITY

The palm of the superior hand contacts the ASIS. The palm of the inferior hand rests on the knee. Envision the thigh lengthening and the tissues reorganizing themselves along the vertical axis running along the center of the thigh. Be sensitive to any subtle movements occurring in the thigh, and let your hands softly follow them. Hold for 30 to 60 seconds.

SHIATSU

With the palms or fists, compress the thigh from the hip to the knee. These compression movements stimulate the stomach and spleen channels, running approximately along the lateral and medial borders of the rectus femoris muscle.

Swedish/Cross Fiber

1. Perform effleurage strokes on the anterior thigh and knee.
2. Perform kneading strokes on the anterior thigh muscles.
3. Perform friction strokes on the anterior thigh and knee.
4. Apply cross-fiber strokes to the quadriceps muscles using the broad side of the thumb and/or the heel of the hand.

Connective Tissue

MYOFASCIAL SPREADING

Place the heels of the hand on the midline of the thigh, just above the patella. Slowly draw the hands apart, spreading the tissues. Continue, working in horizontal strips, to the hip.

Deep Tissue/Neuromuscular Therapy

SEQUENCE

1. Patellar ligament
2. Quadriceps (vastus lateralis, rectus femoris, vastus intermedius, and vastus medialis) ▶
3. Abdominal warm-up
4. Iliacus
5. Psoas ▶

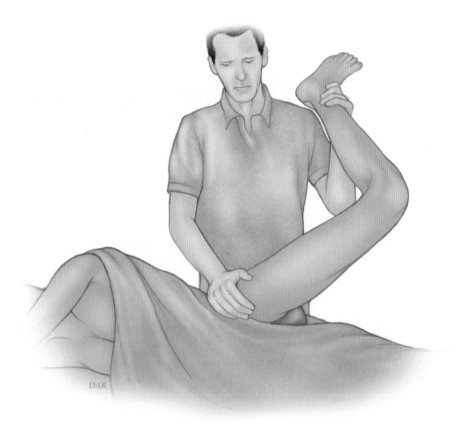

FIGURE 9-53 Stretch for the tensor fascia latae.

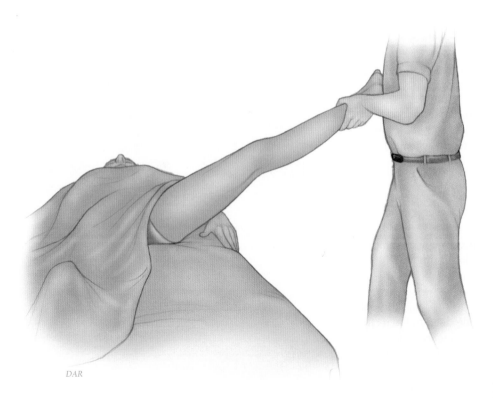

FIGURE 9-54 Stretch for the adductor muscles.

Patellar Ligament

Strokes

- Place your thumbs on the tibial tuberosity below the patella. Do short, up-and-down and side-to-side strokes on the ligament (Fig. 9-55D).

Quadriceps (Vastus Lateralis, Rectus Femoris, Vastus Intermedius, and Vastus Medialis)

Vastus Lateralis

Origin: Intertrochanteric line, greater trochanter, gluteal tuberosity, lateral lip of the linea aspera, lateral intermuscular septum.

Insertion: Lateral border of the patella, patellar ligament to the tibial tuberosity.

Action: Extension of leg at the knee joint.

> Along the anterior portion, a group of trigger points may be found at midthigh level that refers pain along the length of the muscle. The majority of trigger points form along the lateral aspect of the muscle. They may be spaced just above the knee, in the middle of the thigh, and at the attachment on the upper femur.
> Trigger points in the superficial fibers usually fire more locally. Trigger points in the deeper layers refer pain throughout the muscle and down to the side of the knee.

Rectus Femoris

Origin: Anterior head—AIIS. Posterior head—groove of the ilium above the acetabulum.

Insertion: Patella and tibial tuberosity via the patellar ligament.

Action: Extension of the leg at the knee joint, flexion of the thigh at the hip joint.

> The most commonly occurring trigger point in this muscle is found just below its attachment on the AIIS. It refers pain to the knee area.

Vastus Intermedius

Origin: Anterior and lateral surfaces of the upper two-thirds of the shaft of the femur, lower part of the lateral intermuscular septum.

Insertion: Deep aspect of the quadriceps tendon, patella, and tibial tuberosity via the patellar ligament.

Action: Extension of the leg at the knee.

> Trigger points in this muscle are difficult to palpate because of its position deep to the rectus femoris. These trigger points tend to develop in clusters rather than singly. The pain referral zone is most concentrated at midthigh level but may extend down over the knee or to the upper thigh, depending on the location of the trigger point.

Vastus Medialis

Origin: Lower half of the intertrochanteric line, medial lip of the linea aspera, medial intermuscular septum, medial supracondylar line.

Insertion: Medial border of the patella, tibial tuberosity via the patellar ligament.

Action: Extension of the leg at the knee.

> The most frequently occurring trigger point is located in the lower, thick fibers on the medial thigh, slightly above the knee. Pain may be exhibited along the medial side of the muscle. A second trigger point may form about halfway up the thigh. Left untreated, these trigger points may cause a weakening in the quadriceps and bouts of buckling of the knee when the person is walking.

Strokes

- Using the forearm or knuckles, perform elongation strokes from the knee to the AIIS. Cover the area thoroughly between the sartorius muscle and the iliotibial tract (Fig. 9-55A).
- With the thumbs or elbow, trace the lateral and medial borders of the rectus femoris muscle, from the patella to the AIIS (Fig. 9-55B).

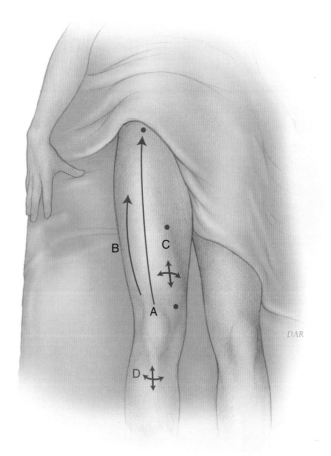

FIGURE 9-55 Sequence of deep tissue strokes on the quadriceps.

• Using the thumbs or elbow, thoroughly work small sections of the muscles with up-and-down and side-to-side strokes (in Fig. 9-55C).

 Massage to the psoas group can be challenging to receive. Before proceeding, describe what will happen next and secure the client's permission.

Abdominal Warm-Up

Position
• The client is lying supine, with a bolster placed under both knees.
• The therapist is standing at the side of the table next to the client's waist.
1. Perform circular effleurage on the abdomen.
2. Wave stroke—Place the heels of both hands against the border of the rectus abdominus muscle on the side of the body you are standing next to, with your fingers curled around the opposite edge of the muscle (Fig. 9-56). Gently push against the abdomen with the heels of the hands, creating a bulge in front of your palms. With your fingers, reach across to the opposite side of the wave, and pull the abdominal tissue back toward you. Repeat several times, creating a fluid, continuous motion.
3. Using the heel of the hand, apply circular friction around the abdomen in a clockwise direction.

Iliacus

Origin: Superior two-thirds of the iliac fossa, inner lip of the iliac crest, anterior sacroiliac and iliolumbar ligaments.

 A trigger point in the iliacus is frequently found in the upper portion of the muscle, slightly superior to the ASIS.

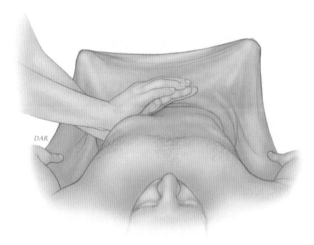

FIGURE 9-56 Beginning hand position for the wave stroke.

Insertion: Lesser trochanter of the femur.
Action: Hip flexion, trunk flexion, hip external rotation (in conjunction with the psoas).

Strokes
• Place your fingers against the inner border of the iliac crest, just above the ASIS (Fig. 9-57). Allow your fingers to melt into the tissues, as if being drawn into quicksand.
• Apply short, side-to-side strokes with your fingers, sinking further into the muscle. Pause at areas of resistance and/or tenderness.

 Remain above the ASIS at all times. Avoid putting pressure on the inguinal ligament, which attaches to the ASIS and the pubis.

Psoas Major

Origin: Inferior borders of transverse processes of the L1–L5 vertebrae, bodies and intervertebral disks of the T12–L5 vertebrae.
Insertion: Lesser trochanter of the femur.
Action: Hip flexion with origin fixed, trunk flexion with insertion fixed (in conjunction with the iliacus), external hip rotation, flexion of the lumbar spine (bilaterally), lateral flexion of the lumbar spine to the same side (unilaterally).

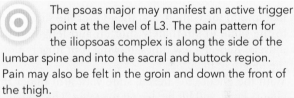 The psoas major may manifest an active trigger point at the level of L3. The pain pattern for the iliopsoas complex is along the side of the lumbar spine and into the sacral and buttock region. Pain may also be felt in the groin and down the front of the thigh.

When pressed, these trigger points usually refer pain to the back of the body. If the trigger points are on one side only, the pain zone is more vertical, along the lumbar spine. If the trigger points are bilateral, pain may refer in a horizontal pattern across the low back.

Strokes
• Place the fingers of both hands against the border of the rectus abdominus muscle. Point your fingers slightly inward, toward the spine, and reach under the edge of the rectus abdominus (Fig. 9-58). Allow your fingers to sink into the tissues. Pause at resistance and/or tenderness, and wait for the musculature to soften.
• Perform short, side-to-side strokes with your fingers, sinking further toward the psoas.
   Note: Check to be sure that you are on the psoas by having the client lift the knee a few inches to contract the muscle. You should be able to feel the muscle contracting under your fingers.
• While maintaining pressure on the psoas, have the client flex the knee and straighten the leg, aiming the

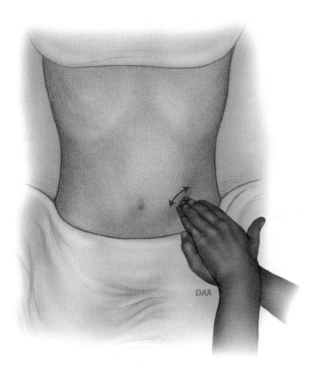

FIGURE 9-57 Contacting the iliacus on the inner rim of the tubercle of the iliac crest.

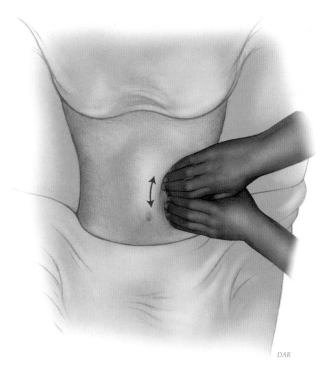

FIGURE 9-58 Contacting the psoas, starting with fingertips along the border of the rectus abdominus.

foot toward the ceiling, and then lower the straight leg to the table to alternately shorten and lengthen the muscle. Repeat a few times, moving your fingers along the length of the psoas.

- With the client's leg flexed, slide your arm under the client's knee, and lift the leg off the table. The fingers of your other hand remain in contact with the psoas. Adduct the client's thigh to access the lateral portion of the psoas. Abduct the thigh to reach the medial fibers of the muscle next to the spine (Fig. 9-59).

STRETCH

The client slides toward the end of the table so that the hips are against the edge of the table. The client then lies back on the table and holds the flexed knee of the nonstretched leg to his or her chest. The leg to be stretched is hanging off the end of the table, with the knee flexed.

Place one hand over the client's hands that are holding the flexed knee. Assist in pressing the client's thigh toward his or her chest as your other hand holds the thigh on the stretched side slightly above the knee. Press the thigh toward the floor (Fig. 9-60). This stretches the psoas muscle.

To stretch the rectus femoris, the client remains in the same position as above. Kneel down, and hold the ankle of the leg to be stretched. Slowly bring the heel in the direction of the

table as the client tucks the hips under. A stretch should be felt in the belly of the rectus femoris muscle.

ACCESSORY WORK

1. This session may be balanced with deep tissue work on the erector spinae, quadratus lumborum, gluteals, and hamstrings.
2. The muscles around the temporomandibular joint are sometimes sensitive to changes to the pelvis and psoas. They should also be massaged to balance the upper pole of the body with the pelvis.
3. On the foot, the heel is the reflex area corresponding to the pelvis. Points in the heel region on the sole of the foot may be pressed with the thumb tip. The therapist may then hold the foot around the metatarsal region with one hand while the other hand cups the heel (Fig. 9-61). With the fingers of the hand supporting the heel, the therapist may reach around to the side of the foot to press points below the malleolus. Switching hand positions allows the therapist to work on the other side of the heel.

CLOSING

Sitting at the foot of the table, lightly hold the heels of the client's feet in your hands for 30 to 60 seconds. Remove your hands slowly to complete the session.

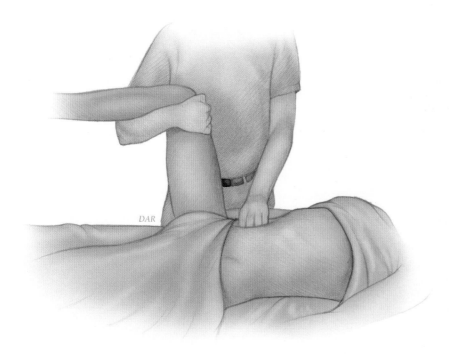

FIGURE 9-59 Position for addressing the psoas with the client's leg flexed.

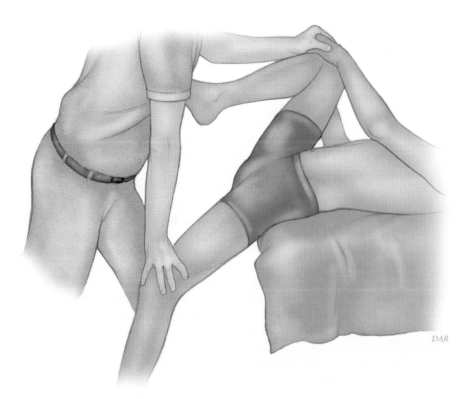

FIGURE 9-60 Stretch for the psoas.

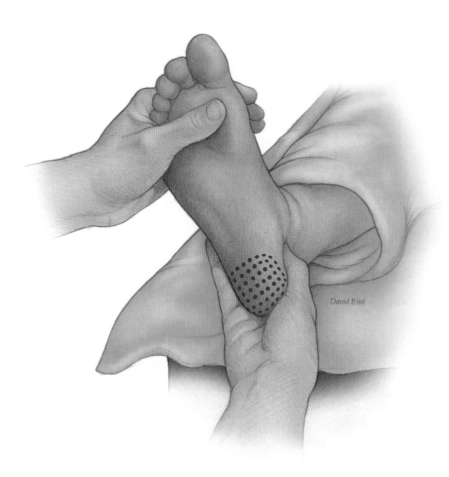

FIGURE 9-61 Reflex zone for the pelvis on the heel.

SESSION IMPRESSION

RECTUS FEMORIS AND ILIOPSOAS

The client is a 27-year-old man named Eric, who is an actor. Eric is in good physical health. He enjoys reading about and becoming involved in activities that contribute to his health and self-improvement. He participates in yoga and dance classes regularly, and he tries to maintain a low-fat diet. Eric enjoys outdoor activities like bicycling and hiking. He has been receiving a series of deep tissue therapy sessions as part of his health and high-level wellness regimen. This case describes the session that focused on his hip flexors.

Eric has a well-balanced musculature overall. His anterior thigh and gluteal muscles, however, appear to be overdeveloped in relation to the rest of his body. He exhibits an anterior pelvic tilt and slight pelvic rotation, with the left iliac crest drawn both forward and downward. Observing his walking pattern reveals that he initiates thigh movements primarily with the rectus femoris muscles. This is apparent on observation because instead of

allowing his thighs to swing from a mobile pelvis when he walks, he lifts his knees toward his chest and remains rigid in the pelvic region.

Eric complains that his thighs become very sore after dance classes and after hiking. He also gets winded sooner than he feels he should during strenuous activities, and he sometimes experiences cramping (a "stitch") under his rib cage. At irregular intervals, he experiences pain in his low back, more concentrated on the left side, near the sacrum.

Eric provides an example of someone who does not move from his core. His rectus femoris muscles overwork during hip flexion movements, and his psoas muscles are underactive. Eric has gained fairly good control of his body, but his movements are not as fluid as they could be if initiated from the pelvic center. His poor stamina reflects the lack of coordinated action between the extrinsic and intrinsic muscles. This is the fourth session dealing with the core; the abdominal and thigh muscles

SESSION IMPRESSION (*continued*)

have been worked on previously. Getting Eric more in touch with the iliopsoas complex will likely provide the missing key for him in understanding how to control his body movements properly.

The rectus femoris muscles were fairly sore. Elongation strokes along the fibers were performed extremely slowly, giving time for Eric to relax and the muscle to lengthen. At least 10 minutes were spent on each rectus femoris muscle, allowing it to soften and lengthen fully. The attachment of the rectus femoris on the anterior inferior iliac spine was particularly sensitive. Initially, the client experienced extreme ticklishness when the attachment was contacted. After being directed to focus on slowing his breathing and to relax into the sensations, however, the ticklishness transformed into extreme pain. The pressure was adjusted to a tolerable level and maintained without any movement until the client reported a considerable diminishing of the sensation. At that point, the therapist began a cross-fiber motion on the tendon to complete the treatment of the rectus femoris.

After warming up the abdominal region, the border of the iliacus was contacted along the rim of the ilium. Surprisingly little discomfort was experienced there. The muscle responded well to the strokes, and it softened considerably. After placing his fingers in the left lower quadrant of the abdominal cavity in the proper location to palpate the psoas, the therapist had the client flex his left thigh to contract the muscle fibers. It was difficult to locate the psoas initially, but when the muscle was finally palpated, the fibers felt extremely taut, like a thin cord. This was an unusual occurrence, because the psoas is a thick, cylindrically shaped muscle. It obviously was extremely contracted, appearing to be frozen in position. The therapist very gradually moved the fingers up the length of the muscle, parallel to the bodies of the lumbar vertebrae. The

client was not experiencing much sensation other than awareness of the presence of the fingers deep in his abdomen. At the level of L3 vertebra, however, he experienced a sharp pain as the therapist rolled across a tight knot of fibers. The pain was radiating into Eric's low back, near the sacrum. This was exactly the area where he had reported experiencing intermittent low back pain. The point was held until Eric reported an almost complete disappearance of the pain in his low back.

After the psoas muscles were worked on both sides, the client expressed feeling a wonderful sense of freedom, almost euphoria. He said he felt much more of a sense of being in his body. He felt light and open in his legs and feet, and he was actually aware of his spinal column, an experience he had never had before. It is not uncommon for clients to have a renewed burst of self-awareness after receiving psoas work. It is often the most profound deep tissue session they experience. ■

Topics for Discussion

1. How would you teach a client to attain greater awareness and function of the psoas muscles?
2. Describe the ideal walking pattern of a person who initiates thigh movements primarily from the psoas muscles.
3. A client's left psoas muscle is stronger than the right psoas. How is the client's pelvic alignment affected by this situation?
4. What is the relationship of the psoas and rectus abdominus muscles in reference to the pelvis when a person is in a standing position?
5. Which exercises stretch the psoas muscles?

REVIEW QUESTIONS

Level 1

Receive and Respond

1. Valgus stress suggests that the knees are. . .
   a. laterally deviated.
   b. hyperextended.
   c. medially deviated.
   d. hypotonic.

2. Varus stress suggests that the knees are. . .
   a. hypotonic.
   b. medially deviated.
   c. hyperextended.
   d. laterally deviated.

3. What is the labrum?
   a. A cartilaginous ring that wraps around the head of the femur
   b. The depression with which the head of the femur articulates
   c. The name for the single structure composed of the ilium, ischium, and pubis
   d. The ligamentous capsule that defines the hip joint

4. Which muscle is NOT a lateral rotator of the femur?
   a. Iliopsoas
   b. Gluteus minimus
   c. Piriformis
   d. Obturator femoris

5. What are the borders of the femoral triangle?
   a. Inguinal ligament, gracilis, vastus medialis
   b. Pectineus, gracilis, sartorius
   c. Sartorius, adductor magnus, rectus femoris
   d. Inguinal ligament, sartorius, medial thigh

6. The lateral edges of the abdominal obliques blend into what structure?
   a. Deep lateral rotators
   b. Abdominal aponeurosis
   c. Lumbodorsal fascia, latissimus dorsi
   d. Iliopsoas

Level 2

Apply Concepts

1. When a body is in best balance, the stride is initiated by the. . .
   a. psoas.
   b. rectus femoris.
   c. hamstrings.
   d. gluteus maximus.

2. If a person's pelvis appears to be tipped anteriorly, what muscles are most likely to be shortened?
   a. Gluteus medius, quadratus lumborum
   b. Rectus abdominus, hamstrings
   c. Iliopsoas, quadratus lumborum
   d. Hamstrings, quadriceps

3. If a person appears to have one iliac crest higher than the other while standing, what is a possible muscular involvement?
   a. Abductors are shortened on the low side
   b. Quadratus lumborum is shortened on the high side
   c. Rectus abdominus is stretched and weak on the low side
   d. Gluteus maximus is stretched and weak on the high side

4. What is an effective position for stretching the iliopsoas?
   a. Side-lying, with the knee in extension as the thigh is pressed toward the floor
   b. Supine, with the knee in flexion and the thigh laterally rotated

   c. Prone, with the knee in flexion as the thigh is lifted up off the table
   d. Supine, with the leg hanging off the end of the table

5. What is the recommended sequence for deep tissue/neuromuscular therapy at the posterior hip?
   a. Superficial gluteal muscles, followed by deep gluteal muscles, followed by deep lateral rotators
   b. Hamstrings, followed by gluteal muscles, followed by deep lateral rotators
   c. Quadriceps, followed by hamstrings, followed by deep lateral rotators, followed by tensor fascia latae
   d. Sacral ligaments, followed by tensor fascia latae, followed by deep lateral rotators, followed by hamstrings

Level 3

Problem Solving: Discussion Points

1. Massage of the abdomen is accompanied by some cautions and concerns for safety and client permission. Since this area is so fraught, why not simply skip it? Discuss this with a classmate; try role-playing a client who is a bit resistant to receiving abdominal work.

2. Some clients may have deep concerns about receiving work to their abdomen or pelvis, even though they may derive great benefit from massage to these areas. With a partner, brainstorm some ideas for how you might make it possible for a nervous person to feel safe to receive work in these areas. Make a list of possible adjustments and accommodations that you might offer.

3. This chapter places a lot of emphasis on increasing awareness of pelvic placement and freedom of movement. What is the benefit of becoming more aware of this area and how our body moves with and around it? Do some of the recommended exercises for pelvic awareness, and describe your experience to a classmate. How might you use this information to help a client?

Balancing the Upper Pole

Having completed homework, classroom instruction, and practice related to Chapter 10 of *The Balanced Body*, the learner is expected to be able to. . .

- Apply key terms and concepts related to integrated deep tissue therapy as related to the neck and head
- Identify anatomical features of neck and head, including
  - Bony landmarks
  - Muscular and fascial structures
  - Endangerments or cautionary sites
- Identify common postural or movement patterns associated with pain or impaired function of the neck and head
- Use positioning and bolstering strategies that provide safety and comfort for clients to receive integrated deep tissue therapy to the neck and head

- Generate within-scope recommendations for client self-care relevant to the neck and head
- Safely and effectively perform the integrated deep tissue therapy routines as described
- Organize a single session to address the neck and head, using the integrated deep tissue therapy approach, customized to individual clients
- Plan a series of sessions to address whole-body incorporation using the integrated deep tissue therapy approach, customized to individual clients

The Neck and Head

▶ GENERAL CONCEPTS

The neck defines the area around the cervical vertebrae. Although it is often considered to be a separate body unit, the neck is actually the upper portion of the spine. Posturally, it serves the important function of balancing the head over the shoulders. The neck also serves as a transitional segment, creating both space and integration between these two body parts. The adult head usually weighs between 13 and 15 pounds. Strong muscles and ligaments, anchored to the neck and shoulder girdle, are required to support it.

The neck sometimes serves as a barometer of tension throughout the body. Reducing tension in contracted neck muscles and repositioning the head for better balance are important elements of integrated deep tissue therapy. When the lower portions of the body are out of ideal alignment, this may be reflected in compensating displacements of the head, neck, and shoulders. In this series, work on the neck and head comes after the abdomen and pelvis sessions, because these two body segments counterbalance each other. If one of these segments is off-center, the other often adjusts its position to attempt integrity and equilibrium.

Correct positioning of the head on the neck is crucial to proper alignment throughout the body. When the bones are stacked correctly, weight transfer from the head to the feet occurs efficiently, with capacity for resilience and shock absorption. When the head is properly poised over the atlas—not tilted to the side, forward, or back, then the body carries a feeling of vertical lift. This sensation is the result of good muscle balance and the body's optimal relationship to gravity.

By contrast, when the head is not carried in an optimal position, problems can develop. Forward head posture describes a pattern in which the head is habitually held anterior to its best position. This can lead to neck strain and pain, an exaggerated thoracic curve, disc problems, and many other issues related to unnecessary tension in the neck and spine. The opposite extreme is sometimes called "military neck": a situation in which the cervical curve is diminished and the neck becomes rigidly vertical. This also creates tension, and interferes with the neck's normal capacity to absorb weight-bearing stress.

The cranium and spine protect the brain and the spinal cord. Sometimes misalignment of these bones may press on or restrict the nerves that pass through the spinal cord, thus inhibiting the function of the nervous system. Correct alignment of the head can occur only when the condyles of the atlas, on which the occiput rests, are on the horizontal plane. If the head deviates from this position, muscles will be called into action to prevent the head from sliding further off-center. Alignment of the head is most functional if the two ears are on the horizontal plane. From a side view, a vertical line should pass from the center of the ear through the center of the shoulder (Fig. 10-1A and B).

The deepest layer of neck muscles, the intervertebral muscles, works to stabilize the cervical vertebrae. More superficial muscles, notably the sternocleidomastoid (SCM), levator scapulae, and trapezius, serve to connect the head to the shoulder girdle. When the head–neck relationship is off, the superficial muscles tend to take over the job of stabilizing the head and the cervical spine; in this situation they may appear to be visibly ropy or tight. This situation occurs because the deeper, intrinsic muscles have become essentially locked as they constantly brace the vertebrae against further misalignment.

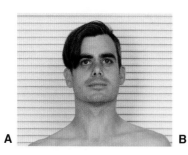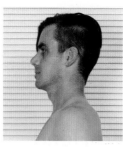

FIGURE 10-1 Optimal alignment in the head: **A.** Are the ears even? **B.** Does the center of the ear rest over the center of the shoulder?

This imbalance of muscle action results in reduced range of motion in the neck, a sensation of tension, and a probability of neck pain and headaches.

Patterns of chronic muscular contraction can become ingrained as the proprioceptors establish inefficient levels of tone as "normal." Tight, painful muscles restrict local blood flow, which reinforces the tightness in a typical ischemia–pain–spasm cycle. As the muscles and fascia become increasingly tight, the neck area shortens further, compressing vertebrae, and raising the risk of spondylosis, bone spurs, and nerve irritation.

▶ MUSCULOSKELETAL ANATOMY AND FUNCTION

The Neck

The cervical spine consists of seven vertebrae. The first two vertebrae (C1 and C2) are uniquely designed to allow support and movement of the head. The other five vertebrae (C3–C7) are similar to those of the thoracic and the lumbar spine, except that their bodies are smaller, with thinner discs between them. This design allows great mobility in the cervical spine. Lateral bending of the vertebrae, however, is limited by the rectangular shape of the bodies and the short, broad, transverse processes that block further lateral movement after they make contact with each other. (See Essential Anatomy Box 10-1 for a summary of muscles, bones, and landmarks.)

As a group, the posterior neck muscles are responsible for extension when acting bilaterally and for lateral flexion and rotation when acting unilaterally. The anterior and posterior triangles of the neck are defined in Fig. 10-2.

BOX 10-1 ESSENTIAL ANATOMY | **The Neck Routines**

MUSCLES
Upper trapezius
Splenius capitis, splenius cervicis, and levator scapula
Longissimus capitis and semispinalis capitis
The transversospinal muscles—semispinalis, multifidus, and rotatores
The suboccipital muscles
Platysma
Sternocleidomastoid
Scalenes
Suprahyoid muscles—digastric, stylohyoid, and mylohyoid
Infrahyoid muscles—omohyoid, sternohyoid, and sternothyroid
Prevertebral muscles—longus capitis and longus colli

BONES AND LANDMARKS
Cervical vertebrae
Occipital ridge
Clavicle
Sternum
Mastoid process
Styloid process
Mandible
Digastric fossa
Hyoid
Greater horns of hyoid
Lesser horn of hyoid
Trachea

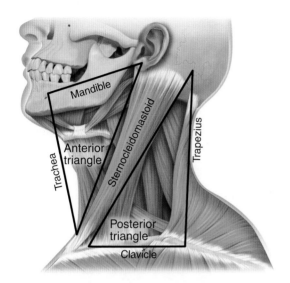

FIGURE 10-2 Anterior and posterior triangles of the neck.

The most superficial muscle, the **trapezius**, extends the head, as does the **splenius capitis** in the intermediate layer. The two other muscles in the intermediate layer, the **splenius cervicis** and the **levator scapula**, extend the cervical spine (Fig. 10-3A). In the first layer of deep muscles, the **longissimus capitis** and the **semispinalis capitis** are capital (head) extensors. The transversospinalis muscles, which link the vertebrae, are cervical extensors. They are the **semispinalis**, **multifidus**, and **rotatores**. The deepest-lying muscles, the **suboccipitals**, extend the head. This alternating of actions throughout the layers provides additional strength and support to neck and head movements.

To varying degrees, all the posterior neck muscles are subject to strain. This can be from a significant trauma like whiplash, or from cumulative day-to-day overuse or minor injuries that may eventually contribute to trigger points and substantial pain in the neck, head, and face.

The **sternocleidomastoid** (or **SCM**) is the largest neck flexor. It has two branches, both originating on the mastoid process and inserting separately on the sternum and clavicle (Fig. 10-3B). This muscle serves several functions. When contracted bilaterally, the SCM flexes the neck and draws the head forward and downward toward the chin. Unilateral contraction produces lateral flexion of the head to the same side and rotation of the head to the opposite side. When the neck is in a straight-up or extended position and the head is still, the SCM can elevate the sternum and clavicle, assisting inspiration.

The SCM also provides an important stabilizing function. It prevents hyperextension of the neck when the head is turned upward, and it resists strong, backward movement of the head during sudden body shifts, such as a backward fall. It aids the trapezius in maintaining a stable head position when the mandible is moving, as in talking and chewing. Active trigger points in the SCM most commonly are felt in

the head rather than in the neck. They can also be responsible for feelings of disequilibrium when standing or moving.

The **scalenes** ▶ have three divisions: anterior, medial, and posterior (Fig. 10-1C). They all originate on the transverse processes of the cervical vertebrae. The anterior and middle scalenes insert on the first rib. The posterior scalene muscle inserts on the second rib.

When contracting unilaterally, all three scalenes contribute to lateral flexion of the cervical spine, particularly the posterior scalene, because of its almost vertical position along the side of the neck. The anterior and middle scalenes are positioned at a forward oblique angle to the cervical spine. When they contract bilaterally, they increase the curve in the neck. They are opposed in this action by the **longus colli** and **longus capitis** ▶, which straighten the cervical spine. All three scalenes aid in respiration by lifting the first two ribs during forced inspiration.

The space formed between the anterior and middle scalenes is known as the thoracic outlet. The brachial plexus (composed of spinal nerves C5–C8 and T1) and the subclavian artery emerge from this opening and then pass through the space between the clavicle and the first rib. The spinal nerves merge into cords to become the median, radial, and ulnar nerves, which continue down the arm to the hand and fingers.

The hyoid bone is a horseshoe-shaped bone that is located on the front of the neck, between the mandible and the larynx. It does not articulate with any other bone; rather, it is suspended in place by a series of muscles and a ligament. The main purpose of the hyoid is to provide an attachment for muscles that control movements of the tongue.

The muscles that attach above the hyoid are called the suprahyoid muscles (Fig. 10-3B). They are the **digastric**, **hyoglossus, geniohyoid, mylohyoid**, and **stylohyoid**. The muscles that attach below the hyoid, on the sternum, clavicle, and scapula, are called the infrahyoid muscles, and they are the **sternohyoid, thyrohyoid**, and **omohyoid**. Restrictions in the hyoid muscles can interfere with the mechanics of sound articulation in speech, and with the function of swallowing.

The longus colli and longus capitis are both located on the anterior side of the spinal column, deep to the trachea (Fig. 10-3C). The longus colli extends from the atlas to the body of the third thoracic vertebra. The longus capitis runs from the transverse processes of the C3–C6 vertebrae to the base of the occiput. The longus colli flexes the cervical spine, while the longus capitis flexes and stabilizes the head. Both muscles contribute to side-bending of the cervical spine.

The first cervical vertebra is called the atlas. It rests on the second cervical vertebra, called the axis. A small, peg-like projection on the axis, called the odontoid process (or dens), fits into the inside of the anterior arch of the atlas above it. The atlas is held in place on the axis by a transverse ligament. This allows the head and atlas to pivot around the dens, providing rotation of the head. The atlas is the only vertebra capable of independent movement; all the other vertebrae

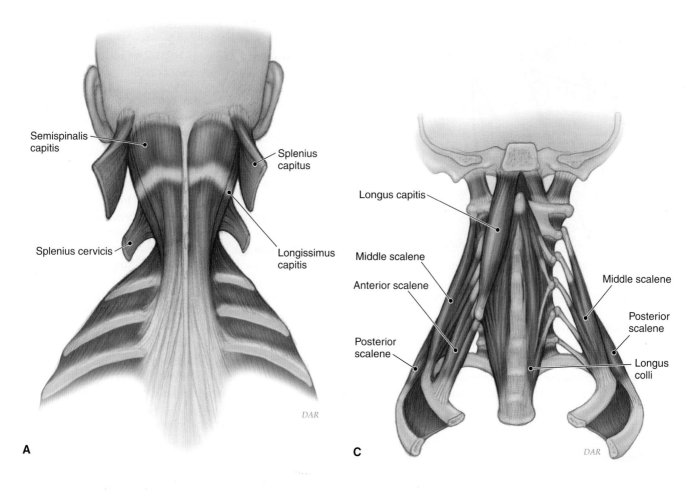

A

Semispinalis capitis

Splenius capitus

Splenius cervicis

Longissimus capitis

DAR

C

Longus capitis

Middle scalene

Anterior scalene

Posterior scalene

Middle scalene

Posterior scalene

Longus colli

DAR

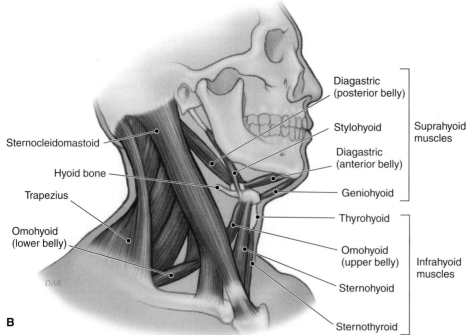

B

Sternocleidomastoid

Hyoid bone

Trapezius

Omohyoid (lower belly)

DAR

Diagastric (posterior belly)

Stylohyoid

Diagastric (anterior belly)

Geniohyoid

Suprahyoid muscles

Thyrohyoid

Omohyoid (upper belly)

Sternohyoid

Sternothyroid

Infrahyoid muscles

FIGURE 10-3 A. Posterior neck muscles, deep layer. **B.** Hyoid muscles, with sternocleidomastoid and trapezius. **C.** Prevertebral muscles.

move together as a unit. This limits the range of motion at each joint of the spine, which protects the spinal cord from damage caused by excessive bending in one place.

The Cranium

The cranium consists of eight bones: the frontal, sphenoid, ethmoid, two temporal bones, two parietal bones, and the occiput. The head shares a design feature with the pelvis, in that it is not a massive singular structure but, rather, is a series of bones connected together to form a bowl, or basin. The cranium has several hollow spaces called sinuses. These both decrease weight of the head bones, and they amplify sound. The bones of the head are joined by sutures that are saw-toothed in shape and fit together like pieces of a jigsaw puzzle. They are supported by fascial tissues and require little muscular reinforcement. In the classic anatomic view, these sutures are immobile in adults. Osteopaths, craniosacral therapy practitioners, and some other clinicians suggest that these sutures are pliable, allowing the cranium to shift subtly and absorb trauma that might otherwise injure the brain.

The occipital bone is located at the posteroinferior portion of the skull. The spinal cord passes through a hole in its base, the foramen magnum, and into the vertical tunnel formed by the stacked vertebrae below. On either side of the foramen magnum are two oval, convex condyles, which fit into two corresponding, concave articular facets on the atlas. The atlas is ring-shaped; it does not have a central body, as the other vertebrae do. This allows the spinal cord to pass through it.

The rounded surfaces of the articulations between the occiput and the atlas form an enarthrosis, which is a ball-and-socket type joint that can perform movements in three planes. The oval shape of the condyles, which are longer than they are wide, favor forward and backward motions, like those of a rocking chair. All this motion occurs on the surface area about the size of two fingertips.

Because of its weight, the head tends to slide forward on the condyles. Many daily activities, such as reading, writing, working at a computer, and looking at a cellphone or tablet can contribute to a forward tilting of the head. The posterior muscles of the neck have to work to prevent the head from sliding further forward in this position, leading to tension and possible trigger point formation. Attaining proper alignment of the head is a primary goal in reducing tension in the neck.

Several muscles play an important role in stabilizing the head on the atlas, especially the multifidus, interspinalis, semispinalis capitis, and semispinalis cervicis. It is essential that these muscles do not become chronically contracted so

the head can subtly adjust its position as needed. This helps to prevent restriction of the arteries, veins, and nerves that pass into the head from the neck, and it helps to maintain whole-body equilibrium by keeping the head in a position where it is supported by the spine rather than by excessive muscular tension.

Maintaining the head in a horizontal balance over the atlas is important for many reasons. Chronically holding the head in off-balanced positions may affect the flow of blood, lymph, and spinal fluid. Inefficient muscular patterns than can become habitual, even though they are not optimal. The vestibular system of the inner ear relies on our orienting our eyes with the horizon to establish our sense of position. When any of these functions are impaired, a host of problems may arise.

▶ HEAD AND NECK ENDANGERMENT SITES

Several structures in the neck need to be considered when performing massage in this area.
- The thyroid gland is located on the anterior surface of the trachea, from the level of the C5–T1 vertebrae. It is deep to the sternothyroid and sternohyoid muscles. The thyroid gland may have nodules or uneven growth that is palpable while working with these muscles (Fig. 10-4).
- The common carotid artery runs along the anterior border and posterior to the SCM muscle. It is important not to exert pressure on the common carotid in this area, as this

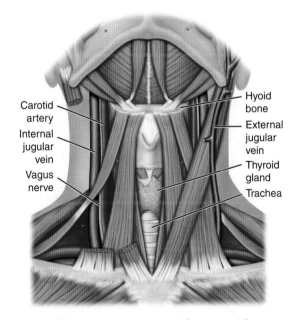

Carotid artery
Internal jugular vein
Vagus nerve

Hyoid bone
External jugular vein
Thyroid gland
Trachea

FIGURE 10-4 Endangerment sites of anterior neck.

can cause a sudden drop in blood pressure to the head. The carotid artery may also house atherosclerotic plaque or small clots that can be loosened. If this happens, the inevitable consequence is a cerebrovascular accident, or stroke.

- The internal jugular vein is located lateral to the common carotid artery, and is vulnerable to external pressure.
- The vertebral artery passes through the foramina of the transverse processes of the cervical vertebrae; it is relatively well protected here, but a person with unstable neck vertebrae may require extra care for this structure.
- The occipital nerves run from the posterior neck over the occipital ridge into the scalp. They can be entrapped by manual pressure in this area, which can contribute to headaches (Fig. 10-5).

▶ CONDITIONS

1. *Torticollis.* This condition is commonly referred to as "stiff neck" or "wryneck." It is an involuntary twisting or a tilt of the head. Torticollis can have many causes, including spasms in the neck muscles. It can be brought about by a neurological problem, trauma to the neck area, or tension. When the cause is neck tension, some precipitating factors include sleeping in an awkward position, allowing the neck to become chilled, unusual activity with the neck, and extended periods in deep neck flexion, as seen with cellphone use. The muscles most often involved are the SCM, the scalenes, the levator scapula, the trapezius, and the posterior cervical muscles.

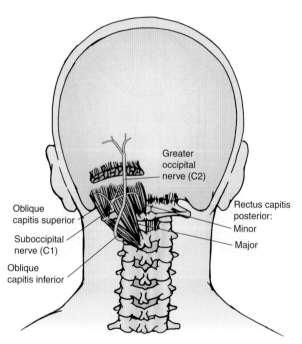

FIGURE 10-5 Endangerment sites of posterior neck.

2. *Whiplash.* This is a general term referring to injuries to the tissues of the neck caused by rapid, front to back or side to side movements of the head; a synonym is cervical acceleration–deceleration. These injuries, usually sustained in a motor vehicle accident, cause the neck muscles to be overstretched and then hypertonic. Damage to the neck can consist of microscopic tears to the muscles and ligaments, as well as damage to the other structures of the cervical region. Vertebral fractures, damage to the esophagus, trachea, and thyroid gland are all possible with a whiplash injury. For this reason, massage therapists should always be sure that a medical doctor has examined the client before attempting any massage work.

3. *Disc Damage.* Damaged discs in the cervical region can create symptoms in a number of ways. Irritated nerves can produce tingling down the arm all the way to the hand. Weakness may be present in the affected arm and hand. To check for disc involvement, have the client perform range-of-motion movements for the neck. If severe pain occurs in one direction of movement but not in the other, this is a common indicator of a disc problem. Clients exhibiting signs of disc problems should be referred to a medical doctor for evaluation.

4. *Ligament Tears.* Damage to neck ligaments can occur from injury or chronic misuse, and from poor alignment of the head and neck, which contributes to weakening and fraying of the ligamentous tissue. This injury is characterized by pain, particularly during passive head movements. Ligament injuries in the neck can also refer pain down the arm, but this symptom is typically much less severe than the pain referral seen with nerve irritation.

5. *Thoracic Outlet Syndrome.* This syndrome is caused by entrapment of the neurovascular bundle that passes through the space between the anterior and middle scalenes and the space between the clavicle and the first rib. Symptoms of nerve compression include pain and paresthesia (tingling) in the neck, shoulder, arm, hand, and fingers. Vascular compression may produce numbness, pain, cold, and fatigue in the shoulder and arm.

   Causes of thoracic outlet syndrome include the development of fascial bands around the scalenes, which decrease the size of the spaces that the nerves and blood vessels pass through. Rounded shoulders accompanied by hyperkyphosis and an increased cervical curve lead to chronic shortness and fascial thickening in the scalenes. Restrictions in the breathing muscles, resulting in shallow upper chest breathing, also strain the scalenes. Treatment includes deep tissue massage to the scalenes, correction of faulty postural and breathing habits, and regular, slow stretching of the scalenes and pectoralis minor.

See Appendix A for more information on these conditions.

HOLISTIC VIEW

The Neck

"Behold the turtle: he only makes progress when he sticks his neck out." (James Bryant Conant)

The neck serves as a channel linking the head with the rest of the body. Passageways in the neck help to transfer food, air, the flow of blood and lymph, and nerve impulses. The neck is also responsible for balancing the head on a surprisingly small surface area. For having so many duties, it is a small, weak region, vulnerable to overuse and stress-related conditions.

The neck can act as a bridge between the intellect and the heart, or the emotions and their expression. When we wish to express a strong emotion, the words sometimes feel trapped in the throat: in this way, the neck determines what communications get through and what do not. Chronic suppression of strong feelings may lead to tightness in the muscles of the anterior neck.

When the muscles of the neck and throat have an appropriate level of tone and tension, this can indicate and facilitate a healthy ability to express feelings.

The neck is a vulnerable area, and manual therapy in this area may provoke a sense of fear. Very likely, someone who has been attacked or raped was grabbed and held at the neck. Having that area touched, particularly the anterior neck region, may elicit feelings of anxiety, rage, or panic. The therapist should always check during the presession interview, and again during the session before touching the anterior neck to ensure that the client is comfortable with receiving massage in this region.

If a client agrees to proceed with the work, the therapist should move slowly and deliberately, allowing the client time to relax and to verbalize any feelings of discomfort. The client must always feel in control and know that he or she can stop the massage at any time, if desired. ■

▶ POSTURAL EVALUATION

Frontal View

1. Does the head appear to be resting on a horizontal base (Fig. 10-6A and B)?
2. Are the two sides of the neck of equal length?
3. Does the head tilt or rotate to one side or to the other?
4. Assess the musculature of the neck.
   - Are one or both of the SCM muscles prominent?
   - Are the tendons of the SCM muscles at the manubrium prominent?
   - Are there hollows above the clavicles? (A hollow area denotes shortness of the scalenes.)

Side View

1. Are the centers of the earlobe, shoulder, hip, knee, and ankle aligned in a straight line (Fig. 10-7A and B)?
2. Check the tilt of the head.
   - Forward?
   - Backward?
   - Neutral?
3. Is there the appearance of vertical lift in the body, a sense of being led upward by the head?
4. Does the body appear to be compressed, with the head pushing down into the neck?

Refer to Table 10-1 for a list of common distortions of the neck and Table 10-2 for range of motion of the neck.

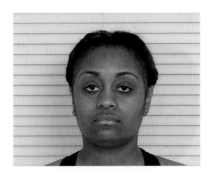

FIGURE 10-6 Postural evaluation: anterior neck and head.

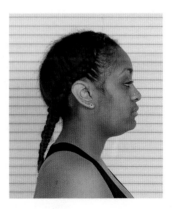

FIGURE 10-7 Postural evaluation: lateral neck and head.

TABLE 10-1 | **Body Reading for the Neck**

Postural Habit	Muscles That May Be Shortened
Lateral tilt of the head	Sternocleidomastoid
	Scalenes
	Upper trapezius
	Levator scapula
Military neck	Sternocleidomastoid
	Longus capitis
	Longus colli
Forward head	Scalenes
	Splenius capitis
	Upper trapezius
	Semispinalis capitis

TABLE 10-2 | **Range of Motion (ROM) for the Neck**

Action	Muscles
Flexion (ROM 45°)	Longus capitis
	Longus colli
	Scalenes
	Sternocleidomastoid
Extension (ROM 55°)	Splenius cervicis
	Splenius capitis
	Upper trapezius
	Semispinalis capitis
	Semispinalis cervicis
Lateral flexion (ROM 40°)	Longus colli
	Scalenes
	Sternocleidomastoid
	Splenius capitis
	Splenius cervicis
	Upper trapezius
Rotation same side (ROM 70°)	Longus colli
	Longus capitis
	Splenius cervicis
	Splenius capitis
Rotation opposite side (ROM 70°)	Scalenes
	Sternocleidomastoid
	Trapezius
	Semispinalis

▶ EXERCISES AND SELF-TREATMENT

1. *Forward Flexion* (stretches the neck extensor muscles—splenius cervicis, splenius capitis, upper trapezius, semispinalis capitis, and semispinalis cervicis). Tilt your head forward, bringing your chin toward the chest. Place your hands on the back of the head, and gently press down until you feel a mild stretch in the back of the neck.
2. *Extension* (stretches the neck flexor muscles—longus capitis, longus colli, scalenes, and SCM). Slowly raise your head to look up toward the ceiling. Reach up from the back of the neck and the front to prevent compression of the cervical vertebrae. Draw your lower teeth up over the upper teeth to further stretch the anterior neck muscles.
3. *Lateral flexion* (stretches scalenes, SCM, splenius capitis, splenius cervicis, and upper trapezius).
   - Looking straight ahead, with your head upright, place your right hand on the left side of your head above the left ear. Slowly move your right ear toward the right shoulder. Press gently against the left side of your head to increase the feeling of stretch. Relax, and imagine breathing into the tight muscles on the left side of your neck.
   - Place your left hand on the right side of your head, above the right ear. Slowly move your left ear toward the left shoulder. Press gently against the right side of your head to increase the stretch. Relax, and imagine breathing into the tight muscles on the right side of your neck.
4. *Relaxation of the Neck and Head.* Lie on your back on the floor, with the knees flexed and both feet on the floor. As you breathe deeply, imagine that your head is a heavy bag filled with sand. Visualize the sand slowly flowing out of the bag from a small hole located just below the external occipital protuberance (EOP), emptying the interior of the head and neck of all stress and tightness. Rest in this position for several minutes.

▶ NECK AND HEAD EXTENSORS ROUTINE

Objectives

- To lengthen the posterior neck
- To begin the process of repositioning the head on the cervical spine
- To relieve tightness in neck muscles, which may be contributing to neck or head pain
- To reduce muscular pulls on cervical vertebrae
- To assist the client in acquiring more effective neck and head alignment in everyday activities to help reduce stress factors

Energy

POSITION

- The client is in side posture. A small pad is placed under the side of the head; a bolster is positioned between the knees.
- The therapist is standing behind the table at the client's neck and head region.

POLARITY

The palm of one hand is placed lightly across the occipital ridge. The palm of the other hand contacts the C7 vertebra. Envision the neck lengthening as the cervical vertebrae decompress and the musculature of the neck relaxes. Maintain contact for at least 1 minute.

SHIATSU

Place one hand on the client's shoulder. Wrap your other hand around the posterior neck, just below the occipital ridge, with the thumb on one side of the trapezius and the fingers on the other. Slowly squeeze the neck, and hold for a few seconds (Fig. 10-8). Let go, slide your hand to the middle of the neck, and repeat. Then, putting your hand at the base of the neck, squeeze again. This move helps to stimulate the points on the portion of the bladder channel that passes through the posterior neck.

Swedish/Cross Fiber

1. Perform effleurage strokes from the acromion to the occipital ridge.
2. Perform one-handed pétrissage:
   - From the shoulder to the base of the neck
   - From the base of the neck to the occiput
3. Perform fingertip raking across the posterior neck, working in horizontal strips, from the C7 vertebra to the occiput.

Connective Tissue

Reaching across the posterior neck, place the fingers of one hand just posterior to the transverse processes of the cervical spine on the opposite side from where you are standing. Allow your fingers to sink into the tissues. As the tissues melt under your touch, let your fingers glide toward you, to the sides of the spinous processes of the cervical spine (Fig. 10-9).

Deep Tissue/Neuromuscular Therapy

SEQUENCE

1. Superficial layer—upper trapezius
2. Intermediate layer—splenius capitis, splenius cervicis, and levator scapula
3. Deep layer—longissimus capitis and semispinalis capitis ▶
   a. Transversospinal muscles—semispinalis, multifidus, and rotatores
   b. Suboccipital muscles—obliquus capitis superior, obliquus capitis inferior, rectus capitis posterior major, and rectus capitis posterior minor ▶

Superficial Layer

Upper Trapezius
Origin: Medial third of the superior nuchal line and EOP, ligamentum nuchae and spinal processes of C1–C5 vertebrae.
Insertion: Lateral third of the clavicle.
Action: Elevation and upward rotation of the scapula, capital extension.

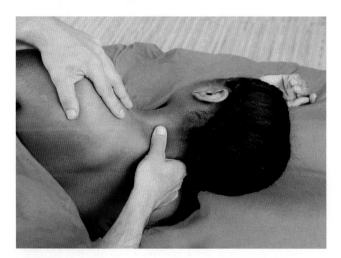

FIGURE 10-8 Shiatsu compression of the posterior neck.

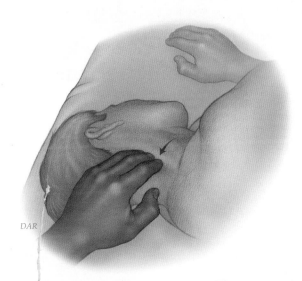

FIGURE 10-9 Connective tissue release of the posterior neck.

Trigger points in this muscle frequently are responsible for tension headaches that may be felt at the temple, behind the eye, and sometimes, at the mastoid process and down the posterior neck. Trigger points are located in the fibers slightly behind the border of the muscle, near where it attaches on the lateral portion of the clavicle. They are best palpated by squeezing the edge of the muscle between the thumb and fingers.

Strokes

- Wrap your hand around the base of the neck, as in the shiatsu procedure above, with the thumb pad at the border of the trapezius. Using the thumb pad, stroke posteriorly, from the border of the trapezius to the spinous process of the C7 vertebra (Fig. 10-10).
- Sliding your thumb a half-inch superior, repeat the stroke. Continue, working in strips, to the occipital ridge.
- Using the thumbs, apply up-and-down and side-to-side strokes to the attachment of the upper trapezius on the superior nuchal line on the occiput.

Intermediate Layer

Splenius Capitis
Origin: Ligamentum nuchae from the C3–C7 vertebrae, spinous processes of the C7–T4 vertebrae.

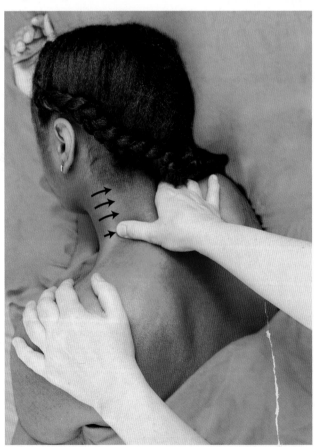

FIGURE 10-10 Deep tissue stroking on the upper trapezius, from C7 to the occiput.

Insertion: Mastoid process of the temporal bone, lateral third of the superior nuchal line of the occiput.
Action: Extension of the head, lateral flexion of the head to the same side.

A trigger point may be found in the upper portion of the muscle, on the occiput, in the space between the trapezius and SCM. It refers pain to the highest point on the head on the same side as the trigger point.

Strokes

- Using your thumb pad, stroke at an oblique angle from the spinous processes of C3 and C4 to the mastoid process. Repeat the stroke, beginning at the C5 vertebra. Continue, working in strips, to T3 (Fig. 10-11).
- Roll your thumb across the fibers of the muscle, and feel for taut bands. Check for trigger points.

Splenius Cervicis
Origin: Spinous processes of the T3–T6 vertebrae.
Insertion: Transverse processes of the C1–C3 vertebrae (varies).
Action: Extension of the cervical spine, rotation of the cervical spine to the same side, flexion of the cervical spine to the same side.

A commonly experienced trigger point can be palpated near the transverse process of C3. It refers pain to the eye on the same side. In some cases, treatment of this trigger point may relieve blurred vision in that eye.

Strokes

- With your fingertips, find the posterior aspects of the transverse processes of the C2–C4 vertebrae. Perform short, up-and-down strokes (Fig. 10-12).
- Pause at trigger points and hold.

Deep Layer

Three areas of trigger point activity form in the line of the lamina groove:

- The first one is found at the level of C4 and C5. Pain can be referred up to the suboccipital area and also down to the upper vertebral border of the scapula.
- The second area of trigger point activity is located at the level of C2. The pain referral zone is around the occiput and upward toward the top of the head.
- The third location of trigger points is right below the occipital ridge at the attachment point of semispinalis capitis. The pain pattern forms a band around the head, with the most severe sensation felt at the temple and forehead over the eye.

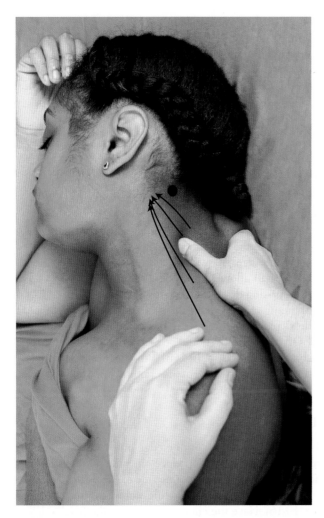

FIGURE 10-11 Deep tissue strokes on the splenius capitis.

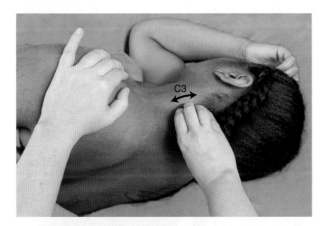

FIGURE 10-12 Working the attachments of the splenius cervicis and levator scapula, from C2–C4.

Longissimus Capitis

Origin: Transverse processes of the T1–T5 vertebrae, articular processes of the C4–C7 vertebrae.

Insertion: Posterior margin of the mastoid process of the temporal bone.

Action: Extension of the head, lateral flexion and rotation of the head to the same side.

Semispinalis Capitis

Origin: Transverse processes of the T1–T7 vertebrae (varies), articular processes of the C4–C6 vertebrae.

Insertion: Occiput between the superior and inferior nuchal lines.

Action: Extension and lateral flexion of the head.

Strokes
- With your thumb, perform combination stroking (up and down and side to side), working in small sections in the space between the spinous processes and the transverse processes of the cervical vertebrae. Begin at the level of the C7 vertebra, and continue to the occiput (Fig. 10-13). Treat trigger points when you find them.
- Work on the attachments of the muscles on the occiput using the combination strokes:
- Longissimus capitis—posterior margin of the mastoid process.
- Semispinalis capitis—the space between the superior and inferior nuchal lines.

Transversospinal Muscles (Semispinalis, Multifidus, and Rotatores)

Origin (Semispinalis cervicis, multifidi, and rotators): Transverse processes of cervical vertebrae.

Insertion:
    Semispinalis cervicis—spinous processes of the C2–C5 vertebrae.
    Multifidi—spinous processes of two to four vertebrae above the origin.
    Rotatores—base of spinous process of the next highest vertebra.

Strokes
- With your thumb, perform the combination stroke in the lamina groove of the cervical spine, from C7 to the occiput (Fig. 10-14). Working in small sections, pay attention to soft tissue dysfunction at the deepest level, next to the bone. Treat trigger points as you find them.

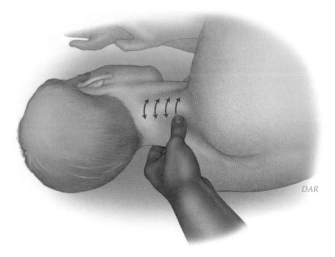

FIGURE 10-13 Deep tissue strokes on the longissimus capitis and semispinalis capitis, from C7 to the occiput.

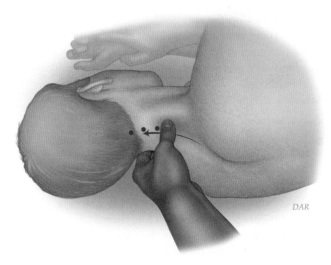

FIGURE 10-14 Deep tissue strokes on the transversospinalis muscles.

Suboccipital Muscles (Obliquus Capitis Superior, Obliquus Capitis Inferior, Rectus Capitis Posterior Major, and Rectus Capitis Posterior Minor)

Obliquus Capitis Superior

Origin: Transverse process and superior surface of the atlas.

Insertion: Occiput between the superior and inferior nuchal lines (lateral to semispinalis capitis).

Action: Extension of the head of the atlas, lateral flexion to the same side.

Obliquus Capitis Inferior

Origin: Apex of the spinous process of the atlas.

Insertion: Inferior and dorsal part of the transverse process of the atlas.

Action: Extension of the head, lateral flexion to the same side.

Rectus Capitis Posterior Major

Origin: Spinous process of the axis.

Insertion: Lateral part of the inferior nuchal line of the occiput.

Action: Extension of the head, rotation of the head to the same side, lateral flexion of the head to the same side.

Rectus Capitis Posterior Minor

Origin: Tubercle on posterior arch of atlas.

Insertion: Medial part of inferior nuchal line of occiput.

Action: Extension of head, lateral flexion of head to same side.

Strokes

- Standing at the head of the table, cup your palm over the back of the cranium, hooking your fingers under the occipital ridge. Allow them to sink in as far as the client's tissues will allow without discomfort (Fig. 10-15A). Do slow, up-and-down and side-to-side strokes.
- Standing at the side of the table and facing the client's head, place the thumbs on the occipital ridge, next to the EOP. The thumbs should be in a horizontal position, one above the other (Fig. 10-15B). Roll the thumbs alternately upward along the base of the cranium and slightly below, on the neck, at the level of C1 and C2.

STRETCH

The client sits upright, on the edge of the table. Sitting or standing behind the client, place one palm on the shoulder and the other palm on the same side of the head, above the ear. Laterally flex the head while stabilizing the shoulder (Fig. 10-16). Have the client slowly rotate the head to bring the chin toward the chest. Pause, and maintain the stretch where tightness and/or tenderness are experienced. Be careful not to overstretch the neck in this position. Direct the client to imagine breathing into the muscles being stretched as they relax and lengthen.

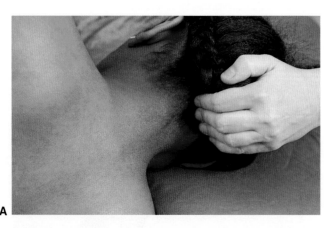

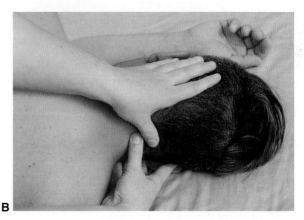

A **B**

FIGURE 10-15 A. Using the fingertips to release the suboccipital muscles. **B.** Deep tissue thumb strokes to release the suboccipital muscles.

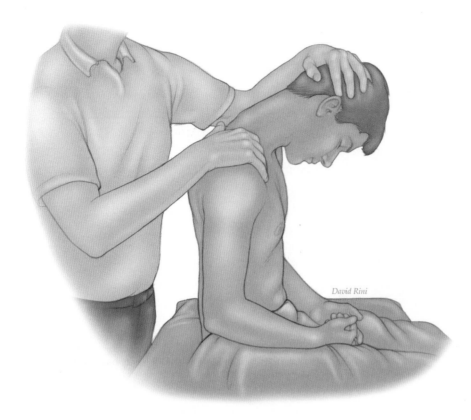

David Rini

FIGURE 10-16 Stretch for posterior neck muscles.

ACCESSORY WORK

1. Work on neck and head extensors in conjunction with the neck and head flexors to balance the musculature of the cervical region.
2. Jaw work should accompany the neck session, because imbalance is almost always reflected in both segments simultaneously.
3. Work on the feet synchronizes the upper and lower poles of the body and grounds the client after neck and head massage.

CLOSING

Sitting at the foot of the table, lightly hold the heels of the client's feet in your hands for 30 to 60 seconds. Remove your hands slowly to complete the session.

▶ NECK AND HEAD FLEXORS ROUTINE

Objectives

- To elongate the muscles of the anterior neck
- To balance the anterior neck muscles with the posterior neck muscles

- To continue the process of balancing the head on the cervical spine
- To relieve painful conditions caused by shortened flexor muscles
- To reduce uneven pulls on the hyoid bone

Energy

POSITION

- The client is lying supine on the table.
- The therapist is sitting at the head of the table.

POLARITY

The therapist holds the client's head by placing his or her right palm (positive pole) across the client's occipital ridge (negative pole) and the left palm (negative pole) across the forehead (positive pole) (Fig. 10-17). This head hold is very relaxing. It is sometimes referred to as the "brain drain" because of its effectiveness in easing excessive mental activity. The position is held for at least 1 minute.

SHIATSU

Press the conception vessel 22 point, which is located in the notch at the base of the throat, just above the sternum

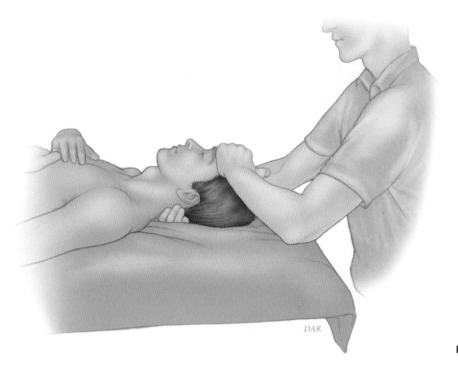

FIGURE 10-17 Polarity balancing head hold.

(Fig. 10-18). This point is intended to open the throat passage and to relieve sore throat and other inflammatory conditions of the throat and chest.

⚠ Keep your finger on the superior edge of the manubrium. Do not press into the soft tissues above it, because nerves and blood vessels are close to the surface here.

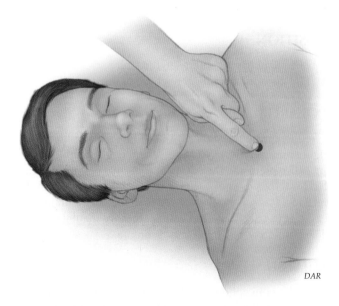

FIGURE 10-18 Contacting conception vessel 22 point.

Swedish/Cross Fiber

1. Perform effleurage strokes down the sides of the neck.
2. Apply circular fingertip friction along both sides of the neck.
3. Perform thumb sweeping on the side of the neck, stroking each side individually.

Connective Tissue

Holding the client's head in one hand, rotate it slightly to the side. Place the fingers of your other hand along the anterior border of the SCM. Allow your finger pads to sink into the muscle. As the tissues yield, let your fingers slowly glide in a posterior direction. Repeat along the length of the neck.

Deep Tissue/Neuromuscular Therapy

SEQUENCE

1. Platysma
2. SCM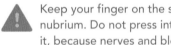
3. Scalenes
4. Suprahyoid muscles—digastric, stylohyoid, and mylohyoid ▶
5. Infrahyoid muscles—omohyoid, sternohyoid, and sternothyroid
6. Prevertebral muscles—longus capitis and longus colli

Platysma

Origin: Fascia covering the upper portion of the chest.

Insertion: Mandible, subcutaneous fascia, and muscles of the chin and jaw.
Action: Depresses lower lip and draws it backward, lifts skin of the chest.

 Active trigger points in this muscle are usually found where it covers the SCM. These trigger points may be palpated best by sifting the platysma between the thumb and fingers. The trigger points refer to the area of the mandible. The sensation of pain is superficial, as if originating in the skin over the jaw.

Strokes
- Place the fingers of one hand on the mandible, just below the corner of the mouth. Perform a slow elongation stroke, following the fibers of the muscle, down the neck, over the clavicle, and onto the upper chest (Fig. 10-19).

Sternocleidomastoid

Origin:
  Sternal head—sternum, ventral surface of the manubrium.
  Clavicular head—superior and anterior surface of the medial third of the clavicle.
Insertion: Mastoid process of the temporal bone, lateral half of the superior nuchal line of the occiput.
Action: Flexion of the cervical spine (both muscles), lateral flexion of the cervical spine to the same side, rotation of the head to the opposite side, capital extension (posterior fibers); lifts the sternum in forced inhalation.

 Trigger points may be found almost anywhere along the length of the sternal and clavicular branches of the muscle.

Sternal Division

A trigger point in the lower portion of the muscle refers pain downward, over the upper part of the sternum.

Trigger points in the middle section tend to shoot pain across the cheek area, around the eye orbit, into the eye, and sometimes, into the external part of the ear canal. Trigger points along the medial border of the middle SCM refer pain into the throat and the back of the tongue, creating the sensation of a sore throat. Trigger points in the upper section refer pain to the occipital ridge and the top of the head.

Eye problems, such as blurred vision and an inability to control eye muscles fully, can be an associated autonomic response to trigger points in the sternal division of the SCM.

Clavicular Division

Trigger points in the middle section refer pain to the forehead.
Dizziness can be an associated autonomic response to trigger points in the clavicular division, particularly after the SCM muscle has been stretched.

Strokes
- Holding the client's head in one hand, rotate the head slightly. Place your thumb pad on the mastoid process. Using the broad side of the thumb, perform an elongation stroke along the fibers of the SCM, ending at the sternum.
- With the thumb or index finger, apply cross-fiber strokes to the SCM attachment on the sternum. Glide your thumb along the top edge of the clavicle to the clavicular attachment of the SCM, and apply cross-fiber strokes to it.
- Grasp the SCM muscle between your fingers and thumbs, and sift the muscle fibers thoroughly, searching for trigger point activity (Fig. 10-20). Begin near the insertion on the mastoid process, and continue down to the origins on the sternum and clavicle.

Scalenes

Scalenus Anterior
Origin: Transverse processes of the C3–C6 vertebrae.
Insertion: Scalene tubercle on the inner border of the first rib.
Action: Flexion of cervical spine, elevation of the first rib on inhalation, rotation of the cervical spine to the opposite side, lateral flexion of the cervical spine to the same side.

Scalenus Medius
Origin: Transverse processes of the C2–C7 vertebrae.
Insertion: Superior surface of the first rib.
Action: Flexion of the cervical spine (weak), elevation of the first rib on inhalation, lateral flexion of the cervical spine to the same side, cervical spine rotation to the opposite side.

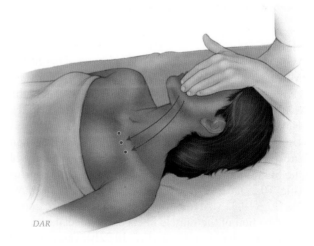

FIGURE 10-19 Direction of deep tissue stroking on the platysma.

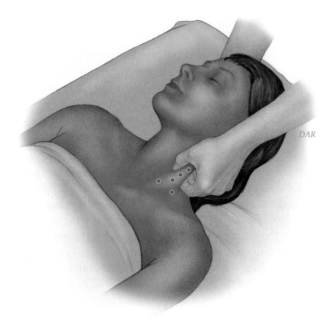

FIGURE 10-20 Sifting the sternocleidomastoid.

Scalenus Posterior
Origin: Transverse processes of the C4–C6 vertebrae (variable).
Insertion: Outer surface of the second rib.
Action: Cervical flexion (weak), elevation of the second rib on inhalation, lateral flexion of the cervical spine (assists), cervical spine rotation to the opposite side.

> The order of frequency of trigger point activity in the scalene muscles is from anterior to medial to posterior. Trigger points in the three scalenes may refer pain to the chest, the upper arm and shoulder, and in the back of the body, to the medial border of the scapula. Trigger points in these muscles often form secondarily to trigger points in the SCM, so it is important to check both muscles together.

Strokes
- With your fingers, find the posterior border of the SCM. Moving it slightly anterior and avoiding the jugular vein, gently press your fingers down on the front portion of the transverse processes of the cervical vertebrae (Fig. 10-21). Hold tender points.
- Using the broad side of your thumb, perform an elongation stroke in the triangle formed by the posterior border of the SCM and the anterior border of the upper trapezius (Fig. 10-22). Move, in an inferior direction, to the clavicle (Fig. 10-22A). Then, with your fingers, stroke across the direction of the muscle fibers of the medial scalene, seeking taut bands of tissue (Fig. 10-22B). Pause to treat trigger points.

> ⚠ Do not apply deep pressure in the posterior triangle area, because the subclavian artery and vein are located here. Light, cross-fiber strokes are sufficient to relax the scalene muscles.

- With your index finger, reach under the superior edge of the clavicle, toward the scalene attachments on the first and second ribs (Fig. 10-22C). Apply cross-fiber strokes to the attachments. Keep your finger against the inside surface of the clavicle to avoid pressing on nerves.

Suprahyoid Muscles (Digastric, Mylohyoid, and Stylohyoid)

Digastric
Origin:
Posterior belly—mastoid notch on the temporal bone.

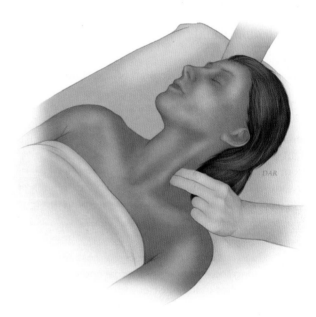

FIGURE 10-21 Contacting the scalene attachments on the transverse processes of C3–C6.

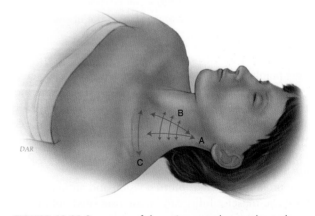

FIGURE 10-22 Sequence of deep tissue strokes on the scalenes.

Anterior belly—inner side of the inferior border of the mandible near the symphysis.

Insertion: Intermediate tendon and to hyoid bone via a fibrous sling.

Action: Mandibular depression, elevation of the hyoid bone during swallowing, anterior belly draws the hyoid forward, posterior belly draws the hyoid backward.

⚠ Take great care in this area of the neck as several structures are vulnerable to damage, and intrusive pressure may feel unsafe.

◎ A trigger point may be found in the digastric muscle near its attachment on the mandible, just under the chin. It refers to the lower front teeth and the alveolar ridge below them.

Strokes

- *Digastric and Mylohyoid Attachments on the Mandible.* Place the pad of your index finger on the underside of the mandible near the center, at the digastric fossa. Slowly stroke across the inside border of the bone, to the angle of the mandible (Fig. 10-23).
- *Belly of Digastric.* Beginning with your index finger at the digastric fossa of the mandible, stroke along the fibers of the muscle on the underside of the chin, to the fibrous loop on the superior border of the hyoid (Fig. 10-24).

Mylohyoid

Origin: Mylohyoid line (from symphysis to molars) on the inside surface of the mandible.

Insertion: Hyoid bone.

Action: Raises the hyoid bone and the tongue for swallowing.

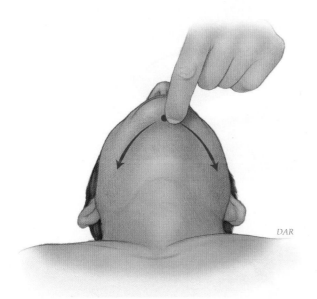

FIGURE 10-23 Working the digastric and mylohyoid attachments on the inside border of the mandible.

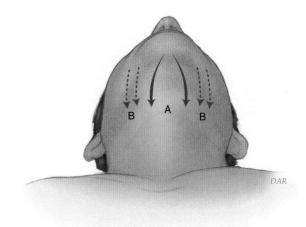

FIGURE 10-24 Direction of deep tissue strokes on the bellies of the digastric (A) and mylohyoid and stylohyoid (B).

Stylohyoid

Origin: Styloid process of the temporal bone.

Insertion: Hyoid bone.

Action: Hyoid bone drawn upward and backward; assists in opening the mouth; possible participation in mastication and speech.

Strokes

- *Belly of Mylohyoid and Stylohyoid.* Place your fingers at the inferior border of the mandible. Stroke in an inferior direction from the mandible to the hyoid bone (see Fig. 10-24). Repeat the stroke, starting more laterally on the mandible and covering the entire surface area of the muscles. Feel for taut bands, and hold at trigger points. This stroke moves across the fibers of the muscles rather than parallel to them.

Note: The mylohyoid muscle forms the floor of the mouth.

⚠ Be careful to avoid moving off the mylohyoid muscle fibers on the lateral side, because the submandibular lymph nodes are located here.

- *Attachments on the Hyoid Bone.* To locate the hyoid bone, slide the fingers of one hand downward from the inferior border of the mandible until they touch the superior border of the hyoid bone (Fig. 10-25). To stabilize the hyoid, keep the index finger on the superior border of the bone while placing your thumb on the tip of the greater horn of the hyoid on one side and your middle finger on the tip of the greater horn on the other. To relax the muscles that attach to the hyoid bone, remove your index finger from the superior border. Maintaining the hold on the ends of the bone, slowly shift the hyoid from side to side. To work the suprahyoid muscle attachments, place the index finger of your other hand on the superior border of the hyoid while you continue to hold on to the ends of the bone (Fig. 10-26). Move your finger across the edge of the bone, getting client feedback about tenderness. Pay special

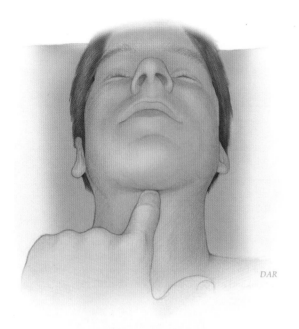

FIGURE 10-25 Palpating the superior border of the hyoid bone.

attention to the fibrous loop on the lesser horn of the hyoid that connects the digastric muscle to the bone.

 The hyoid bone is fragile. Do not squeeze it tightly or apply strong pressure.

Infrahyoid Muscles

Strokes
- Still stabilizing the hyoid with one hand, place the index finger of your other hand on the body of the hyoid, and slowly stroke side to side. Hold sensitive points.
- Slide your finger down slightly, and stroke side to side on the inferior border of the hyoid.
- Slide the pad of your index finger onto the inner surface of the clavicle, and stroke side to side on the medial end to contact the attachment of the sternohyoid.

Prevertebral Muscles (Longus Capitis and Longus Colli)

Longus Capitis
Origin: Transverse processes of the C3–C6 vertebrae.
Insertion: Inferior basilar part of the occiput (anterior to the foramen magnum).
Action: Capital flexion, rotation of the head to the same side.

Longus Colli
Superior Oblique Part
Origin: Transverse processes of the C3–C5 vertebrae.
Insertion: Tubercle of the anterior arch of the atlas.

Inferior Oblique Part
Origin: Anterior bodies of the T1–T3 vertebrae (variable).
Insertion: Transverse processes of the C5–C6 vertebrae.

Vertical Portion
Origin: Anterior bodies of the C5–C7 and T1–T3 vertebrae.
Insertion: Anterior bodies of the C2–C4 vertebrae.
Action of all three parts: Cervical flexion (weak), cervical rotation to opposite side (inferior oblique), lateral flexion (superior and inferior oblique).

Strokes
- Place the fingers of both hands lengthwise along the borders of the trachea. Slowly and lightly slide the fingers medial, under the trachea, toward the anterior bodies of the cervical vertebrae (Fig. 10-27).

Do not press on the top of the trachea so that the thyroid gland can be avoided. Move slowly and sensitively in this area, because the vertebral artery runs parallel to the trachea. If you feel a pulse as you slide under the trachea, lift your fingers slightly, and move them more medial to take pressure off the artery.

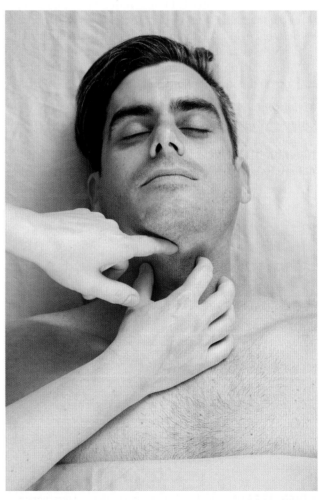

FIGURE 10-26 Hand position for contacting muscle attachments on the hyoid bone.

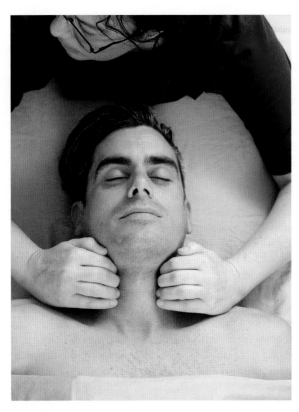

FIGURE 10-27 Contacting the prevertebral muscles underneath the trachea.

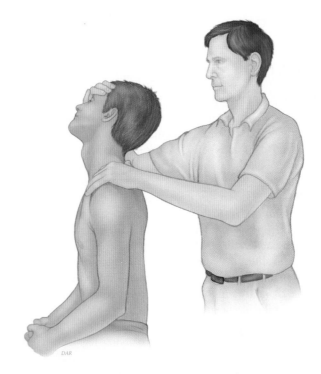

FIGURE 10-28 Stretch for the anterior neck muscles.

- Slowly move the fingers of one hand at a time up and down and side to side along the prevertebral muscles, feeling for knots and taut bands. Work each side individually. Get client feedback about tenderness. Hold trigger points.

Note: A cough reflex may be encountered at the base of the neck, near the sternal attachment of the SCM.

STRETCH

The client sits upright, on the edge of the table. Sitting or standing behind the client, place one palm on the shoulder and the other palm on the same side of the head, above the ear.

Laterally flex the head while stabilizing the shoulder. Slowly turn the client's head toward extension (Fig. 10-28). Move in small increments, pausing to hold as the various muscle groups just worked on are stretched.

ACCESSORY WORK

1. *Suboccipital Relaxation.* Sitting at the head of the table, slide your fingers under the client's occipital ridge. Let them sink into the tissues under the base of the cranium. Hold for 1 or 2 minutes.
2. *Reflex Zone.* The zone on the foot that tradition suggests corresponds to the neck is the shaft of the big toe. To access this connection, hold the sides of the big toe near the base with your

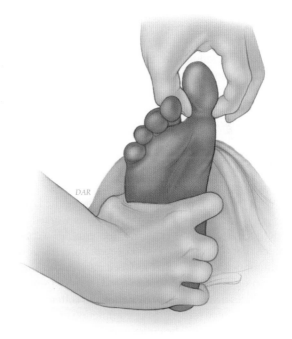

FIGURE 10-29 Contacting the neck reflex zone on the big toe.

thumb and index finger (Fig 10-29). Glide the fingers up and down in small movements. Repeat on the other foot.

CLOSING

Sitting at the foot of the table, lightly hold the heels of the client's feet in your hands for 30 to 60 seconds. Remove your hands slowly to complete the session.

SESSION IMPRESSION

THE NECK

The subject is a 20-year-old woman named Chloe, who is a college student. Chloe is not a regular massage client. She schedules appointments sporadically, usually during high-stress periods in her life. Her reason for seeking deep tissue therapy at this time is that for the past week, she has been experiencing severe pain in her posterior neck. It radiates down her upper back to the level of the T12 vertebra and up to the occiput. She is experiencing pain in the temporal region of her head, which she feels is being generated by the tight muscles in her neck. It is difficult for her to study, because the act of leaning forward at a desk to read causes shooting pains to radiate to the top of her head and throughout the posterior neck and upper back.

Chloe has been involved in several car accidents over the last 5 years. She has never been seriously injured, but she has experienced whiplash to varying degrees as a result of each accident. She has received medical treatment for neck injuries sustained from these accidents and currently visits a chiropractor twice a month.

Although she has a history of neck injuries, Chloe feels that the source of the pain is as much psychological as it is physical. The pain is always much worse during times of high stress. In addition to studying for exams, she is experiencing relationship problems that have her concerned to the point that she is not sleeping well at night. She often wakes in the morning with a stiff, painful neck.

The focus of this session will be deep tissue work on the posterior and anterior neck, the muscles of the upper back (particularly the trapezius), and the cranium. Some work will also be done on the jaw muscles, along with stimulation of spinal reflex points on the feet.

With the client lying in a prone position, the layers of posterior neck muscles were meticulously worked, from superficial to deep. As expected, the muscles were very tender. Trigger points were discovered along the borders of the upper trapezius that radiated pain to the anterior portion of the temporal muscle, where she frequently experiences headache pain. A significant softening of the region was noted following the completion of deep tissue therapy on the neck. The entire upper back was massaged, with careful attention paid to the entire trapezius.

Immediately after the client turned supine, the suboccipital relaxation procedure was applied. When the therapist initially placed the fingers under her occipital ridge, Chloe reported feeling a throbbing pain near the top of her head. This pain was triggered by pressure to the fibers of the upper portion of splenius capitis, between the borders of the trapezius and SCM. The therapist reduced pressure, to check in with Chloe. She was willing to continue with the work in this area, and the therapist reintroduced pressure here more gradually. During approximately the first 30 seconds of the procedure, Chloe's head was held suspended, away from the palms of the therapist's hands, because of constrictions in the neck muscles. After about 1 minute of holding, her head began to sink toward the therapist's palms. Within another minute of holding, the back of her head was resting in the therapist's palms, and she was smiling broadly. She reported that the pain at the top of her head was completely gone and that her head felt light and free.

Massage to the cranium and facial muscles was followed by deep tissue therapy to the SCM, scalenes, and prevertebral muscles. All these muscles were tender and elicited dull pain, particularly the attachments to the scalenes on the anterior side of the transverse processes of the cervical vertebrae. After clarifying that the pain was not electrical or zapping (to rule out nerve compression), the therapist applied Swedish and cross-fiber strokes to the pectoralis major to balance the work done on the upper and midback. The session was completed with foot massage accompanied by reflexology and polarity.

After the session, the client reported feeling "like a new person." She said it felt as if someone had lifted her head off her shoulders. Because of the extreme tenderness in some of the neck muscles and the high incidence of radiating pain that was uncovered, Chloe decided to schedule another massage for the following week. She was shown neck stretches to perform whenever she began to feel strain in her neck muscles. The benefits of purchasing a portable editor's desk or bookstand to use when studying so that she does not have to flex her neck and head was discussed. She also agreed to consider using a smaller pillow when she sleeps so that her head is not elevated so much, causing her neck to remain flexed all night. ▪

Topics for Discussion

1. Why is examination by a medical doctor crucial before massage therapy is applied to a client who has experienced a neck injury?
2. Describe the head and neck displacements characterized by the "forward head" and "military neck" positions. Which muscles are likely to be shortened in each of these patterns?
3. Name all the muscles that are directly affected by the suboccipital relaxation procedure.
4. Create a self-care program to aid a client who regularly experiences tension headaches.
5. Why is it advantageous to perform some neck work at the beginning of every massage session?

The Facial Muscles and Temporomandibular Joint

▶ GENERAL CONCEPTS

Probably more than any other part of the body, the head and face tend to define a person's identity. Many people have the image of themselves as a head carrying around the body like baggage. When asked the question, "Where do you feel yourself to reside in your body?" many people will answer, "In my head." One of the greatest benefits of deep tissue bodywork is the reconnection of the head with the rest of the body.

In our society, the values most appreciated are those associated with the head. In many workplaces, people are generally valued more for their mental abilities than for their physical prowess. Most occupations rely on mental and sensory acuity for success and advancement. Partly because of these factors, the head and face become a focal point for the awareness of stress. Headaches related to tension are common and often debilitating. Massage to the scalp and facial muscles has a relaxing, rejuvenating quality that does much to counteract the effects of mental and emotional tension.

The temporomandibular joint (TMJ) of the jaw is one of the most frequently used joints in the body. Its movement accompanies talking and eating, two of the most common functions in which we engage. Therefore, the muscles that control the TMJ need to have strength and stamina. These muscles are subject to stress and dysfunction because of overuse and emotional factors. Tightening the jaw by clenching the teeth is a frequent response to tension and is often done unconsciously, even while a person is asleep. Chronically shortened jaw muscles can generate painful trigger points and misalign the TMJ. Fortunately, careful massage therapy can often improve the muscular component of jaw pain.

Dysfunction of the TMJ is a problem that is often misdiagnosed and untreated. In addition to muscle overuse and fatigue, other factors in in TMJ disorder include trauma to the jaw, keeping the mouth open for long periods of time (as during a dental examination), cartilage damage and inflammation within the joint capsule, and malocclusion of the jaw.

TMJ disorders can create many symptoms. Pain may occur around the joint itself, in the jaw muscles, and in or above the ears. Dizziness is also common. Referred pain patterns may be perceived as toothache or neck pain. It may be difficult to open or close the mouth, and a clicking sound may be heard. Dysfunction of the TMJ may affect the position of the facial and cranial bones. They can become compressed, resulting in ringing in the ears, vision disorders, headaches, and/or chronic sinus inflammation.

Often, a correspondence is found between tension areas in the jaw and the pelvis. The two are reflections of each other, being at either end of the spinal column. In polarity terms, the head and jaw represent the positive pole, and the pelvis acts as the negative pole. The balance of both poles helps to integrate the entire body.

▶ MUSCULOSKELETAL ANATOMY AND FUNCTION

The TMJ is the articulation of the mandible with the temporal bone of the cranium. This joint is unique in the body in that the lower portion hangs from the upper portion, requiring muscular action to keep the jaw shut (Fig. 10-30). The joint consists of the convex-shaped mandibular condyle, the concave

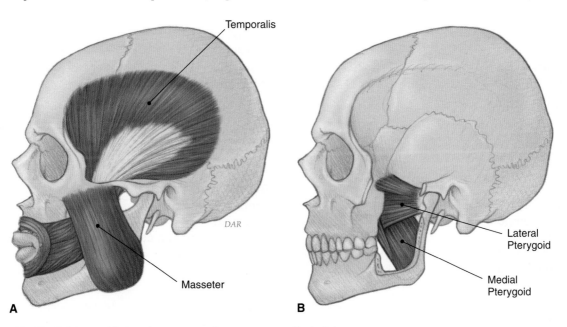

A   **B**

FIGURE 10-30 A and **B.** Muscles acting on the temporomandibular joint.

articular eminence of the temporal bone, and a disc between these bony surfaces. Each TMJ is really two joints: an upper and a lower portion. The articulation of the temporal bone and disc form the upper joint, while the mandible and disc form the lower joint. Complete opening and closing of the mouth along with side flexion, protraction, and retraction are dependent on coordinated action of these two joints. (See Essential Anatomy Box 10-2 for a summary of muscles, bones, and landmarks of the cranium and face and Essential Anatomy Box 10-3 for those of the TMJ.)

The disc between the temporal bone and the mandible is called the meniscus. It is irregularly shaped, narrower in the center than at the two ends, so its center is concave at both the top and bottom surfaces. This allows a great adaptability of fit against differently shaped bony surfaces. Each meniscus is attached to the medial and lateral sides of the condyle of the mandible. The anterior end of the disc is attached to both the joint capsule and the *lateral pterygoid* muscle. ▶ At the posterior end, bands of fibers stabilize the disc so that it can cushion and move with the bones, but cannot move out of place.

The mandible is a U-shaped bone that articulates with the temporal bone on both ends. Its fitting in the TMJ allows it to be capable of depression and elevation (opening and closing the mouth), protraction and retraction (jutting the jaw forward and backward), and lateral deviation (sliding from side to side). The mandible can also move asymmetrically around its condyles, a motion that is used in chewing. The TMJ is called into action during chewing, talking, and swallowing. The contacting bony surfaces are covered with dense, slick fibrocartilage to allow for smooth movement. Unlike other symmetrical joints, it is impossible to engage one TMJ without also using the other side.

When the jaw first opens, the mandibular condyle rotates on the inferior surface of the disc, allowing between 11 and 25 mm of opening. To open the mouth further, the disc and condyle unit glide anteriorly, along the articular eminence of the temporal bone. The normal vertical span of a fully open mouth is between 40 and 50 mm. To close the mouth, these actions occur in reversed order.

Mandibular depression is accomplished primarily by the digastric muscle. The lower portion of the lateral pterygoid also assists in this action. Elevation of the mandible is performed by the *masseter*, *temporalis*, and *medial pterygoid* as well as the upper portion of the lateral pterygoid muscle.

Because of its prominent role in closing the jaw and chewing, the masseter is prone to dysfunction, including trigger point formation. Eating hard, fibrous foods, or habitually chewing gum can cause the masseter to overwork. Biting down hard on ice or frequently holding things between the teeth can also aggravate this muscle. Emotional distress often is reflected in chronic contraction of the masseter, accompanied by gritting the teeth. Shortness in the masseter can be assessed by a person's inability to fully open the mouth vertically.

BOX 10-2 ESSENTIAL ANATOMY | **The Cranium and Facial Routines**

MUSCLES	**BONES AND LANDMARKS**
Temporalis	Occipital
Occipitalis	Temporal
Galea aponeurotica	Parietal
Auricularis	Frontal
Frontalis	Orbital ridge
Procerus	Maxilla
Orbicularis oculi	Mandible
Masseter	Zygomatic arch
Buccinator	

BOX 10-3 ESSENTIAL ANATOMY | **The TMJ Routine**

MUSCLES	**BONES AND LANDMARKS**
Temporalis	Temporal
Tendon of temporalis	Sphenoid
Masseter	Lateral pterygoid plate
Lateral pterygoid	Mandible
Medial pterygoid	Ramus of mandible
Digastric	Condyle of mandible
	Coronoid process

The temporalis assists the masseter in mandibular elevation. The posterior section of the muscle assists in retraction of the jaw and lateral deviation of the mandible to the same side. Dysfunction in this muscle as a result of trigger points may manifest as local hypersensitivity and tension headaches caused by referred pain patterns. Sometimes, pain in the upper incisor teeth originates from trigger points in the temporalis muscle.

The lateral pterygoid consists of two segments that work in opposition to each other. The upper portion, which is attached to the anterior end of the disc and to the condyle of the mandible, acts in unison with the temporalis and masseter to elevate the mandible. It also maintains traction on the disc when the jaw closes. When the upper lateral pterygoid becomes chronically short, it pulls the disc forward of the condyle as the jaw closes, causing a clicking sound and making the mouth difficult to close.

The lower portion of the lateral pterygoid acts to open the jaw, to protract the jaw when both sides of the muscle are contracting, and to pull the jaw to the opposite side when contracting unilaterally. Pain felt in the TMJ frequently comes from a shortened lateral pterygoid muscle.

▶ CONDITIONS

1. *Bell Palsy.* This is a result of damage to cranial nerve VII, also known as the facial nerve. Several factors, including viral infections like cold or flu, cause the nerve to swell and become impinged. Symptoms include loss of muscle tone on the affected side. This can look like a drooping mouth or eye, and in some cases severe, one-sided facial distortion. It is a temporary paralysis, but recovery may take several months. Massage treatments may help to relieve some of the stress accompanying the condition, and because the paralysis does not cause numbness, massage therapy may also help to keep the facial muscles healthy during the recovery process.
2. *Trigeminal Neuralgia.* This is an irritation of cranial nerve V, the trigeminal nerve. This is the primary source of sensation for the face, and when the nerve is aggravated the result is extreme, sharp, shooting, electrical pain on one side. Episodes can last from a few seconds to a few minutes. Triggers can be difficult to predict, but they include a cold breeze or resting the face on a cold surface (i.e., the window of a car or other vehicle), having hair touch the face, or other very minor stimuli. Many people with trigeminal neuralgia cannot tolerate touch on their face, but they may benefit from massage to the neck and shoulders.
3. *Headaches.* Many types of headaches have been identified; some of the most common are described here:
   a. *Tension headaches.* Tension headaches are the most common form of headache. They are triggered by chronic contraction or spasm of the muscles of the neck, face, and head. Contributing factors include postural habits, ergonomics, eyestrain, and stress. Tension headaches are frequently described as feeling like a tight band around the head, or diffuse bilateral pain. Massage to tight muscles in the head and neck frequently provides relief.
   b. *Chemical headaches.* Chemical headaches are brought on by the body's reaction to foods or environmental factors. Monosodium glutamate (MSG), nitrites, and other additives frequently trigger chemical headaches. They can also occur with dehydration (this is usually the case with a hangover), and as a part of withdrawal symptoms, especially for nicotine and caffeine. Rebound headaches, that occur when headache medication is halted, are a form of chemical headache.
   c. *Migraine.* A migraine headache is characterized by sharp and debilitating pain on one side of the head, sometimes behind the eye, and a clear sense of throbbing. It may be accompanied by visual disturbances, such as seeing lights or ropes floating in front of the eyes, and possibly by nausea and vomiting. The headache may last from several hours to several days. Migraine headaches have many precipitating factors, including stress, exposure to bright light, hormone cycle, and allergic reactions.
4. *Sinus Congestion.* This may be a result of seasonal allergies, in which case it can be relieved through a combination of heat, massage, and acupressure treatment to the appropriate areas of the face. Congestion due to a sinus infection, however, needs to be treated differently and may require a doctor's care.

▶ EVALUATION OF THE FACIAL AREA

1. Observe the overall shape and contours of the head.
2. Check for symmetry in the face (Fig. 10-31).
   - Imagine a vertical line dividing the face into right and left segments.
   - Compare the two sides.
3. Observe the eyes.
   - Are they the same size?
   - Are they on the same horizontal plane?
   - Where are they looking?
4. Make note of any lines of stress on the face.
   - Across the forehead?
   - Between the eyebrows?
   - Outside corners of the eyes and mouth?
5. Observe any muscular tension in the face and neck region.

Refer to Table 10-3 for a description of common tension manifestations in the facial area and the muscles involved.

HOLISTIC VIEW

"The face is the mirror of the mind" (Saint Jerome)

The face projects our persona: the part of us that we consciously or subconsciously choose to present to the world. A person's face is often the first impression we use to assess his or her quality of character. We can frequently deduce a person's emotional state by interpreting his or her facial features.

The face can be the mask we take off to reveal ourselves, or the one we put on to hide what we are thinking or feeling. It has been said that a person's soul can be seen through the eyes. In the same way, we can block or limit what we reveal about ourselves by controlling our facial expression with tight, rigid muscles.

The conflict between our outer facade and our inner state is often a source of tension. It can be frightening and confrontational to have one's face closely scrutinized. Make-up and glasses are sometimes used as a means to shield the face, in an attempt to hide or protect the person inside. Taut, unmoving facial muscles can serve the same purpose: they provide a barrier, and they also inhibit the spontaneous sharing of nonverbal communication.

It is fairly common to encounter people who do not want their faces massaged, or even touched. Therefore, the massage therapist needs to obtain permission both in the presession interview and again during the session before assuming that touch in this area will be welcomed.

A lot of information about our mood and stress levels can be conveyed through the set of the jaw. The jaw is used in eating and speaking, as well as in helping to create our facial expression. The jaw and teeth are strong and capable of tearing and grinding. Animals frequently use the jaw and teeth as weapons, and we assert ourselves through the use of the jaw, claiming what we want through speech and through nonverbal facial gestures.

Tightness in the jaw muscles often denotes a withholding of feeling or expression. A person who is contracting the jaw muscles might be blocking the communication of strong emotion. It is a common experience for many of us to "swallow my feelings" or "hold my tongue." This bottling up of expression can lead to habitual tightness and secondary problems.

Bruxism, or teeth-grinding, is a condition that dentists see frequently. The reduction of tension in the jaw might be accompanied by a desire to express what one has been holding inside, whether it is words or simply sounds that convey our feelings. We often limit our vocal expression to words, but sounds like grunting, hissing, or screaming can tap into our unspoken feelings, and, when expressed in a suitable setting, can be very therapeutic. Ultimately the goal is to find an appropriate way to convey our feelings, so that our facial muscles and jaw muscles may be relaxed and tension-free. ■

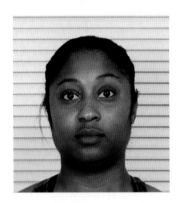

FIGURE 10-31 Postural evaluation: look for symmetry and asymmetry of the facial features.

TABLE 10-3 | Body Reading for the Face

Postural habits	Muscles
Furrowed brow—lines on the forehead and/or between the eyebrows	Frontalis
	Temporalis
	Procerus
Constant frown—the corners of the lips are turned down	Platysma
	Digastric
Facial misalignment—asymmetry of the features and/or bone structure of the face	Treat the tight muscles that seem to be distorting the face
	Some imbalances may be permanent

▶ EVALUATION OF THE TMJ

1. Have the client open and close his or her mouth a few times.
   - Observe the motion of the jaw. It should move symmetrically on both sides.
   - The bone at the TMJ junction should not jut out on either side when the mouth opens and closes.
   - Observe the alignment of the upper and lower teeth. The teeth should not shift laterally as the mouth opens and closes.

2. Place your fingers on both sides of the client's jaw, at the TMJ. Have the client slowly open and close the mouth a few times.
   - Feel for a smooth, gliding motion on both sides. Note any deviations.
   - Listen for any clicking or popping sounds.

Note: A number of injuries can cause TMJ problems. These include blows to the jaw and whiplash injuries that cause the cervical spine and jaw to hyperextend. Biting down on hard food and overindulgence in chewing gum may also be culprits.

▶ EXERCISES AND SELF-TREATMENT

1. *Eye Exercises.*
   - Slowly look straight up, toward the eyebrows, then down, toward the cheeks. Perform the movement three times. Close the eyelids, and rest for a few moments.
   - Slowly look across a horizontal path to the right corners of the eyes. Look across a horizontal path to the left corners of the eyes. Perform the movement three times. Close the eyelids, and rest for a few moments.
   - Look around the eye sockets in a clockwise direction, making a full circle. Begin by looking up, toward the eyebrows, and then continue around the eye orbit to the left. Perform the movement three times. Rest for a few moments and then trace three slow circles in a counterclockwise direction.
   - Lie down on your back. Rub both palms together vigorously to generate heat and then rest the palms over your closed eyes. Allow the warmth and energy to penetrate into the eyes and cheeks, and feel the entire area around the eyes relaxing. Rest, with the eyes closed, for several minutes.

2. *Facial Tension Reducer.* This exercise may be performed either sitting or lying down. As you inhale, expand the face by slowly making a look of surprise. Open the eyes very wide and the mouth as far as you can, and flare the nostrils. Hold for a few moments. Exhaling, pull all the features of the face toward the center by closing the eyes tight, draw the cheeks in, and pucker the mouth. Squeeze and hold for a few moments. Repeat both facial expressions two more times and then rest, allowing all the tension to flow out of the facial muscles.

3. *Jaw and Tongue Tension Reducer.*
   - Place the pads of both thumbs on the underside of your chin. Slowly begin to yawn as you press against the underside of the chin with the thumbs, creating resistance to the opening of the mouth. Repeat a couple of times, and then rest the jaw muscles.
   - With the mouth closed, circle your tongue in a clockwise direction over the upper and lower teeth. Repeat nine more times. Reverse the direction of the tongue circling, and complete 10 repetitions counterclockwise.

SESSION IMPRESSION

TMJ DISORDER

The subject is a 29-year-old woman named Rachel, who works as a part-time secretary. Her experience with massage therapy is limited. She has received several relaxation-style massages as gifts. She moved to the Southeast from the West Coast about 8 months ago, and since moving, she has been experiencing sinus headaches on a weekly basis, which she attributes to allergic reactions to the vegetation. She is also experiencing severe jaw pain and some restriction when opening her mouth wide. The jaw pain seems to be worse when she wakes in the morning. Rachel's dentist has informed her that she is clenching and grinding her teeth at night. She is going to be fitted with a night guard this week. The dentist also recommended that she receive massage therapy for the cranial and jaw muscles to reduce tension in those areas.

Rachel was asked if she had a history of TMJ dysfunction. She said that she did not, that her problems began after her move. She has never been struck in the face, and she has never suffered whiplash. About 5 years ago, however, as she was biting into an apple, her jaw momentarily stuck in an open position. It scared her quite a bit, but the mandible immediately slipped back into place. The incident has not recurred.

To evaluate movement of the jaw, Rachel was asked to slowly open and close her mouth as the therapist lightly held his fingers on her right and left TMJs. When her mouth reached about a 0.75-inch opening, the mandible slipped to the left, and a clicking sound was heard. When the mouth reached an opening of 1.25 inches, the client began to experience pain in the jaw muscles.

The session focused on the TMJ and related muscles. The neck massage was performed first, followed by the cranial massage. The temporalis muscles were sore, but the client said that pressure on the muscles felt good. Therefore, the therapist held points on both sides simultaneously for several seconds. After the entire cranial area was relaxed, the facial muscles were addressed. Focused attention was paid to the tendon of the temporalis muscle above the zygomatic bone. It was quite tender. The masseter muscles were bulky and unyielding to pressure. Circular friction strokes helped to relax the muscles. Numerous trigger points were found in the masseters.

The lateral pterygoids were the final muscles in the facial area to be massaged. Because the mandible pulled to the left, the right lateral pterygoid most likely was the more contracted. The therapist explained the intraoral

(continued)

SESSION IMPRESSION (*continued*)

procedures to the client and put on a protective glove. (Latex gloves are typical, but they are also associated with allergic reactions. Nitrile gloves are well tolerated by most people.) The left lateral pterygoid was massaged first, both to accustom the client to the protocol and to induce relaxation in the less-involved muscle before the more problematic right side was contacted. Even though both lateral pterygoid muscles had much tenderness, the client handled the procedure very well.

The procedure was done slowly to allow the client to breathe and relax throughout. The therapist removed his finger from inside the client's mouth several times during the procedure to allow her to relax and assimilate the change as well as to report her feelings toward the work. She said that, amazingly, when the therapist touched the lateral pterygoids, it triggered the pain in her sinus cavities that she had been attributing to allergies. Her eyes watered a little during the work, so she was given a tissue to wipe away the tears. She said the tears were not from pain or emotions but more of a reflexive reaction.

After the completion of the session, Rachel observed her face in a mirror. She noted that she looked like she had shed about 5 years of age in her face. She felt completely relaxed and elated at gaining some insight regarding her sinus pain as well as feeling pain relief in her jaw muscles. When her jaw movement was evaluated after the session, the click was minimal, and the mandible barely shifted. It was agreed that she should receive more TMJ work,

along with deep tissue therapy to other areas of her body.

Rachel had a realization that much of her TMJ problem was a stress reaction to her moving to a new part of the country and starting her life over again. She also realized that she had been holding back from saying some important things to certain people in her life, and that the suppression of those feelings was contributing to her jaw pain. She greatly appreciated the support she was receiving through massage therapy and from her dentist. As part of a home care plan, she was taught deep abdominal breathing to incorporate as a stress reduction technique to help minimize nighttime teeth clenching. ■

Topics for Discussion

1. What are some common indications that a person may have a TMJ problem?
2. What suggestions to minimize aggravating TMJ discomfort could you offer to a client?
3. Explain to a client why his or her jaw clicks when opening or closing the mouth.
4. List several kinds of activities that may contribute to TMJ misalignment and pain.
5. Practice putting an apprehensive client at ease by fully explaining the purpose and methodology of intraoral procedures.

▶ HEAD/FACE/JAW ROUTINE

Objectives

- To reduce tightness in the cranial muscles, which can be a major stress reliever
- To help alleviate aggravating factors in headaches and facial pain
- To reduce tension in muscles affecting the jaw and TMJ
- To reduce muscular stresses in the facial muscles

Energy

POSITION

- The client is lying supine on the table. A bolster may be placed under the knees for comfort.
- The therapist is sitting at the head of the table.

POLARITY

Place your right palm (positive pole) under the client's occipital ridge (negative pole) and your left palm (negative pole) across the client's forehead (positive pole). Imagine your hands drawing all the tension out of the head. Breathe deeply and relax fully as you maintain the contact. Hold for 1 to 2 minutes.

SHIATSU

Place your fingers on the sides of the client's head, above the ears. With your fingers curved and separated, press in against the cranium. Move your fingers to several different places on the sides of the head, and repeat. This move stimulates points on the gallbladder and triple heater channels.

Swedish/Cross Fiber

1. Perform circular friction with the fingertips on the scalp. Start from the back of the head, and work forward to the forehead.

2. Perform effleurage strokes with the fingertips across the forehead, cheeks, and chin.
3. Perform circular friction with the fingertips under the cheekbones and down the sides of the jaw.

Deep Tissue/Neuromuscular Therapy

SEQUENCE

1. Cranium—temporalis, occipitalis, and galea aponeurotica
2. Facial muscles—frontalis, procerus, and orbicularis oculi
3. Jaw—tendon of temporalis, masseter, and lateral pterygoid

Cranium

Temporalis
Origin: Temporal fossa, temporal fascia.
Insertion: Coronoid process and anterior border of the ramus of the mandible.
Action: Elevates the mandible, clenches the teeth; posterior fibers retract the mandible; assists in lateral grinding motion.

Several trigger points may form in this muscle. They usually occur in an arc around the section where the muscle fibers join the tendon. These trigger points often account for headache pain in the temple region and for pain around the eyes into the upper teeth.

The first trigger point, which is in the lower anterior portion of the muscle, refers pain along the supraorbital ridge and inferiorly into the upper front teeth. The second and third trigger point regions, which are in the middle lower portion of the muscle, send pain to the temple and into the maxillary teeth. The fourth section of trigger point formation, which is in the posterior aspect of the muscle, has a referral zone located behind and above the trigger point.

Strokes
- Place your fingertips or thumb on the side of the client's head, slightly above the ear (Fig. 10-32). To stabilize the head, put the palm of your other hand against the temporalis muscle on the other side.
- Move up and down and side to side, working on small sections of the muscle, and feel for stringy fibers and points of tenderness. Cover the entire muscle, and treat trigger points as you find them. Repeat on the other side.

Occipitalis
Origin: Lateral two-thirds of the superior nuchal line on the occipital bone, mastoid process on the temporal bone.
Insertion: Galea aponeurotica.
Action: Draws back the scalp, helps the frontalis to raise the eyebrows and wrinkle the forehead.

Trigger points in this muscle are common culprits in the formation of headaches that shoot pain over the top of the head and into the eye.

Strokes
- From the external occipital protuberance, slide your fingers laterally, along the superior nuchal line to the mastoid process part of the temporal bone.
- Move your fingers up and down and side to side, working on small sections of the muscle (Fig. 10-33). Feel for taut bands and points of tenderness, and treat trigger points as you find them. Both sides may be worked simultaneously, or each side may be worked separately.

Galea Aponeurotica (Tendinous Sheet Connecting the Occipitalis and Frontalis)

Strokes
- Positioning the fingers of both hands above the occipitalis muscles, move the scalp up and down, working in small

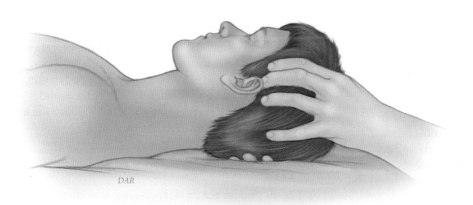

FIGURE 10-32 Hand position for releasing the temporalis.

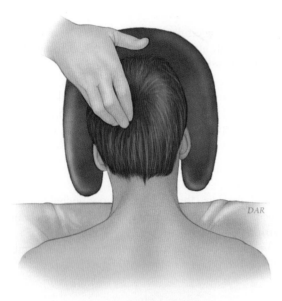

FIGURE 10-33 Palpating the occipitalis above the superior nuchal line.

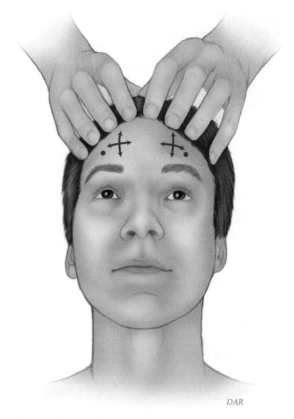

FIGURE 10-34 Reducing tone in the frontalis muscle.

sections and sliding it over the cranium. Pay attention to sections of tissue that are immobile. Hold trigger points until they become less sensitive.

- Continue, moving up over the top of the head to the frontalis. Be thorough, and cover the galea aponeurotica completely.

Facial Muscles

Frontalis
Origin: Fascia of the facial muscles above the nose and eyes and the skin.
Insertion: Galea aponeurotica.
Action: Along with the occipitalis, draws the scalp back, raises the eyebrows, and wrinkles the forehead; working alone, raises the eyebrow on the same side.

 A trigger point may be found about halfway between the eyebrow and the hairline, toward the midline of the forehead. It refers pain over the forehead on the same side that the trigger point is located.

Strokes
- Place the fingers of both hands on the front portion of the scalp, above the hairline. Move the fingers up and down and side to side, working in small sections, over the fibers of the muscle (Fig. 10-34). Feel for taut, stringy fibers and for painful, stuck areas.
- Continue the stroke in an inferior direction, covering the entire forehead to the eyebrows.

Procerus
Origin: Nasal bone and nasal cartilage.
Insertion: Skin of the forehead between the eyebrows.
Action: Wrinkles the skin between the eyebrows, draws the medial part of the eyebrows downward.

Strokes
- Place your thumbs horizontally and parallel to each other on the bridge of the nose, in the space between the eyebrows (Fig. 10-35).
- Alternately roll the thumbs over each other, in the direction of the forehead, in a small, continuous motion but without moving them off the space between the eyebrows.

Orbicularis Oculi
Origin: Nasal part of the frontal bone, frontal process in front of the lacrimal groove of the maxilla.
Insertion: All around the orbit of the eye, blends with the occipitofrontalis and corrugator, skin of the eyelid.
Action: Closes the eyelids gently or forcibly, draws the eyelids and lacrimal canals medially.

 Trigger points along the upper ridge of the eye socket may refer pain to the nose.

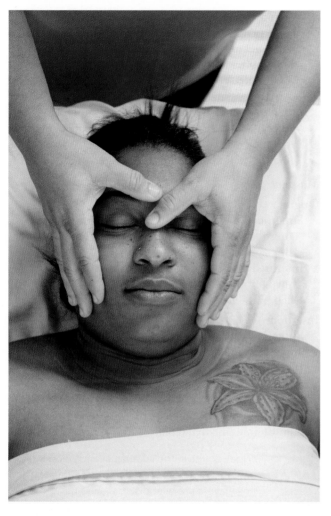

FIGURE 10-35 Deep tissue stroke on the procerus.

Strokes
- Place the pads of your index fingers against the medial side of the upper portion of the eye sockets (supraorbital ridge). Both sides may be worked simultaneously.
- Slowly trace the border of the bone with your finger to the lateral side of the upper part of the eye socket, pausing at areas of tenderness (Fig. 10-36). Repeat several times.

Jaw (Tendon of Temporalis, Masseter, and Lateral Pterygoid)

Tendon of Temporalis

Strokes
- Place your fingers or thumb slightly above the lateral portion of the superior border of the zygomatic process of the temporal bone.
- Pressing your fingers against the tendon, slowly move side to side, and feel for taut bands and trigger points. Having the client open the mouth stretches the tendinous fibers, making them easier to palpate.

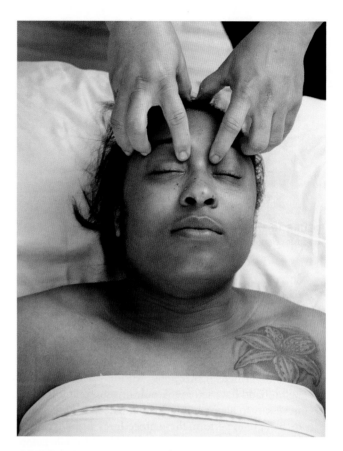

FIGURE 10-36 Pressing against the supraorbital ridge to work with the orbicularis oculi muscles.

- With the client's mouth open, place your index finger in the space between the zygomatic bone and the coronoid process. Stroke side to side across the tendon.
- Stroke side to side on the top edge of the coronoid process. Pause and hold on points of tenderness (Fig. 10-37).

Procedures and Precautions for Performing Intraoral Techniques
1. Check local ordinances to ascertain whether performing intraoral procedures is legal where you practice massage therapy.
2. Obtain the client's permission before attempting this work.

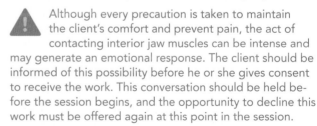 Although every precaution is taken to maintain the client's comfort and prevent pain, the act of contacting interior jaw muscles can be intense and may generate an emotional response. The client should be informed of this possibility before he or she gives consent to receive the work. This conversation should be held before the session begins, and the opportunity to decline this work must be offered again at this point in the session.

3. Always describe the procedure to your client beforehand. Explain how releasing the masseter and, especially, the lateral pterygoid muscles can alleviate many of the symptoms of TMJ syndrome and relax the jaw area in general. To ease any feelings of apprehension, explain

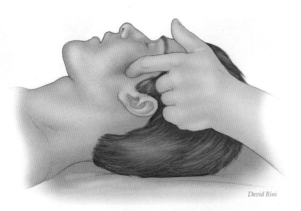

David Rini

FIGURE 10-37 Contacting the insertion of the temporalis on the superior edge of the coronoid process.

where your fingers will be placed inside of the mouth and which muscles will be addressed. Showing clients an illustration of the jaw muscles may be helpful in furthering their understanding of the procedure.

4. Do the necessary preparatory work before performing intraoral techniques. These procedures are the final ones described in this book. All the sessions learned beforehand have led to this culmination point. It is not necessary to have completed all the deep tissue sessions on a client to perform these procedures, but the client's body should be in a fairly relaxed and healthy state before attempting this work. Intraoral massage procedures are always preceded by massage of the neck, cranial, and facial muscles.

5. The therapist always wears a protective glove or finger cot when performing intraoral techniques. These items may be purchased at massage or medical supply stores. Rinse away any powder on the surface with water before putting your finger in the client's mouth. The glove should always be moistened before placing your finger against the tissues inside the mouth. This can be accomplished by dabbing your finger on the client's tongue to coat the working surface of the glove with a layer of saliva. Dry gloves can stick to the delicate tissues inside the mouth and cause minor abrasions.

6. Communication with the client is extremely important throughout the procedure; however, it may be difficult for the client to speak with your finger in his or her mouth. A system of finger signals may be incorporated to allow the client to communicate his or her reactions to the work. For instance, explain to the client that raising the thumb means more pressure can be applied. Forming a circle with the thumb and index finger means the pressure is adequate and comfortable. Turning the thumb down means the pressure is too intense and needs to be reduced. Raising the entire hand signals that the client needs to have the work halted immediately and the therapist's finger removed from the mouth. The therapist

should remind the client of the meaning of each signal while performing the procedure so that the client does not forget or become confused.

7. The approach to treating the internal jaw muscles is very gentle. The tissues are contacted only to the point of mild resistance and then held without applying any further pressure until a softening of the muscles is sensed. Proceed slowly, maintaining your full attention on where your finger is placed, the response of the tissues, and the client's reaction to what is occurring.

Masseter

Origin:

Superficial part—zygomatic process of the maxilla, maxillary process, and inferior border of the arch of the zygomatic bone.

Intermediate part—inner surface of the anterior two-thirds of the zygomatic arch.

Deep part—posterior one-third of the zygomatic arch.

Insertion:

Superficial part—angle and lower half of the lateral surface of the ramus of the mandible.

Intermediate part—central part of the ramus of the mandible.

Deep part—superior half of the ramus and coronoid process of the mandible.

Action: Elevates the mandible.

 Trigger points in the superficial and deeper layers of this muscle have different referral zones. These layers are best distinguished using the sifting technique.

Trigger points in the superficial layer send pain to the lower jaw, maxilla, molars, and gums. Trigger points along the anterior border, in the upper portion, refer to the maxilla, upper molars, and the gums around them. Pain coming from these trigger points often is misinterpreted by the client as inflammation of the sinus cavities.

Trigger points along the base of the mandible send pain in an arc across the temple and eyebrow.

The deeper layer trigger points can send pain into the cheek, around the lateral pterygoid, and sometimes, into the ear, which is perceived as a ringing sensation.

Strokes

• Place your fingers or thumbs on the anterior fibers of the muscle at the inferior border of the zygomatic arch (Fig. 10-38). Do an elongation stroke downward, to the base of the mandible. Press both sides simultaneously.

 Avoid pressing on the most posterior fibers of the muscle, because the parotid gland covers them.

• Have the client open the mouth to stretch the masseter. Place your thumbs or index fingers on the anterior borders

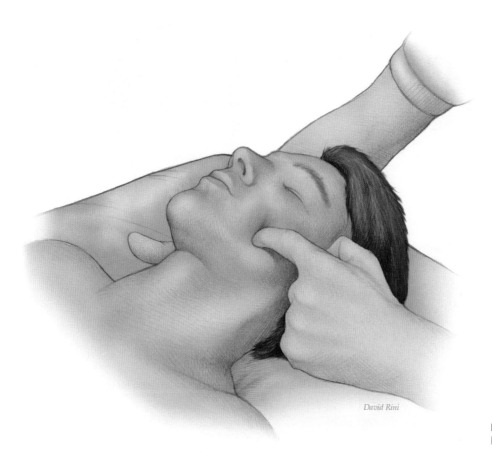

David Rini

FIGURE 10-38 Palpating the anterior border of the masseter muscle.

of the masseter, at the origin. Press in and up, toward the zygomatic bone, and hold for a minimum of 10 seconds. This is an excellent tension reduction point. Continue to stroke along the border, inferiorly, to the base of the mandible.

Note: The remaining strokes are performed inside the client's mouth and require the therapist to wear a latex glove or finger cot.

- Sift the muscle by squeezing the fibers between your thumb and index finger, one of which is placed on the cheek and the other inside the mouth (Fig. 10-39). As you roll the fibers, check for trigger points.

Lateral Pterygoid

Origin:
  Superior head—lateral surface of the greater wing of the sphenoid.
  Inferior head—lateral surface of the lateral pterygoid plate of the mandible.
Insertion: Condylar neck of the mandible, anterior margin of the articular capsule and disc of the TMJ.
Action: Aids opening the mouth by protracting the mandibular condyle and disc of the TMJ joint forward while the mandibular head rotates on the disc; protracts the jaw, bringing the lower teeth forward of the upper teeth; acting on the same side with the medial pterygoid,

causes the mandible and jaw to rotate to the opposite side (chewing motion).

 Trigger points in this muscle are a major source of TMJ pain. They can also refer to the maxillary sinus.

Strokes
- Have the client open the mouth slightly. Slide the pad of your index finger along the upper gum, fitting it into the pocket formed between the inside surface of the mandible and the lateral pterygoid plate on the sphenoid bone, behind the back upper molars.
- Press inward and upward, along the roof of the cheek and aiming the finger toward the condylar neck of the mandible, where the lateral pterygoid inserts (Fig. 10-40). Move slowly, because extremely painful trigger points may be encountered.

STRETCH

The client places both thumbs under the center of the chin. The client then yawns, pressing up against the base of the chin to apply resistance to the downward movement of the mandible (Fig. 10-41). This stretch helps to relieve tension in the muscles of the jaw.

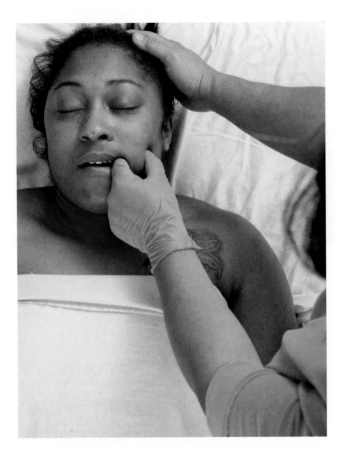

FIGURE 10-39 Sifting the fibers of the masseter.

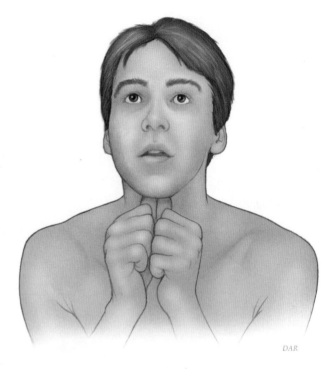

FIGURE 10-41 Tension reduction exercise for the temporomandibular joint muscles.

ACCESSORY WORK

1. Posterior and anterior neck work should accompany any work done on the jaw.
2. Pain and restriction in the jaw often corresponds to restriction in the pelvis. Simultaneously contacting both areas, with one hand on the face and the other on the pelvis, may provide relief of pain and restore balance to these indirectly but intricately connected areas of the body.
3. Working on the feet completes a session focusing on the cranium.

CLOSING

Sitting at the foot of the table, lightly hold the heels of the client's feet in your hands for 30 to 60 seconds. Remove your hands slowly to complete the session.

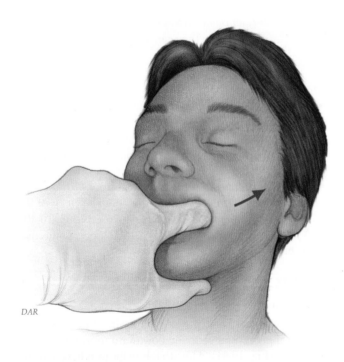

FIGURE 10-40 Palpating the lateral pterygoid.

REVIEW QUESTIONS

Level 1

Receive and Respond

1. What is the primary function of the suboccipital muscles?
   a. Lateral flexion of the neck
   b. Rotation of the head
   c. Flexion of the head and neck
   d. Extension of the head and neck

2. Trigger points in the sternocleidomastoid usually create pain in the. . .
   a. chest.
   b. neck.
   c. head.
   d. arm.

3. What type of joint is formed between the occiput and C1?
   a. Modified ball and socket
   b. Hinge
   c. Modified cartilaginous
   d. Gliding

4. This structure may be encountered during work on the anterior neck. It may have nodules or other anomalies that are palpable during massage. What is it?
   a. Thymus
   b. Thyroid
   c. Parotid
   d. Pineal

5. Where is the hyoid bone?
   a. Inferior posterior neck
   b. Inferior anterior neck
   c. Superior posterior neck
   d. Superior anterior neck

Level 2

Apply Concepts

1. What is a common consequence of chronically shortened deep neck muscles?
   a. Headaches
   b. TMJ disorders
   c. Subluxations
   d. Forward head posture

2. If a person has symptoms of brachial plexus entrapment, what is one possible factor?
   a. Ligament laxity at the glenohumeral joint
   b. TMJ disorder that refers into the arm
   c. Compression between the anterior and middle scalenes
   d. Hypertonicity of pectoralis major

3. If a person has a "military neck," what muscles are likely to be shortened?
   a. Scalenes, upper trapezius
   b. Sternocleidomastoid, longus capitus
   c. Elevator scapulae, rhomboids
   d. Splenius cervicis, splenius capitus

4. If a person reports dizziness, facial and ear pain, and a clicking sound when they chew, what condition might be present?
   a. TMJ disorder
   b. Migraine headache
   c. Trigger points of the masseter
   d. Bell palsy

5. What is the first step in performing intraoral work during a massage session?
   a. Obtain the client's permission
   b. Make sure this is within the legal scope of practice
   c. Put on gloves
   d. Prepare facial muscles

6. What is the recommended sequence for deep tissue massage to the posterior neck?
   a. Splenius capitus, followed by suboccipital muscles, followed by levator scapulae
   b. Suboccipital muscles, followed by levator scapulae, followed by upper trapezius
   c. Sternocleidomastoid, followed by upper trapezius, followed by infrahyoid muscles
   d. Upper trapezius, followed by levator scapulae, followed by semispinalis capitus

Level 3

Problem Solving: Discussion Points

1. Work to the anterior neck is fraught with cautions and endangerments. Why is it not preferable simply to skip this area? Discuss with a classmate the benefits and risks of treating or ignoring this area.

2. Your client had surgery on his jaw 3 years ago. He would like to receive some work in this area to help with his jaw clenching and headaches. What adaptations will you make for this client?

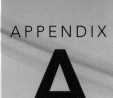

APPENDIX A

Conditions

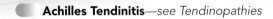

Achilles Tendinitis—*see Tendinopathies*

Acute Bronchitis (Chapter 6)
Pronunciation: ah-KYUTE brong-KY-tis

• What Is It?

Acute bronchitis is inflammation of the bronchial tree anywhere between the trachea and the bronchioles. If inflammation extends into the bronchioles and alveoli, it is called bronchopneumonia.

• How Is It Recognized?

The hallmark of acute bronchitis is a persistent, productive cough along with sore throat, nasal congestion, fatigue, and fever. Although other symptoms generally subside within 10 days, the cough may last for several weeks while the bronchi heal.

• Massage Risks and Benefits

RISKS: When a bronchial infection is acute, rigorous massage is not the best choice: not only because of the risk of communicability from the client to the practitioner, but because the person with an infection is metabolically dedicated to solving this problem—the extra challenge of a massage that demands an adaptive response is an unnecessary addition. Even when a person is in recovery, being flat on a table may be irritating, so accommodations may need to be made in positioning.

BENEFITS: During acute bronchitis, gentle, supportive bodywork may be helpful for improving sleep. When a person is in recovery, massage may be useful in dealing with tension in the breathing muscles and improving general energy levels.

Ankle Sprain—*see Sprains*

Asthma (Chapter 6)
• What Is It?

Asthma is the result of airway inflammation, intermittent airflow obstruction, and bronchial hyper-responsiveness.

• How Is It Recognized?

Asthma attacks are sporadic episodes involving coughing, wheezing, and difficulty with breathing, especially exhaling.

• Massage Risks and Benefits

RISKS: A client in the midst of an acute asthma attack is not a good candidate for massage. It is important to prepare the session room for clients with a tendency toward asthma by avoiding scents, candles, and essential oils that might exacerbate symptoms, and by using a hypoallergenic lubricant.

BENEFITS: Clients with asthma or other breathing problems, who are not in the midst of an acute episode, typically have extremely tight breathing muscles: the diaphragm, intercostals, and scalenes can benefit from any work that improves their efficiency.

Bell Palsy (Chapter 10)
• What Is It?

Bell palsy is flaccid paralysis of one side of the face caused by inflammation or damage to CN VII, the facial nerve.

• How Is It Recognized?

Symptoms of Bell palsy include a sudden onset of weakness in the muscles of the affected side of the face. Ear pain, headaches, hypersensitivity to sound, and drooling may also occur.

• Massage Risks and Benefits

RISKS: It is important to identify the cause of cranial nerve damage if possible, since some factors that contribute to Bell palsy may contraindicate massage. Otherwise, because sensation is intact so the client can give accurate feedback, massage has no specific risks for this condition.

BENEFITS: Massage may help to keep facial muscles flexible and nourished during the period of nerve repair that follows an episode of Bell palsy.

Bunions (Chapter 8)
Pronunciation: BUN-yunz

• What Are They?

A bunion is a protrusion at the metatarsophalangeal joint of the great toe that occurs when the toe is laterally deviated.

• How Are They Recognized?

Bunions are recognizable by the large bump on the medial aspect of the foot. When they are inflamed, they are red, hot, and painful.

• Massage Risks and Benefits

RISKS: Bunions locally contraindicate deep specific massage, which may exacerbate inflammation and pain.

BENEFITS: Lymphatic work to reduce local inflammation may help with some bunion pain, and work elsewhere on the foot and with other gait compensation patterns may be helpful for a client with this painful condition.

Bursitis (Chapter 7)

• What Is It?

A bursa is a fluid-filled sac that acts as a protective cushion, eases the movement of tendons and ligaments moving over bones, and cushions points of contact between bones. Bursitis is the inflammation of a bursa.

• How Is It Recognized?

Acute bursitis is painful and is aggravated by both passive and active motion. Muscles surrounding the affected joint often severely limit range of motion. It may be hot or edematous if the bursa is superficial.

• Massage Risks and Benefits

RISKS: Acute bursitis locally contraindicates any massage that is deep or specific. Bursitis due to infection contraindicates massage until the infection has been treated and eradicated.

BENEFITS: Lymphatic work to reduce local inflammation may help with some bursa pain, but does not address the root of the problem. Massage elsewhere on the body during an acute phase and directly to the muscles around the affected joint (within pain limits) in a subacute phase is appropriate.

Chronic Obstructive Pulmonary Disease—*see Emphysema*

Compartment Syndrome (Chapter 8)

• What Is It?

Compartment syndrome is a situation in which a fascial compartment is under so much pressure that oxygen and nutrients can no longer reach cells. It can be acute, which is a medical emergency, or chronic and less severe. It usually happens in the lower leg, but can occur in any fascially contained space.

• How Is It Recognized?

Acute compartment syndrome usually follows a trauma (a crushing injury, arterial damage, a long bone fracture). It is extremely painful, especially when tissues are passively stretched, and patients often report a tight, full feeling.

Chronic compartment syndrome is typically connected to a specific repetitive athletic activity. Cramping, pain, weakness, and numbness are all possible symptoms. Exercise makes it worse, but symptoms subside when the activity is suspended.

• Massage Risks and Benefits

RISKS: Any modality that manipulates soft tissues during an acute phase of compartment syndrome may make a bad situation worse by drawing more fluid to an area that is already impacted.

BENEFITS: Massage and stretching (or both simultaneously) may help to delay the onset of pain with chronic compartment syndrome. Massage may also be an effective preventive measure for athletes at risk for this condition.

Disc Disease (Chapters 6, 10)

• What Is It?

Disc disease refers to any situation in which the intervertebral disc is damaged in such a way that it puts pressure on nerve roots, the cauda equine, or the spinal cord.

• How Is It Recognized?

Symptoms of nerve pressure include local and radicular pain, specific muscle weakness, paresthesia, and numbness.

• Massage Risks and Benefits

RISKS: Many problems can cause nerve pain that looks similar to disc disease. Before bodywork can be conducted safely, it is important to have as clear a diagnosis as possible. Acutely inflamed discs may do best with gentle work that does not irritate surrounding muscles or other tissues. Muscle splinting around a weakened area must be treated with great care because reducing tone prematurely may aggravate symptoms. Any type of positioning that exacerbates symptoms should be avoided, of course.

BENEFITS: A person with a damaged disc may derive great benefit from careful bodywork that focuses on decompressing the spine, reducing the muscle splinting (when the area is stable), and addressing compensatory postural patterns that often accompany nerve pain.

Diverticulitis (Chapter 9)
Pronunciation: dy-ver-TICK-yu-lar dih-ZEZE

• What Is It?

Diverticulosis is the development of small pouches that protrude from the colon or small intestine. Diverticulitis is the inflammation that develops when these pouches become infected. Collectively, these disorders are known as diverticular disease.

• How Is It Recognized?

Diverticulosis is often silent. When inflammation (diverticulitis) is present, lower left side abdominal pain, cramping, bloating, constipation, or diarrhea may occur.

• Massage Risks and Benefits

RISKS: If the client knows that he or she has diverticulosis, abdominal massage must be done with care because the colon is structurally compromised. During a flare of diverticulitis, it is safest to delay massage until the infection has passed.

BENEFITS: Massage has no specific benefits for diverticular disease, but if the condition is well controlled and care is taken not to exacerbate symptoms, a client with this condition can enjoy the same benefits from massage as the rest of the population.

Dysmenorrhea (Chapter 9)
Pronunciation: dis-men-o-RE-ah

• What Is It?

Dysmenorrhea is the technical term for menstrual pain that is severe enough to limit the activities of women of childbearing age. It may be a primary problem or secondary to some other pelvic pathology.

• How Is It Recognized?

The symptoms of dysmenorrhea are dull aching or sharp, severe lower abdominal pain preceding and/or during menstruation. Nausea and vomiting may accompany very severe symptoms. Secondary dysmenorrhea may cause pelvic pain outside normal periods as well.

• Massage Risks and Benefits

RISKS: If extreme menstrual pain is being generated by an underlying problem, that must be identified before doing any intrusive abdominal massage. Most women would probably also rather avoid deep abdominal work during their periods.

BENEFITS: Massage can have a profoundly positive effect for primary dysmenorrhea, and it can be a helpful coping strategy for pain caused by underlying problems.

Dystonia (Chapter 10)
• What Is It?

Dystonia is a movement disorder resulting in repetitive, predictable, but involuntary muscle contractions. Torticollis is one type of dystonia.

• How Is It Recognized?

The primary symptom of dystonia is repetitive involuntary muscle contractions, especially during stress or in relation to specific tasks. Some forms involve only the head or face, the vocal cords, or one limb, but other forms are progressive or involve the whole body. The contractions themselves are not always painful, but they can lead to painful tissue changes including arthritis, muscle strains, and contractures.

• Massage Risks and Benefits

RISKS: Some of the drugs used to treat dystonia may have implications for massage, so therapists should be aware of how clients with dystonia treat their condition.

BENEFITS: This condition does not affect sensation, so any bodywork that is comfortable to receive is safe. Some dystonia patients may seek massage to help with fatigue and to reduce stress.

Emphysema (Chapter 6)
Pronunciation: em-fih-ZEE-mah

• What Is It?

Emphysema is a condition in which the alveoli of the lungs become stretched out and inelastic. They merge with each other, decreasing surface area, destroying surrounding capillaries, and limiting oxygen–carbon dioxide exchange. Emphysema and chronic bronchitis are part of chronic obstructive pulmonary disease (COPD).

• How Is It Recognized?

Symptoms of emphysema include shortness of breath with mild or no exertion, a chronic dry cough, rales, cyanosis, and susceptibility to secondary respiratory infection.

• Massage Risks and Benefits

RISKS: Emphysema patients may have serious circulatory complications, difficulty lying flat, and a high risk of respiratory infection. All of these require adjustments in bodywork choices.

BENEFITS: If an emphysema patient is resilient enough to receive massage, attention to the breathing muscles can help with anxiety, fatigue, and efficiency of function. Gentle, reflexive work is always appropriate, as long as the client is comfortable and the therapist is not at risk for picking up a communicable infection.

Fractures (Chapter 6)
• What Are They?

A fracture is any kind of cracked or broken bone.

• What Do They Look Like?

Most fractures are painful and involve loss of function at the nearest joints, but some may be difficult to diagnose without imaging technology.

• Massage Risks and Benefits

RISKS: Acute fractures locally contraindicate massage, until the bones are stabilized and other soft tissue damage is addressed.

BENEFITS: Swelling is a frequent complication of casting. Any lymphatic work to decrease fluid retention may help with both comfort and efficiency of circulatory turnover in the compromised area. Massage elsewhere to the body while a fracture is healing can help address the challenge of having impaired movement, as well as any limping or other compensations that may occur. A person who has fully recovered from a fracture can enjoy the same benefits from massage as the rest of the population.

Golfer's Elbow—see Tendinopathies

Hammertoe (Chapter 8)
• What Is It?

Hammertoe is a type of foot deformity that affects the lateral toes.

• How Is It Recognized?

Hammertoe involves a characteristic contracture that puts the proximal interphalangeal joint into flexion, and both the metatarsal-phalangeal and the distal interphalangeal joints into hyperextension. It can be passively flexible, or completely rigid.

• Massage Risks and Benefits

RISKS: This condition can involve acute and painful inflammation; any massage or manipulation that exacerbates this should be avoided.

BENEFITS: If the condition is treated while tissues are still soft and malleable, and other environmental factors are changed, massage with stretching and support could help to slow the progression of a hammertoe situation. Massage may also help with postural or gait distortions.

Headaches (Chapter 10)
• What Are They?

Headaches are pain caused by any number of factors. Muscular tension, nerve irritation, vascular spasm and dilation, and chemical imbalances can all contribute to headache. They can sometimes indicate a serious underlying disorder.

• How Are They Recognized?

Headache pain can range from being mild to debilitating; it can involve the whole head or be isolated to a particular area; it can be described as dull, aching, or sharp, electrical, and agonizing.

• Massage Risks and Benefits

RISKS: Headaches due to infection or CNS injury contraindicate massage. Many clients with migraine avoid massage and other stimulus during a headache, but might pursue it as a way to reduce frequency or intensity when the condition is not acute.

BENEFITS: Tension-type headaches, which are the most common variety of headaches, often respond beautifully to massage, which can address both stress and the mechanical imbalances in muscle tension that are so often involved.

Joint Disruptions (Chapter 7)

• **What Are They?**

Joint disruptions include any situation that interferes with the proper alignment between bones in a joint. A dislocation means that the articulating bones within a joint capsule are separated. A subluxation involves bones that are incompletely dislocated: the joint can function, but has limited range of motion. Shoulder separations are a type of subluxation. Hip dysplasia involves abnormalities in the shape of the acetabulum or femoral head that prevents a fully functioning hip joint.

• **What Do They Look Like?**

Traumatic joint disruptions are obvious and painful, with swelling, loss of function, and obvious displacement of the bones. Chronic subluxations and dysplasia can be more subtle.

• **Massage Risks and Benefits**

RISKS: Massage at the site of an acute situation may exacerbate symptoms and inappropriate joint manipulations may lead to a dislocation or subluxation episode.

BENEFITS: Massage for subacute dislocations or subluxations may be appropriate and helpful if the compromised range of motion is respected. Massage elsewhere on the body is safe, and may help to address some of the compensation patterns that develop with chronic musculoskeletal problems.

Ligament Tears—*see Sprains*

Menstrual Cramps—*see Dysmenorrhea*

Morton Neuroma (Chapter 8)

• **What Is It?**

Morton neuroma is not a neuroma; it is a fibrotic growth on the perineurium of the common digital nerve in the distal foot.

• **How Is It Recognized?**

Shooting electrical pain from the ball of the foot to the 3rd and 4th toes is the hallmark of this condition.

• **Massage Risks and Benefits**

RISKS: Massage that compresses the area of the thickening may exacerbate symptoms.

BENEFITS: Massage at the foot to increase space between the affected metatarsals, and to the leg to relieve any fascial restrictions on the rest of the nerve may help to mitigate some Morton neuroma symptoms.

Muscle Strains—*see Strains*

Nerve Impingement Syndrome—*see Thoracic Outlet Syndrome*

Osteoarthritis (Chapter 7)
Pronunciation: os-te-o-arth-RY-tis

• **What Is It?**

Osteoarthritis is joint inflammation brought about by wear and tear causing cumulative damage to articular cartilage.

• **How Is It Recognized?**

Affected joints are stiff, painful, and occasionally palpably inflamed. Bony deformation may be easily visible or palpable. Osteoarthritis most often affects knees, hips, and distal joints of the fingers.

• **Massage Risks and Benefits**

RISKS: Acutely inflamed arthritis (which is not typical) at least locally contraindicates massage that may promote local fluid flow and exacerbate inflammation.

BENEFITS: Full body and specific massage for painful joints can reduce stiffness and pain, and improve the quality of life for people with osteoarthritis, even though it is unlikely to contribute to any internal joint repair process.

Patellofemoral Syndrome (Chapter 8)
Pronunciation: pah-tel-o-FEM-or-al sin-drome

• **What Is It?**

Patellofemoral syndrome (PFS) is an overuse disorder that can lead to damage of the patellar cartilage.

• **How Is It Recognized?**

PFS causes pain at the knee, stiffness after immobility, and discomfort in walking down stairs.

• **Massage Risks and Benefits**

RISKS: Massage carries no particular risks for PFS.

BENEFITS: If damage has already occurred to the patellar cartilage, massage is unlikely to reverse that process. However, both general and specific massage can help deal with discomfort and muscular tension that may develop when the knee is stiff and painful.

Pes Planus (Chapter 8)
Pronunciation: pes PLANE-us, pes KAV-us

• **What Are They?**

These are the technical terms for flat feet or jammed arches.

• **How Are They Recognized?**

In pes planus, the feet lack arches. Eversion of the ankle, sometimes referred to as pronation, may also be present. Persons with pes cavus have extremely high arches that do not flatten with weight bearing.

• **Massage Risks and Benefits**

RISKS: Massage carries little risk for a client with pes planus or cavus, unless the foot problems are brought about by an underlying condition that requires some adjustment with bodywork.

BENEFITS: In some cases, the health of intrinsic foot muscles and ligaments can be improved through bodywork, especially if it is combined with increased awareness of posture and movement patterns. If the ligaments are lax through genetic or other problems, then massage may not correct the situation, but it could work with other factors to reduce pain and improve function.

Plantar Fasciitis (Chapter 8)
Pronunciation: PLAN-tar fah-she-Y-tis

• What Is It?

Plantar fasciitis is a condition caused by repeated microscopic injury to the plantar fascia of the foot.

• How Is It Recognized?

Plantar fasciitis is acutely painful after prolonged immobility. Then the pain recedes when the foot is warmed up, but comes back with extended use. It feels sharp and bruiselike, usually at the anterior calcaneus.

• Massage Risks and Benefits

RISKS: If the plantar fascia is acute inflamed (which is unlikely), local deep massage should be delayed. Massage to the plantar fascia for a client who has recently had a cortisone injection may increase the risk of rupture.

BENEFITS: Massage can help release tension in deep calf muscles that put strain on the plantar fascia; it can also help to affect the quality of scar tissue at the site of the injury.

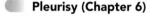 **Plantar Warts**—see Warts

 Pleurisy (Chapter 6)
• What Is It?

Pleurisy refers to inflammation of the pleural lining of the thoracic cavity. As a synonym, it is pleuritis.

• What Does It Look Like?

Stabbing chest pain that is made worse with inhalation is the hallmark of pleurisy. It is typically unilateral, and has a relatively sudden onset in conjunction with a respiratory with an underlying disorder.

• Massage Risks and Benefits

RISKS: Pleurisy is sometimes a sequence of serious underlying diseases that have implications for massage: these must be explored before safety is assured.

BENEFITS: A client whose pleurisy is identified and being treated may be a good candidate for any bodywork that he or she can tolerate, as long as infections are no longer communicable. Massage that focuses on breathing muscles and awareness may be welcomed. A client who has fully recovered from pleurisy can enjoy the same benefits from massage as the rest of the population.

Pneumonia (Chapter 6)
Pronunciation: nu-MO-ne-ah

• What Is It?

Pneumonia is an infection in the lungs brought about by bacteria, viruses, or fungi.

• How Is It Recognized?

The symptoms of pneumonia include coughing that may be dry or productive, high fever, pain on breathing, and shortness of breath. Extreme cases may show cyanosis, or a bluish cast to the skin and nails.

• Massage Risks and Benefits

RISKS: Pneumonia can be a life-threatening event, so a person with an acute infection is not a good candidate for any kind of rigorous massage that demands an adaptive response. Further, pneumonia can be contagious, so a therapist working with a client who is ill must take appropriate precautions.

BENEFITS: A client who is in recovery from pneumonia may benefit from percussive massage that aids the expulsion of mucus from the lungs. Gentle massage that promotes relaxation and sleep is also useful during this time. A client who has fully recovered from pneumonia can enjoy the same benefits from bodywork as the rest of the population.

 Postural Deviations (Chapter 6)
• What Are They?

Postural deviations are overdeveloped thoracic or lumbar curves (hyperkyphosis and hyperlordosis, respectively), or a lateral curve, possibly with a twist, in the spine (scoliosis, rotoscoliosis).

• How Are They Recognized?

Extreme curvatures are easily visible, although radiography is used to pinpoint exactly where the problems begin and end.

• Massage Risks and Benefits

RISKS: Extreme postural deviations are sometimes connected to serious underlying diseases that influence the growth patterns of bone and soft tissues. Severe compression of the rib cage may lead to respiratory or cardiac impairment, along with a risk of pneumonia and rib fragility.

BENEFITS: As long as underlying factors are addressed and bodywork is well tolerated, massage may have a powerfully positive effect on postural deviations, helping to balance soft tissue stress and improve alignment, efficiency of posture, and ease of movement.

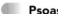 **Psoas Strain**—see Strain

 Rib Fractures—see Fractures

 Rotator Cuff Injuries—see Tendinopathies

 Sciatica (Chapter 9)
• What Is It?

Sciatica refers to a group of signs and symptoms related to irritation of the sciatic nerve, a large nerve that runs down the posterior aspect of the thigh. Contributing factors can include spinal stenosis, disc disease, spondylolisthesis, and muscle spasm in the deep lateral rotators.

• How Is It Recognized?

Symptoms of sciatica vary, depending on where and how seriously the sciatic nerve is impinged. They can include unilateral low back and hip pain, pain in the buttocks that is worse with sitting, paresthesia (burning, tingling, pins and needles) in the affected leg, weakness, numbness, or pain that shoots or zaps down the leg.

• Massage Risks and Benefits

RISKS: Undiagnosed back pain with a nerve-like quality (i.e., zapping, shooting, electrical pain) can suggest nerve impingement. It is possible for careless massage to exacerbate this problem if the practitioner does not know where the impingement is.

BENEFITS: If the practitioner can identify the site of sciatic nerve irritation, it may be possible to reduce mechanical disruption and to create the potential for healthy nerve functioning.

Shin Splints (Chapter 8)
• **What Are They?**

The term "shin splints" refers to a collection of lower leg injuries, including muscle injuries, periostitis, hairline fractures, and other problems. They are usually brought about by overuse and/or misalignment at the ankle.

• **How Are They Recognized?**

Pain along the tibia may be superficial or deep, mild or severe. The pattern of pain differs with the specific structures that are injured.

• **Massage Risks and Benefits**

RISKS: Some shin splint situations may contraindicate massage until more information is gathered, or the acute stage has passed. Compartment syndromes (discussed elsewhere) can be a serious complication, and bone fractures need different treatment options and healing times than other injuries.

BENEFITS: Massage therapy can be helpful to treat uncomplicated muscle injuries around the tibia, and it can also be a useful strategy to augment training and reduce the risk of injury to the lower leg muscular and fascial structures.

Shoulder Separation—see Joint Disruptions

Sinus Congestion—see Sinusitis

Sinusitis (Chapter 10)
Pronunciation: sy-nus-I-tis

• **What Is It?**

Sinusitis is inflammation of the paranasal sinuses from infection, allergies, or physical obstruction.

• **How Is It Recognized?**

Signs and symptoms include headaches; tenderness over the affected area; runny or congested nose; facial or tooth pain; headache; fatigue; and, if it's related to an infection, thick, opaque mucus, fever, and chills.

• **Massage Risks and Benefits**

RISKS: Acute sinus infections contraindicate any bodywork that could exacerbate symptoms. If the client has fever, chills, and other signs of systemic infection, it is best to delay any rigorous massage until this has passed. A client with a tendency toward inflamed sinuses may have problems lying flat on a table, especially, face down. It is important to be able to make accommodations for this problem.

BENEFITS: Very gentle massage around the face, as long as no infection is present, may help the sinuses to drain, and for sinus pain to diminish. A client with inflamed sinuses who does not have an infection can benefit from bodywork as long as he or she is comfortable on the table.

Spasm, Cramps (Chapter 8)
• **What Are They?**

Spasms and cramps are involuntary contractions of skeletal muscle. Spasms are considered to be low-grade, long-lasting contractions, while cramps are short-lived, very acute contractions.

• **How Are They Recognized?**

Cramps are extremely painful, with visible shortening of muscle fibers. Long-term spasms are painful and may cause inefficient movement but may not have acute symptoms.

• **Massage Risks and Benefits**

RISKS: Muscles in acute, painful contraction do not invite rigorous massage on the belly; this may be more irritating or even damaging than not. Some underlying pathologies may cause muscle cramping; these must be ruled out or accommodated if this is a frequent event.

BENEFITS: Stretching along with massage at attachment sites of contracting muscles are often effective strategies for reducing tone. Muscles that have been in involuntary contraction respond well to massage, which can reduce residual pain and improve local circulation.

Sprains (Chapters 8, 10)
• **What Are They?**

Sprains are injured ligaments. Injuries can range in severity from a few traumatized fibers to a complete rupture.

• **How Are They Recognized?**

In the acute stage pain, redness, heat, swelling, and loss of joint function are evident. Later, these symptoms are less extreme, although perhaps not entirely absent. Passive stretching of the affected ligament is painful until all inflammation has subsided.

• **Massage Risks and Benefits**

RISKS: Acutely inflamed sprains locally contraindicate intrusive work until the inflammation has subsided, but lymphatic work to decrease edema may be safe and appropriate. Sprains can sometimes mask symptoms of minor fractures; if symptoms are not significantly relieved within a few days, this possibility should be pursued with a medical professional.

BENEFITS: Damaged ligaments that are not acutely inflamed respond well to specific massage along with passive stretching and full use within pain tolerance.

Strains (Chapter 9)
• **What Are They?**

Strains are injuries to muscles involving torn fibers.

• **How Are They Recognized?**

Pain, stiffness, and occasionally palpable heat and swelling are all signs of muscle strain. Pain may be exacerbated by passive stretching or resisted contraction of the affected muscle.

• **Massage Risks and Benefits**

RISKS: Rigorous massage to an acute muscle injury may exacerbate inflammation and tissue damage.

BENEFITS: Massage after the acute stage of inflammation has passed can powerfully influence the production of useful scar tissue, reduce adhesions and edema, and reestablish range of motion.

Tendinopathies (Chapters 7, 8)
Pronunciation: ten-dih-NOP-ath-ez

• What Are They?

Tendinopathies are injuries or damage to tendons and their fascial sheaths. While it is possible for these injuries to involve acute inflammation (as indicated in the traditional terms *tendinitis* or *tenosynovitis*), most long-term tendon injuries are related to collagen degeneration rather than inflammation. The term for this condition is *tendinosis*. Tennis elbow, golfer's elbow, Achilles tendinitis, and rotator cuff injuries are all types of tendinosis.

• How Are They Recognized?

Pain and loss of range of motion are often present with tendinopathies. Pain is exacerbated by resisted exercise of the damaged muscle-tendon unit. Damage to the tenosynovial sheath may also create pain, resistance to movement, and crepitus: a grinding texture as the tendon moves through its fascial covering.

• Massage Risks and Benefits

RISKS: Tendinopathies with true inflammation are rare, but when they occur, bodywork is best delayed until the acute phase has completed. An exception to this is lymphatic work, which may help to limit some of the negative aspects of swelling.

BENEFITS: Most tendinopathies indicate massage, which aims to help improve the quality and function of the affected connective tissues.

Tennis Elbow—*see Tendinopathies*

Thoracic Outlet Syndrome (Chapters 7, 10)
Pronunciation: thor-AS-ik OUT-let SIN-drome

• What Is It?

Thoracic outlet syndrome (TOS) is a collection of signs and symptoms brought about by occlusion of nerve and blood supply to the arm. It is a typical form of nerve impingement syndrome.

• How Is It Recognized?

Depending on what structures are compressed, TOS shows shooting pains, weakness, numbness, and paresthesia (pins and needles) along with a feeling of fullness and possible discoloration of the affected hand and arm from impaired circulation.

• Massage Risks and Benefits

RISKS: Care must be taken not to exacerbate pressure on delicate structures, either with massage or with positioning on the table. Outside of this limitation, massage has no specific risks for clients with thoracic outlet syndrome.

BENEFITS: Massage that works to create space for unimpeded blood and nerve impulse flow can have a profound positive impact on thoracic outlet syndrome. If the problem arises from structural anomalies, massage may not make much difference beyond temporary symptomatic relief. Muscular imbalances must be addressed from multiple dimensions and directions to achieve lasting change.

Torticollis—*see Dystonia*

Trigeminal Neuralgia (Chapter 10)
Pronunciation: try-JEM-ih-nul nur-AL-je-ah

• What Is It?

Trigeminal neuralgia (TN) is a condition involving sharp electrical or stabbing pain along one or more branches of the trigeminal nerve (CN V), usually in the lower face and jaw.

• How Is It Recognized?

The pain of TN is very sharp and severe. Patients report stabbing, electrical, or burning sensations that occur in brief episodes, but that repeat with or without identifiable triggers. A tic is often present as well.

• Massage Risks and Benefits

RISKS: TN contraindicates massage to the face unless the client can guide the therapist into what feels safe and comfortable. Clients may not be comfortable lying face-down if the face cradle of the table elicits symptoms.

BENEFITS: Massage elsewhere to the body, especially to the neck and shoulders, may offer great relief to TN patients.

Varicose Veins (Chapter 9)
Pronunciation: VARE-ih-kose vanez

• What Are They?

Varicose veins are distended veins, usually in the legs, caused by venous insufficiency and retrograde blood flow.

• How Are They Recognized?

Varicose veins are ropy, bluish, elevated veins that twist and turn out of their usual course. They are most common in branches of the great saphenous veins on the medial side of the calf, although they are also found on the posterior aspects of the calf and thigh. Varicose veins can also develop at other locations, in which case they have other names.

• Massage Risks and Benefits

RISKS: Extreme varicose veins, especially with compromised skin, contraindicate any massage that might disrupt or irritate them. Milder varicose veins locally contraindicate deep specific work, but are safe for superficial massage as long as the skin is healthy. It is important to note that people with varicose veins are at increased risk for deep vein thrombosis, so massage therapists need to be knowledgeable about both conditions.

BENEFITS: Massage is unlikely to change or improve varicose veins. As long as they are accommodated, clients with varicose veins can enjoy the same benefits from bodywork as the rest of the population.

Warts (Chapter 8)
• What Are They?

Warts are growths caused by slow-growing viral infections of keratinocytes in the epidermis.

• How Are They Recognized?

The most common warts (verruca vulgaris) look like hard, cauliflower-shaped lumps. When they grow on the bottom of the feet, they are called plantar warts. Warts can affect anyone, but children and teenagers are especially prone to them.

• Massage Risks and Benefits

RISKS: Warts locally contraindicate massage. The risk of communicability is low but not zero, and the growths may shed virus in sloughing skin cells and local bleeding.

BENEFITS: Massage has no direct benefit for warts, but a client with a history of this infection can enjoy the same benefits from bodywork as the rest of the population.

Whiplash (Chapter 10)
• What Is It?

Whiplash is a collective term referring to a collection of soft tissue injuries that may occur with cervical acceleration followed by deceleration. These injuries include sprained ligaments, strained muscles, damaged joint capsules, and temporomandibular joint problems. Although whiplash technically refers to soft tissue injury, damage to other structures, including vertebrae, discs, and nerve tissue, frequently occurs at the same time.

• How Is It Recognized?

Symptoms of whiplash vary according to the nature of the injuries. Posttrauma pain at the neck and referring into the shoulders and arms, along with chronic headaches, are the most frequent indicators.

• Massage Risks and Benefits

RISKS: Acute injuries, along with those that have not been fully diagnosed, contraindicate any but the gentlest bodywork. The risks of exacerbating inflammation or of disrupting unstable bones or joints are important to respect.

BENEFITS: Postacute and mature whiplash injuries can benefit from massage that focuses on restoring healthy muscle tone and movement patterns, along with improving the quality of any connective tissue scarring that may have occurred.

Trigger Point Locations and Pain Referral Patterns

Chapter 6: Breath & Support

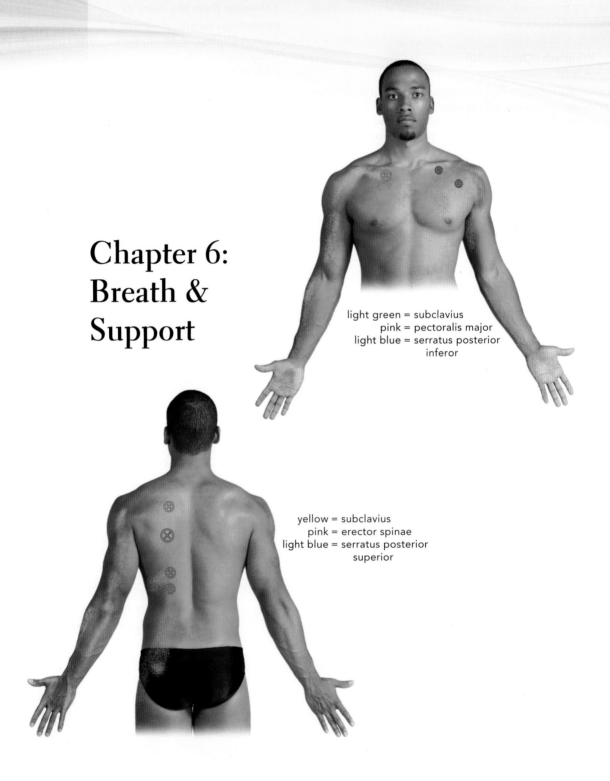

light green = subclavius
pink = pectoralis major
light blue = serratus posterior inferor

yellow = subclavius
pink = erector spinae
light blue = serratus posterior superior

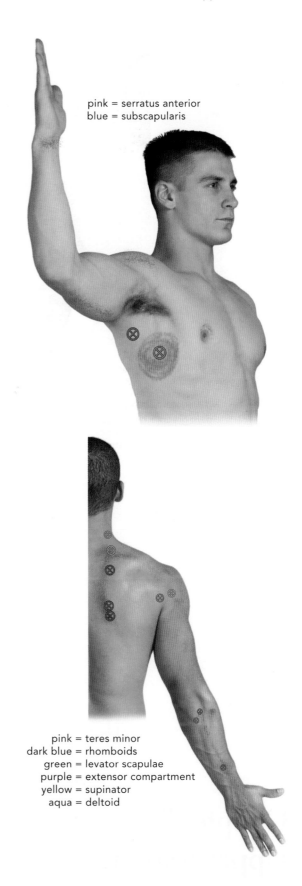

pink = serratus anterior
blue = subscapularis

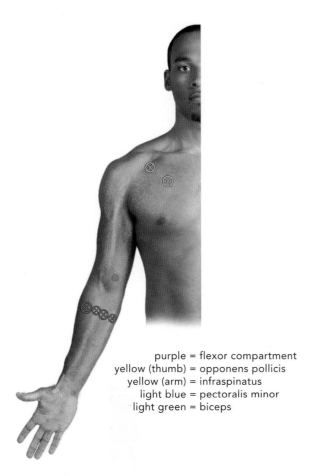

purple = flexor compartment
yellow (thumb) = opponens pollicis
yellow (arm) = infraspinatus
light blue = pectoralis minor
light green = biceps

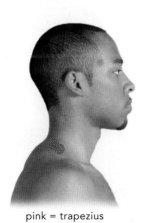

pink = trapezius

pink = teres minor
dark blue = rhomboids
green = levator scapulae
purple = extensor compartment
yellow = supinator
aqua = deltoid

Chapter 7:
Upper Extremity

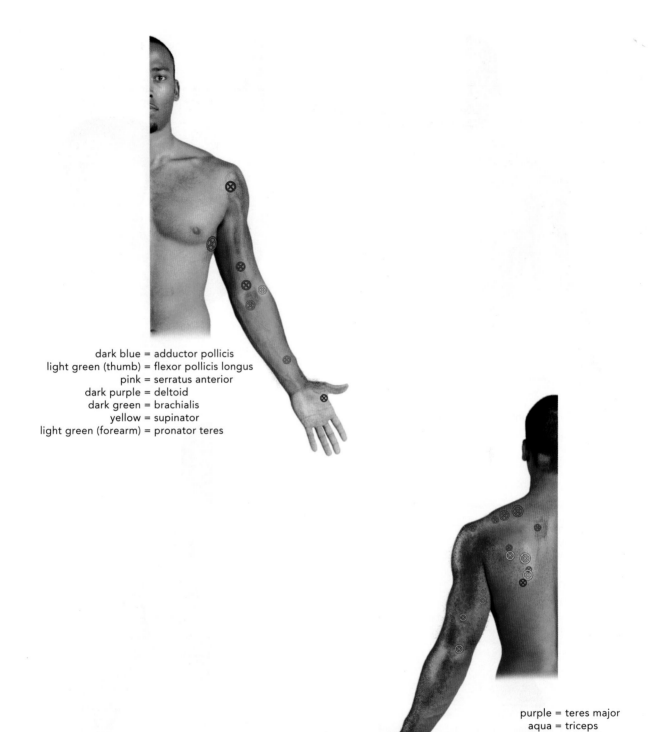

dark blue = adductor pollicis
light green (thumb) = flexor pollicis longus
pink = serratus anterior
dark purple = deltoid
dark green = brachialis
yellow = supinator
light green (forearm) = pronator teres

purple = teres major
aqua = triceps
yellow = infraspinatus
pink shoulder and arm = supraspinatus
pink neck and shoulder = trapezius
dark blue = subscapularis

Chapter 7:
Upper Extremity

Chapter 8: Foot

light green = tibialis anterior

purple = extensor digitorum brevis
aqua = peroneus brevis

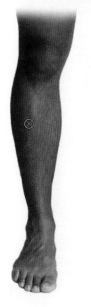

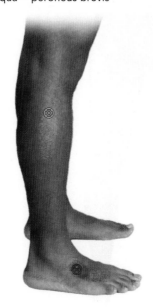

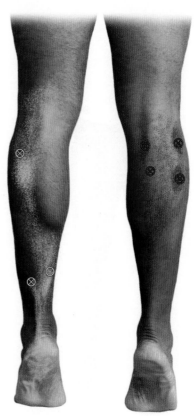

blue = gastrocnemius
yellow = soleus

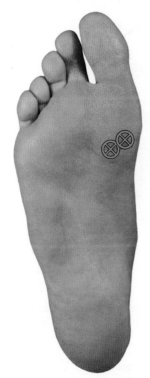

green = flexor hallucis brevis

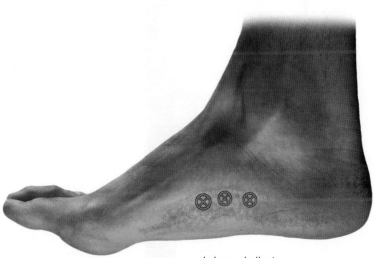

green = abductor hallucis

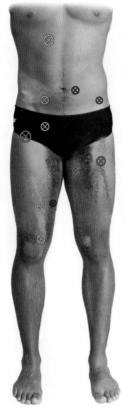

aqua = rectus abdominis
pink = rectus femoris
dark green = adductor magnus
bright green = adductor longus
dark purple = psoas, iliacus
blue = vastus intermedius
yellow = vastus medialis

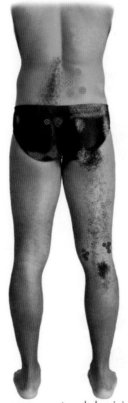

aqua = rectus abdominis
yellow = quadratus lumborum
dark blue = hamstrings
pink = glutues maximus
purple = psoas, iliacus

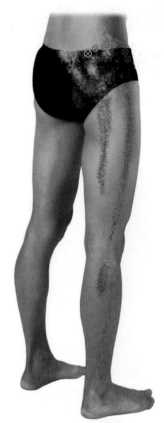

aqua = gluteus medius
dark blue = gluteus maximus

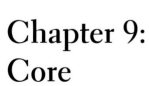

yellow = pectineus
blue = gracilis

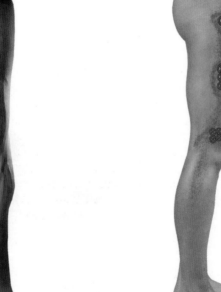

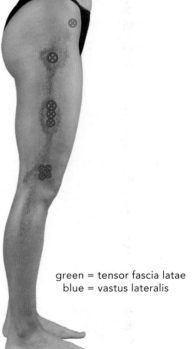

green = tensor fascia latae
blue = vastus lateralis

Chapter 9: Core

Chapter 10: Upper Pole

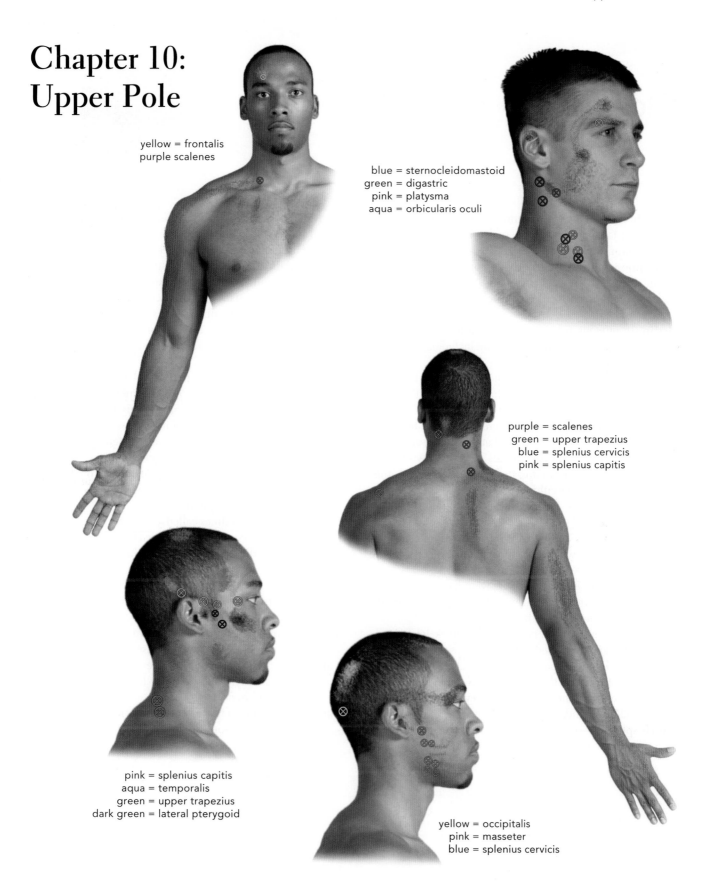

yellow = frontalis
purple scalenes

blue = sternocleidomastoid
green = digastric
pink = platysma
aqua = orbicularis oculi

purple = scalenes
green = upper trapezius
blue = splenius cervicis
pink = splenius capitis

pink = splenius capitis
aqua = temporalis
green = upper trapezius
dark green = lateral pterygoid

yellow = occipitalis
pink = masseter
blue = splenius cervicis

Glossary

acetylcholine—a common neurotransmitter that, when it attaches to a cell membrane, makes it highly permeable to sodium.

adenosine triphosphate (ATP)—a compound that stores and releases energy in cells.

collagen—a protein fiber found in connective tissue, cartilage, and bone.

elastin—a mucoprotein fiber that is elastic in nature. It is found in pliable structures of the body, including connective tissue, ligaments, and tendons.

endorphin—an opiate polypeptide produced in the brain that binds to opiate receptor sites, thus raising the threshold for pain perception.

enkephalin—an opiate polypeptide produced in the brain that binds to opiate receptor sites and acts as a pain analgesic.

facilitated nerve pathways—routes developed within the neural structures from areas of hyperirritation to other segments of the musculoskeletal system.

fibrils—minute fibers located in the sarcoplasm of muscle fibers.

interoception—any sense that is normally stimulated from within the body, includes proprioception, hunger, digestive upset, and others.

meridians—also known as channels. Meridians are energetic pathways often associated with the organs. Meridians distribute *qi* throughout the body.

motor unit—a single motor neuron and all the skeletal muscle fibers that are innervated by that neuron's axon terminals.

mucopolysaccharide—polysaccharides that chemically bond with water. They are thick, gelatinous substances that form intercellular ground substance. They are also found in synovial fluids and mucous secretions.

muscle splinting—increased tonus in muscle tissue surrounding injury to provide protection by limiting movement.

phasic—a term applied to the muscles primarily responsible for movement of the body through space.

qi—a Chinese word referring to the vital life force.

referred pain zone—a site within the myofascial tissues that registers pain, numbness, weakness, or paresthesia from a stimulus originating in another area.

reflex arcs—nerve feedback loops operating through the spinal cord that link the sensory and motor systems. They monitor and direct muscle actions, mostly at an unconscious level.

sarcomere—the contractile unit of skeletal muscle.

stress–tension–pain cycle—a self-perpetuating, dysfunctional cycle in which increased demand on the body/mind system causes a condition of stress, heightening the activity of the sympathetic nervous system. This leads to increased muscular tension, which diminishes the ability of the muscles to eliminate waste materials from the cells, resulting in stimulation of nociceptive nerve receptors and increased pain perception.

stretch reflex—sometimes called a myotatic reflex, an involuntary muscle contraction triggered by sudden stretching.

tensile—the ability to withstand stretching tension without breaking.

tonic—a term referring to muscles with the primary function of supporting the body in static positions (i.e., postural muscles).

trigger point—hyperirritable areas in muscles where compression may elicit a twitch response and/or referred pain.

valgus—a condition of the lower extremity in which the bones deviate laterally from the longitudinal axis. Also called bow-legged.

varus—a condition of the lower extremity in which the bones deviate medially from the longitudinal axis. Also known as knock-kneed.

Index

Page numbers in *italics* denote figures; those followed by a "t" denote tables; and those followed by a "b" denote boxes.